T0383328

Emergency Ultrasound

Editors

MICHAEL BLAIVAS
SRIKAR ADHIKARI

ULTRASOUND CLINICS

www.ultrasound.theclinics.com

Consulting Editor
VIKRAM S. DOGRA

April 2014 • Volume 9 • Number 2

ELSEVIER

1600 John F. Kennedy Boulevard • Suite 1800 • Philadelphia, Pennsylvania, 19103-2899

http://www.theclinics.com

ULTRASOUND CLINICS Volume 9, Number 2
April 2014 ISSN 1556-858X, ISBN-13: 978-0-323-29020-3

Editor: John Vassallo
Developmental Editor: Stephanie Carter

Ultrasound Clinics (ISSN 1556-858X) is published quarterly by Elsevier, Inc., 360 Park Avenue South, New York, NY 10010-1710. Months of publication are January, April, July, and October. Business and editorial offices: 1600 John F. Kennedy Boulevard, Suite 1800, Philadelphia, Pennsylvania 19103-2899. Accounting and circulation offices: 6277 Sea Harbor Drive, Orlando, FL 32887-4800. Periodicals postage paid at New York, NY, and additional mailing offices. Subscription prices are $270 per year for (US individuals), $327 per year for (US institutions), $130 per year for (US students and residents), $305 per year for (Canadian individuals), $369 per year for (Canadian institutions), $325 per year for (international individuals), $369 per year for (international institutions), and $155 per year for (Canadian and foreign students/residents). To receive student/resident rate, orders must be accompanied by name of affiliated institution, date of term, and the signature of program/residency coordinator on institution letterhead. Orders will be billed at individual rate until proof of status is received. Foreign air speed delivery is included in all Clinics subscription prices. All prices are subject to change without notice. **POSTMASTER:** Send address changes to *Ultrasound Clinics,* Elsevier Health Sciences Division, Subscription Customer Service, 3251 Riverport Lane, Maryland Heights, MO 63043. **Customer Service (orders, claims, online, change of address): Telephone: 1-800-654-2452 (U.S. and Canada); 314-447-8871 (outside U.S. and Canada). Fax: 314-447-8029. E-mail: journalscustomerservice-usa@elsevier.com (for print support); journalsonlinesupport-usa@elsevier.com (for online support).**

Reprints: For copies of 100 or more, of articles in this publication, please contact the Commercial Reprints Department, Elsevier Inc., 360 Park Avenue South, New York, NY 10010-1710. Tel.: +1-212-633-3874; Fax: +1-212-633-3820; E-mail: reprints@elsevier.com.

Contributors

CONSULTING EDITOR

VIKRAM S. DOGRA, MD
Professor of Radiology, Urology, and
Biomedical Engineering, Associate Chair for
Education and Research, Director of
Ultrasound, Department of Imaging Sciences,
University of Rochester School of Medicine,
Rochester, New York

EDITORS

MICHAEL BLAIVAS, MD
Professor, Department of Internal Medicine,
University of South Carolina School of
Medicine, Columbia, South Carolina;
Department of Emergency Medicine,
St. Francis Hospital, Columbus,
Georgia

SRIKAR ADHIKARI, MD, MS
Chief, Section of Emergency Ultrasound,
Associate Professor, Department of
Emergency Medicine, University of Arizona
Medical Center, Tucson, Arizona

AUTHORS

SRIKAR ADHIKARI, MD, MS
Chief, Section of Emergency Ultrasound,
Associate Professor, Department of
Emergency Medicine, University of Arizona
Medical Center, Tucson, Arizona

KARIM ALI, MD
Ultrasound Fellow, Clinical Instructor,
Department of Emergency Medicine, Emory
University School of Medicine, Emory
University, Atlanta, Georgia

RICHARD AMINI, MD
Assistant Professor of Emergency Medicine,
Department of Emergency Medicine,
University of Arizona, Tucson, Arizona

JOHN BAILITZ, MD
Emergency Medicine Ultrasound Fellowship
Director, Cook County Emergency Medicine
Residency, Chicago, Illinois

SIERRA BECK, MD, RDMS, RDCS
Ultrasound Fellowship Director, Assistant
Professor, Department of Emergency
Medicine, Emory University School of
Medicine, Emory University, Atlanta, Georgia

MICHAEL BLAIVAS, MD
Professor, Department of Internal Medicine,
University of South Carolina School of
Medicine, Columbia, South Carolina;
Department of Emergency Medicine,
St. Francis Hospital, Columbus, Georgia

JEREMY S. BOYD, MD
Division of Emergency Ultrasound,
Department of Emergency Medicine,
Vanderbilt University Medical Center,
Nashville, Tennessee

ERIC H. CHOU, MD
Research Fellow, Department of Emergency
Medicine, Maimonides Medical Center,
Brooklyn, New York

EITAN DICKMAN, MD, RDMS, FACEP
Vice Chair of Academics, Director,
Division of Emergency Ultrasound,
Department of Emergency Medicine,
Maimonides Medical Center, Brooklyn,
New York

ROBINSON M. FERRE, MD, FACEP
Division of Emergency Ultrasound, Department
of Emergency Medicine, Vanderbilt University
Medical Center, Nashville, Tennessee

SAMA GHALI, MD
Carolinas Medical Center, Charlotte,
North Carolina

MICHAEL GOTTLIEB, MD
Emergency Medicine Resident, Cook County
Emergency Medicine Residency, Chicago,
Illinois

NADIM MIKE HAFEZ, MD, RDMS
Ultrasound Director, Department of
Emergency Medicine, Rush University
Medical Center, Chicago, Illinois

DANIELLE HALLETT, MD
Resident Physician, Emergency Medicine,
Department of Emergency Medicine,
University of Arizona, Tucson, Arizona

JENNIFER HASHEM, MD
Resident, Department of Orthopaedic Surgery,
Maimonides Medical Center, Brooklyn,
New York

JAMES HWANG, MD, MPH
Director of Emergency Ultrasound, Scripps
Memorial Hospital, La Jolla, California

PARISA P. JAVEDANI, MD
Resident Physician, Emergency Medicine,
Department of Emergency Medicine,
University of Arizona, Tucson, Arizona

MARLA C. LEVINE, MD, RDMS
Attending Physician, Department of
Emergency Medicine, Maimonides Medical
Center, Brooklyn, New York

JENNIFER R. MARIN, MD, MSc
Director of Emergency Ultrasound, Division of
Pediatric Emergency Medicine, Assistant
Professor of Pediatrics and Emergency
Medicine, Children's Hospital of Pittsburgh,
Pittsburgh, Pennsylvania

JARED T. MARX, MD
Assistant Professor, Emergency Medicine,
University of Kansas Hospital, Kansas City,
Kansas

JEHANGIR MEER, MD, RDMS
Director of Emergency Ultrasound,
Assistant Professor, Department of
Emergency Medicine, Emory University School
of Medicine, Emory University, Atlanta,
Georgia

JAMES MOAK, MD, RDMS
Assistant Professor of Emergency Medicine,
School of Medicine, University of Virginia,
Charlottesville, Virginia

JARROD MOSIER, MD
Director of Emergency Medicine/Critical
Care, Assistant Professor of Emergency
Medicine, Department of Emergency
Medicine; Assistant Professor of Medicine,
Section of Pulmonary, Critical Care, Allergy
and Sleep, Department of Medicine, University
of Arizona, Tucson, Arizona

JOHN MUNYAK, MD
Attending Physician, Department of
Orthopaedic Surgery, Maimonides Medical
Center, Brooklyn, New York

LORRAINE NG, MD
Assistant Professor of Pediatrics, Division of
Pediatric Emergency Medicine, Columbia
University Medical Center (CUMC),
New York Presbyterian - Morgan Stanley
Children's Hospital of New York, New York,
New York

REFKY NICOLA, MS, DO
Assistant Professor, Department of
Imaging Sciences and Emergency Medicine,
University of Rochester Medical Center,
University of Rochester, Rochester,
New York

AHMED SALEH, MD
Resident, Department of Orthopaedic
Surgery, Maimonides Medical Center,
Brooklyn, New York

SHIDEH SHAFIE, MD
Attending Physician, Department of
Emergency Medicine, Maimonides Medical
Center, Brooklyn, New York

SHANNON B. SNYDER, MD, FACEP
Division of Emergency Ultrasound,
Department of Emergency Medicine,
Vanderbilt University Medical Center,
Nashville, Tennessee

LORI A. STOLZ, MD
Assistant Professor, Department of Emergency
Medicine, University of Arizona, Tucson,
Arizona

CHRISTOPHER VAUGHN, MD
Assistant Professor of Emergency Medicine,
University of Wisconsin School of Medicine
and Public Health, Madison, Wisconsin

ANTHONY J. WEEKES, MD
Director, Emergency Ultrasound Fellowship;
Associate Professor, Emergency Medicine,
Carolinas Medical Center, Charlotte,
North Carolina

Contents

The use of point-of-care ultrasound by emergency physicians is rapidly becoming standard of care. With the incorporation of ultrasound training into emergency medicine residency core curriculum and inclusion of emergency ultrasound into emergency medicine milestones, it has become a mandatory skill for graduating emergency medicine residents. In addition, there is growing interest to integrate ultrasound into medical school curriculum and in many institutions emergency physicians are leading the way in providing emergency ultrasound education to students throughout 4 years of medical school.

Clinicians in different medical specialties now use point-of-care sonography (POCS) to improve the efficiency and safety of patient care. For nearly 2 decades, POCS has been used in the emergency and critical care settings. This article reviews challenging pitfalls and key pearls to help the busy clinician use Emergency POCS in a safe and efficient manner.

 Videos of abnormal chambers, pericardial disease, myocardial and valve dysfunction, dissection, and other interesting findings accompany this article

Focused cardiac ultrasonography provides emergency and critical care providers with a bedside modality to assess for immediate life threats and to gather essential, time-sensitive information. The clinical usefulness of focused cardiac ultrasonography is greatest in patients with dyspnea/hypoxia, hypotension/shock, tachycardia, and periarrest states. The core applications of focused cardiac ultrasonography include assessing left and right ventricular function, detecting the presence or absence of pericardial fluid, and assessing volume status/volume responsiveness. Routine practice and clinical integration of these applications is critical. Understanding the various limitations of focused cardiac ultrasonography is important and a key step toward realizing its many benefits.

Point-of-care (POC) pelvic ultrasonography by emergency physicians allows for a rapid and safe diagnosis of a multitude of abnormalities, and allows for constant monitoring of both obstetric and nonobstetric patients without mobilization during the acute phase of disease. Assessment of intrauterine pregnancy, ectopic pregnancy, subchorionic hemorrhage, and fetal heart rate is possible with POC pelvic ultrasonography in the obstetric patient, in addition to diagnosis of pathologic

transvenous pacing, ultrasound provides a means for success. The use of ultrasound reduces the number of attempts, the complication rates, and the amount of anesthetic used.

Symptom-based ultrasonography describes 2 approaches to point-of-care ultrasonography for emergency department patients who present with chest pain and dyspnea, or abdominal pain. The aim of this article is provide a framework to rule in or out life-threatening causes rapidly at the bedside and allow narrowing down of a large list of differential diagnosis while additional tests are being ordered. Although this article is primarily written for the emergency physician, it can also be used in other care settings. In the hands of trained clinicians, bedside ultrasonography is a truly valuable tool.

High-resolution sonography is ideal for the evaluation of many oropharyngeal and neck structures because of their superficial nature. Clinicians can use point-of-care ultrasonography to evaluate for different types of infectious and inflammatory conditions in this area, including cellulitis and/or abscess formation of the superficial soft tissues, peritonsillar abscess, cervical lymphadenitis, salivary gland inflammation and sialolithiasis, dental abscess, inflammation of the thyroid gland, internal jugular thrombosis and thrombophlebitis, and sinusitis.

Ultrasonography has been shown to be an effective imaging modality for the detection of a variety of musculoskeletal conditions, which has led emergency physicians to increasingly use this technology when assessing patients for possible fractures, joint effusions, tendinopathies, joint dislocations, and soft tissue infections. Clinical sonography is performed at the patient's bedside, and in many cases obviates other imaging studies, including radiography and magnetic resonance imaging. However, future studies will likely further delineate the role of musculoskeletal ultrasonography in the acute setting.

The use of bedside ultrasound for evaluation and resuscitation of hemodynamically unstable patients in the emergency department has become increasingly common. It is supported by a growing number of clinical studies and statement publications from various societies. Several ultrasound protocols have been proposed for the assessment of the unstable patient. This article reviews how ultrasound is used by emergency physicians to guide resuscitation of unstable patients and describes different rapid bedside ultrasound protocols that have been proposed.

ULTRASOUND CLINICS

PROGRAM OBJECTIVE:
The goal of the *Ultrasound Clinics* is to keep practicing radiologists and radiology residents up to date with current clinical practice in ultrasound by providing timely articles reviewing the state of the art in patient care.

TARGET AUDIENCE
Practicing radiologists, radiology residents and other healthcare professionals who provide care based on radiologic findings.

LEARNING OBJECTIVES
Upon completion of this activity, participants will be able to:
1. Review symptom based ultrasound.
2. Discuss focused cardiac ultrasound in the emergent patient.
3. Describe ultrasound in the patient with musculoskeletal disorders.

ACCREDITATION
The Elsevier Office of Continuing Medical Education (EOCME) is accredited by the Accreditation Council for Continuing Medical Education (ACCME) to provide continuing medical education for physicians.

The EOCME designates this enduring material for a maximum of 15 *AMA PRA Category 1 Credit*(s)™. Physicians should claim only the credit commensurate with the extent of their participation in the activity.

All other health care professionals requesting continuing education credit for this enduring material will be issued a certificate of participation.

DISCLOSURE OF CONFLICTS OF INTEREST
The EOCME assesses conflict of interest with its instructors, faculty, planners, and other individuals who are in a position to control the content of CME activities. All relevant conflicts of interest that are identified are thoroughly vetted by EOCME for fair balance, scientific objectivity, and patient care recommendations. EOCME is committed to providing its learners with CME activities that promote improvements or quality in healthcare and not a specific proprietary business or a commercial interest.

The planning committee, staff, authors and editors listed below have identified no financial relationships or relationships to products or devices they or their spouse/life partner have with commercial interest related to the content of this CME activity:
Srikar Adhikari, MD, MS; Karim Ali, MD; Richard Amini, MD; John M. Bailitz, MD, FACEP, RDMS; Sierra Beck, MD, RDMS, RDCS; Michael Blaivas, MD; Jeremy S. Boyd, MD; Stephanie Carter; Eric H. Chou, MD; Joseph Daniel; Eitan Dickman, MD, RDMS, FACEP; Vikram S. Dogra, MD; Sama Ghali, MD; Michael Gottlieb, MD; Danielle Hallett, MD; Nadim Mike Hafez, MD, RDMS; Jennifer Hashem, MD; Kristen Helm; Brynne Hunter; James Hwang, MD, MPH; Parisa P. Javedani, MD; Sandy Lavery; Marla C. Levine, MD, RDMS; Jennifer R. Marin, MD, MSc; Jared T. Marx, MD; Jill McNair; Jehangir Meer, MD, RDMS; James H. Moak, MD, RDMS; Jarrod Mosier, MD; John Munyak, MD; Lorraine Ng, MD; Refky Nicola, DO, MS; Ahmed Saleh, MD; Shideh Shafie, MD; Shannon B. Snyder, MD, FACEP; Lori A. Stolz, MD; Christopher Vaughn, MD; Anthony J. Weekes, MD.

The planning committee, staff, authors and editors listed below have identified financial relationships or relationships to products or devices they or their spouse/life partner have with commercial interest related to the content of this CME activity:
Robinson M. Ferre, MD, FACEP received a research grant from Soma Access Systems.

UNAPPROVED/OFF-LABEL USE DISCLOSURE
The EOCME requires CME faculty to disclose to the participants:
1. When products or procedures being discussed are off-label, unlabelled, experimental, and/or investigational (not US Food and Drug Administration (FDA) approved); and
2. Any limitations on the information presented, such as data that are preliminary or that represent ongoing research, interim analyses, and/or unsupported opinions. Faculty may discuss information about pharmaceutical agents that is outside of FDA-approved labelling. This information is intended solely for CME and is not intended to promote off-label use of these medications. If you have any questions, contact the medical affairs department of the manufacturer for the most recent prescribing information.

TO ENROLL
To enroll in the *Ultrasounds Clinic* Continuing Medical Education program, call customer service at 1-800-654-2452 or sign up online at http://www.theclinics.com/home/cme. The CME program is available to subscribers for an additional annual fee of USD 212.

METHOD OF PARTICIPATION
In order to claim credit, participants must complete the following:
1. Complete enrollment as indicated above.
2. Read the activity.
3. Complete the CME Test and Evaluation. Participants must achieve a score of 70% on the test. All CME Tests and Evaluations must be completed online.

CME INQUIRIES/SPECIAL NEEDS
For all CME inquiries or special needs, please contact elsevierCME@elsevier.com.

Preface
Emergency Ultrasound

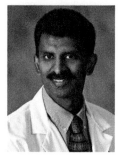 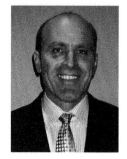

Srikar Adhikari, MD, MS   Michael Blaivas, MD
Editors

Emergency ultrasound has been in existence for well over twenty years. The earliest use of ultrasound by emergency physicians dates back to the late 1980s. In the last decade, bedside ultrasound has become an integral part of all emergency medicine training and has been thoroughly integrated into modern practices. While utilization is based on need and has regional variation, the growth of new applications never previously conceived of or attempted, such as lung ultrasound or many of the new ultrasound-guided procedures, means there will soon be no emergency medicine without emergency ultrasound.

Almost any patient presenting with an emergency complaint can benefit from ultrasound at their bedside. Whether it is therapeutic guidance or more accurate assessment through focused diagnostic ultrasound, sonologists have capabilities other clinicians do not. Unstable patients arriving with life-threatening processes, but no obvious signs, no longer wait for hours before computed tomography results or vague laboratory values that may or may not be helpful. Instead, a patient can now be evaluated on presentation, and perhaps even before registration in the department.

Applications range from ocular to musculoskeletal or soft tissue evaluation of toe complaints and everything in between. Given the realization that health care costs must be contained and medical radiation poses greater risks than ever previously discussed, ultrasound is a natural fit into emergency practice as it is in most other clinical settings. The following articles are designed to show some of the breadth of emergency ultrasound, discuss the current state-of-the-art, and also educate on what emergency ultrasound is capable of today.

Srikar Adhikari, MD, MS
Section of Emergency Ultrasound
Department of Emergency Medicine
University of Arizona Medical Center
1501 North Campbell Avenue
Tucson, AZ 85724, USA

Michael Blaivas, MD
Department of Internal Medicine
University of South Carolina School of Medicine
Columbia, SC, USA

Department of Emergency Medicine
St. Francis Hospital
2122 Manchester Expy
Columbus, GA 31904, USA

E-mail addresses:
sradhikari11@gmail.com (S. Adhikari)
mike@blaivas.org (M. Blaivas)

Ultrasound Clin 9 (2014) xiii
http://dx.doi.org/10.1016/j.cult.2014.01.013
1556-858X/14/$ – see front matter © 2014 Elsevier Inc. All rights reserved.

History, Progress, and Future of Emergency Ultrasound

Srikar Adhikari, MD, MS[a], Michael Blaivas, MD[b,c],*

KEYWORDS

- Point-of-care ultrasound • Emergency ultrasound • Three-dimensional ultrasound
- Ultrasound education • Medical education • Resuscitation • Patient evaluation • Trauma ultrasound

KEY POINTS

- The use of point-of-care ultrasound by emergency physicians is rapidly becoming standard of care.
- The scope of emergency ultrasound will continue to expand, to fill multiple voids and needs but also as available technology continues to improve and emergency physicians grow increasingly more comfortable with a wide variety of applications that can benefit their patients.
- In particular, once approved, ultrasound contrast for body imaging is likely to make a significant impact for a variety of patients seen in the emergency department, but especially those suffering from blunt abdominal trauma.
- Three-dimensional ultrasound is only now entering the emergency ultrasound world, but researchers are confident that multiple applications will migrate to emergency ultrasound practice and that new ones will be developed.
- It is clear that emergency ultrasound will be ubiquitous throughout emergency practice within the next 10 to 20 years.

The primary use of bedside ultrasound is to answer focused clinical questions in a timely manner to direct appropriate treatment. When applied in their setting, physicians often have attached a specialty label to their ultrasound practice and emergency physicians refer to it as Emergency Ultrasound. Emergency ultrasound has numerous advantages: it is safe, rapid, noninvasive, and repeatable; can be performed at bedside; and is therefore is ideal in the emergency department (ED) setting, especially in the management of a critically ill patient. The history of clinician—performed ultrasound dates back to the 1980s when ultrasound was used for the evaluation of the trauma patient. Rozycki[1] introduced the term FAST (Focused Abdominal Sonography in Trauma) for the use of bedside ultrasound by physicians to assess trauma patients. Since then, ultrasound has rapidly expanded in the hands of emergency physicians to include a wide variety of point-of-care ultrasound applications. The unique advantages to ultrasound performed by emergency physicians include rapid assessment of critically ill patients presenting with variety of symptoms, such as chest pain, shortness of breath, or undifferentiated hypotension. It decreases time to consultation or additional diagnostic testing and length of stay in the ED. The use of ultrasound guidance for performing emergent procedures has also been shown to improve patient safety and is revolutionizing the way procedures are performed in the ED as well as allowing emergency physicians to perform procedures that were not previously possible.

The clinical applications of emergency ultrasound have grown rapidly in recent years. The

---

The authors have nothing to disclose.
[a] Section of Emergency Ultrasound, Department of Emergency Medicine, University of Arizona Medical Center, 1501 North Campbell Avenue, Tucson, AZ 85724, USA; [b] Department of Internal Medicine, University of South Carolina School of Medicine, Columbia, SC, USA; [c] Department of Emergency Medicine, St Francis Hospital, 2122 Manchester Expy, Columbus, GA 31904, USA
* Corresponding author. Department of Emergency Medicine, St Francis Hospital, 2122 Manchester Expy, Columbus, GA 31904.
E-mail address: mike@blaivas.org

Ultrasound Clin 9 (2014) 119–121
http://dx.doi.org/10.1016/j.cult.2014.01.005

ultrasound.theclinics.com

gamut of emergency ultrasound has expanded from assessment of trauma patient to very advanced ultrasound applications. Although a novice clinician sonologist may focus on identifying free fluid in the trauma patient, more experienced emergency physicians are performing advanced echocardiograms, and testicular, ocular, and airway ultrasounds. Several factors contributed to the growth of emergency ultrasound, including improved ultrasound technology, advanced ultrasound education, acquisition of advanced skills, and endorsement of emergency ultrasound by multiple societies. Ultrasound technology is rapidly evolving and ultrasound systems are becoming more compact, affordable, and easy to use with good image resolution. Multiple studies have shown that with appropriate training, emergency physicians can accurately perform bedside ultrasound examinations. The rapid proliferation of emergency ultrasound fellowship programs in the United States has also driven expansion because these fellowships provide highly trained educators and ultrasound program leasers. Although only one fellowship existed 20 years ago, that number has grown to more than 80 at last tally. With many academic positions filled for fellowship-trained physicians, more and more are venturing out to community practice where their skills are translating to ultrasound utilization by "boots on the ground physicians." The most recent American College of Emergency physicians (ACEP) Emergency Ultrasound Guidelines published in 2008 explains the scope of practice of emergency ultrasound, training pathways, credentialing, documentation, ultrasound equipment, and the quality assurance process and other societies such as American Institute of Ultrasound in Medicine recognized ACEP Emergency Ultrasound Guidelines as meeting the qualifications for performing ultrasound in the emergency setting.[2]

Recent highlight developments include incorporation of ultrasound into emergency medical services, austere environment, telesonography, and medical student education. Ultrasound's portability, ease of use, and accuracy make it an ideal tool for rapid screening, triage, and resuscitation in disaster situations. Prior studies have shown that screening ultrasonography is very reliable in the assessment of victims of mass casualty incidents.[3] Telesonography is a rapidly developing area that allows transfer of ultrasound data from remote locations through the phone or Internet. With the ongoing development of the Internet and other information technologies, telesonography is an ideal tool in under-resourced regions to obtain consultation and treatment recommendations. Prior studies have reported the feasibility of real-time wireless transmission of ultrasound images from remote locations.[4] The use of telesonography in austere environments and the international space station has also been explored and will continue to expand. Ultrasound can play an important role in the austere environment to make complex triage decisions. Because laboratory and radiology services are often very limited in this setting, ultrasound can be extremely useful to determine which patients need medical evacuation.[5]

The use of point-of-care ultrasound by emergency physicians is rapidly becoming standard of care. With the incorporation of ultrasound training into emergency medicine residency core curriculum and inclusion of emergency ultrasound into emergency medicine milestones, it has become a mandatory skill for graduating emergency medicine residents. In additional, there is growing interest to integrate ultrasound into medical school curriculum and in many institutions emergency physicians are leading the way in providing emergency ultrasound education to students throughout 4 years of medical school. The scope of emergency ultrasound will continue to expand, to fill multiple voids and needs but also as technology available continues to improve and emergency physicians grow increasingly more comfortable with a wide variety of applications that can benefit their patients. In particular, once approved, ultrasound contrast for body imaging is likely to make a significant impact for a variety of patients seen in the ED, but especially for those suffering from blunt abdominal trauma. Three-dimensional ultrasound is only now entering the emergency ultrasound world, but researchers are confident that multiple applications will migrate to emergency ultrasound practice and that new ones will be developed. It is clear that emergency ultrasound will be ubiquitous throughout emergency practice within the next 10 to 20 years and in time emergency physicians will look back and wonder how they functioned blindly, without being able to actually see the heart, gallbladder, or lung movement, or track their needle to its target.

REFERENCES

1. Rozycki GS. Abdominal ultrasonography in trauma. Surg Clin North Am 1995;75:175–91.

2. American College of Emergency Physicians. Emergency ultrasound guidelines. Ann Emerg Med 2009;53(4):550–70.

3. Beck-Razi N, Fischer D, Michaelson M, et al. The utility of focused assessment with sonography for trauma as a triage tool in multiple-casualty incidents during the second Lebanon war. J Ultrasound Med 2007;26(9):1149–56.

4. Blaivas M, Kuhn W, Reynolds B, et al. Change in differential diagnosis and patient management with the use of portable ultrasound in a remote setting. Wilderness Environ Med 2005;16(1):38–41.

5. Russell TC, Crawford PF. Ultrasound in the austere environment: a review of the history, indications, and specifications. Mil Med 2013;178(1): 21–8.

Pitfalls and Pearls in Emergency Point-of-Care Sonography

Nadim Mike Hafez, MD, RDMS[a],*, Michael Gottlieb, MD[b],
John Bailitz, MD[b]

KEYWORDS

- Point-of-care • Ultrasound • Clinical pearls • Clinical pitfalls

KEY POINTS

- Emergency point-of-care sonography (POCS) is a versatile diagnostic and procedural tool that has improved patient care in the fast- paced world of the emergency department for nearly 2 decades.
- As utilization further increases, so will the risk of liability.
- Knowledge about the numerous pitfalls and key pearls can help the busy clinician use emergency POCS in a safe and efficient manner.

FAST

Focused Assessment with Sonography in Trauma (FAST) is one of the most commonly performed Emergency point-of-care sonography (POCS) core applications. Brought to the forefront by Dr Grace Rozycki in the 1990s, FAST now includes evaluation for pneumothorax (PTX) as part of the Extended FAST examination (EFAST).[1] Although many clinicians are already proficient in EFAST, avoiding these pitfalls and recalling these pearls will help both the novice and the expert sonographer.

Pitfalls

- Mistaking a pericardial fat pad for a hemopericardium. A pericardial fat pad appears as an anterior hypoechoic layer. Septations may be noted in the adipose tissue on close inspection. By contrast, an acute hemopericardium is typically a more circumferential anechoic layer, with increasing echogenicity if clot develops.
- Incorrectly equating a normal pericardial sac as negative for pericardial injury in a penetrating trauma patient with a large

hemothorax. A significant injury to the pericardial sac may allow immediate exsanguination into the hemothorax without the retention of blood in the pericardial sac.[2]
- Failing to recognize the double-line sign. Anechoic areas surrounded entirely by hyperechoic lines that may mimic free fluid. Common causes include perinephric fat within Gerota fascia, renal cysts, bowel containing liquid, the gallbladder, and abdominal vasculature.[3,4] By contrast, free fluid is often described as "pointy" and partially bordered by only one hyperechoic line. For example, blood in the Morison pouch appears anechoic in relation to the liver, with a hyperechoic border only along the Gerota fascia (**Figs. 1 and 2**).

Pearls

- Select a transducer that matches the patient's body habitus. An all-purpose convex transducer is often the first choice. However, in thin and pediatric patients, a smaller footprint phased-array transducer facilitates scanning between the ribs for the right upper quadrant and left upper quadrant views. In addition,

The authors have nothing to disclose.
[a] Department of Emergency Medicine, Rush University Medical Center, 1653 W Congress Parkway, Chicago, IL, USA; [b] Cook County Emergency Medicine Residency, 1900 West Polk, Chicago, IL 60612, USA
* Corresponding authors.
E-mail address: nhafezmd@gmail.com

Ultrasound Clin 9 (2014) 123–141
http://dx.doi.org/10.1016/j.cult.2014.01.002
1556-858X/14/$ – see front matter Published by Elsevier Inc.

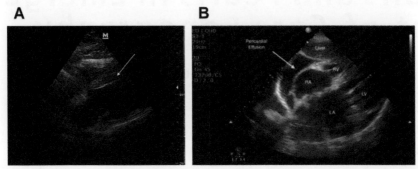

Fig. 1. Pericardial fat pad versus effusion in the subxiphoid view. The arrow in (*A*) is pointing to a pericardial fat pad, which shows some internal echoes. (*B*) The same subxiphoid view shows a positive pericardial effusion that appears completely anechoic.

the phased-array transducer is a better choice for obtaining a parasternal long (PSL) axis view of the pericardium when the subxiphoid view cannot be obtained because of obesity.

- Distinguish hemopericardium from hemothorax by identifying the descending aorta on the PSL view of the heart. Hemopericardium can be seen as an anechoic space in between the left ventricle and the pericardium tapering into an anechoic "rat's tail" anterior to the descending aorta. Hemothorax will only be seen posterior to the descending aorta.[5]

Identify the junction of the right atrium and inferior vena cava (IVC) by directing the transducer from the subxiphoid scanning plane caudad toward the abdomen. Then rotate the transducer indicator 90° clockwise into a longitudinal scanning plane to visualize the posterior pericardium and long axis of the IVC. This action will further distinguish an anterior fat pad from a posterior hemopericardium. In addition, free fluid and a flat IVC supports significant blood loss while hemopericardium and large IVC supports tamponade. A large IVC without a hemopericardium suggests volume overload,

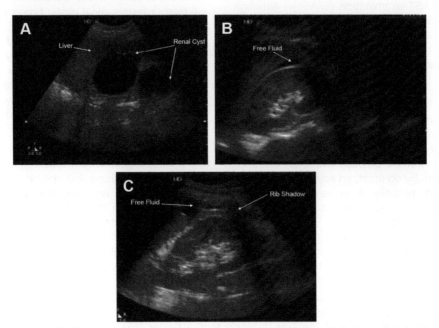

Fig. 2. Renal cyst double-line sign versus free fluid in right upper quadrant at inferior pole of right kidney. (*A*) The appearance of 2 large renal cysts that may be mistaken for free fluid. However, unlike the hypoechoic free fluid seen at the inferior pole of the right kidney in (*B*), these areas are flanked by hyperechoic lines (double-line sign) and have no acute angles. Both (*B*) and (*C*) show fluid collecting at the inferior poles of the right and left kidney, respectively.

impaired cardiac function, or obstructive shock from tension pneumothorax, pulmonary embolism (PE), or other conditions (**Figs. 3–5**).[6–8]

- Evaluate both paracolic gutters to detect early hemoperitoneum. From the right or left upper quadrant views, slide the transducer caudad to visualize the inferior pole of the kidney.[9,10] This action may allow the detection of blood just beginning to spill over from the pelvis into the Morison pouch (see **Fig. 2**B, C).
- Perform serial examinations. Repeating the FAST examination after fluid boluses or a change in clinical condition will improve diagnostic accuracy while providing a dynamic assessment of response to therapy. With continued bleeding, anechoic fluid collections will increase in size. Likewise, the bladder will continue to fill, providing an acoustic window for the detection of pelvic bleeding. Alternatively, placing a Foley catheter, filling the bladder with sterile saline, then clamping during the FAST examination rapidly creates an acoustic window.[9,10]

THORACIC POCS

Thoracic ultrasonography for pneumothorax is now routinely included in the EFAST examination. Portions of both the FAST and EFAST examinations are critical components of numerous POCS shock protocols.[8,11] More detailed thoracic ultrasound techniques are helpful in the evaluation of dyspnea, chest pain, and other medical complaints. Because thoracic ultrasonography relies primarily on the detection of artifacts, this application has unique pitfalls and pearls.

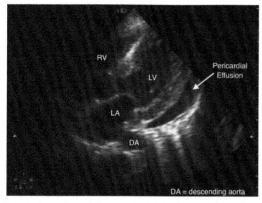

Fig. 3. Parasternal long-axis (PSL) view with pericardial effusion. The pericardial fluid seen in this image layers out above the descending thoracic aorta. LA, left atrium; LV, left ventricle; RV, right ventricle.

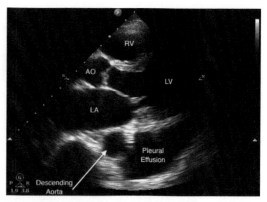

Fig. 4. PSL view with pleural effusion. Pleural effusion borders but does not extend superior to or beyond the descending thoracic aorta. AO, aorta; LA, left atrium; LV, left ventricle; RV, right ventricle.

Pitfalls

- Assuming that loss of normal B-mode lung sliding is diagnostic of a PTX. When lung sliding is not easily visualized, adjust depth to approximately 6 cm. Then use power Doppler or M-mode to improve detection of motion at the pleural line. On M-mode of normal lung sliding, the straight lines above the pleural lines represent the normal chest wall. The granulose appearance below the pleural line represents air artifact in the alveoli. Together the straight lines create the waves above the sand comprising a normal "Sea shore" sign. When lung sliding is indeed absent, remember that the loss of lung sliding may occur in several conditions including shallow reparations, acute respiratory distress syndrome (ARDS), mainstem intubation, and previous pleural injury.[12,13]
- Misinterpretation of the back-and-forth vibrations of the pleura synchronous with the heart beat as sliding lung sign. Rhythmic motion of the pleura caused by cardiac oscillations transmitted through a motionless lung is called lung pulse sign.
- Relying on the presence of lung point to rule in a PTX. A lung point is visualized as the loss of lung sliding at the point where the visceral and parietal pleura are no longer apposed. The lung point is the only 100% specific sign for PTX. However, with a large PTX, the lung point is often no longer present owing to lung collapse, resulting in complete loss of pleural apposition (**Fig. 6**).[12–14]
- Evaluating the lung at only a superficial depth and without turning off the ultrasound system processing features that purposely remove diagnostic artifacts. When evaluating the

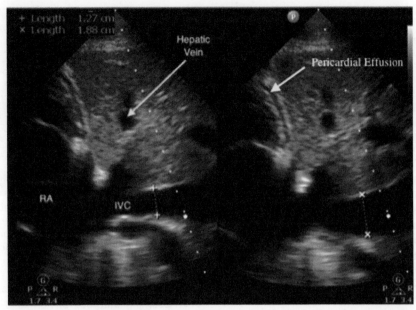

Fig. 5. Split-screen view of the inferior vena cava (IVC) in long axis with a positive pericardial effusion.

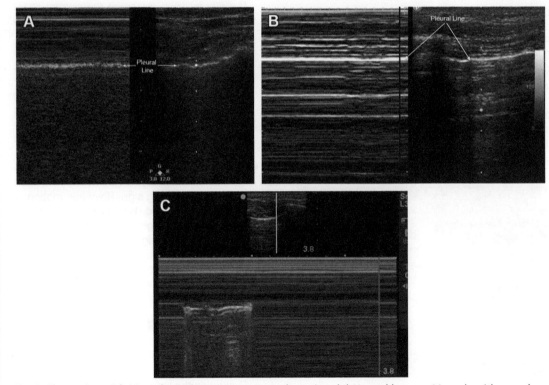

Fig. 6. Pleura view with M-mode seashore versus stratosphere sign. (*A*) Normal lung on M-mode with a seashore sign confirming pleural movement. By contrast, (*B*) shows no pleural movement (barcode or stratosphere sign), which raises the suspicion for a pneumothorax. (*C*) A lung point that is 100% specific for the presence of a pneumothorax.

lung, begin by increasing depth to 18 cm. Then turn off postprocessing features such as harmonics to examine the lungs for the presence of B-line and A-line artifacts. B lines are typically thin hyperechoic, laser-like, reverberation artifacts that originate from the pleural line in the near field before streaking down through the far field. Scattered B lines may often be seen in the supine patient in the posterior lateral lung fields. By contrast, A lines are horizontal mirror-image artifacts of the pleural line. When present, B lines always erase A lines.[13,15]

Pearls

- When subcutaneous emphysema is present, both chest wall anatomy and lung artifacts are lost. Air in the soft tissues will result in ring-down artifact originating immediately below the footprint of the probe, obliterating normal anatomy and artifacts throughout the scanning field.[12,14]
- The presence of B lines has 100% negative predictive value for PTX. In addition, the presence of 3 or more B lines in one lung zone is pathologic.[11,12] When present in at least 2 of 4 anterior lateral lung zones on each hemithorax, an alveolar interstitial syndrome (AIS) is present. Acute AIS often results from congestive heart failure (CHF) or ARDS. Acute

CHF is confirmed by poor function of the left ventricle, a large IVC, and AIS on lung ultrasonography. As preload increases, the volume of interstitial thin alveolar fluid increases. Thin B lines thicken and ultimately coalesce. For both CHF and PTX, POCS has now been demonstrated to be more accurate than plain radiography (**Fig. 7**).[13,15,16]

AORTA POCS

Consistent anatomy within commonly understood anatomic planes makes evaluation of the abdominal aorta a core application in emergency POCS that is easy to learn. For the low-risk stable patient with new back pain, emergency POCS often reduces the need for computed tomography (CT) screening for abdominal aortic aneurysm (AAA). For the high-risk unstable patient, Emergency POCS often confirms the diagnosis of AAA and speeds the time to operative intervention. Even in this seemingly straightforward examination, there are important pitfalls to avoid and pearls to remember to ensure appropriate emergency POCS utilization.

Pitfalls

- Failing to visualize the entire abdominal aorta. Most AAAs are fusiform and are evident throughout the mid to distal aorta. However,

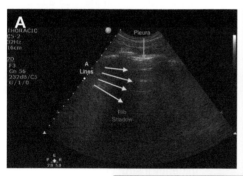
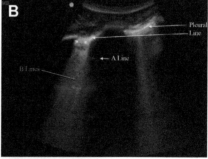
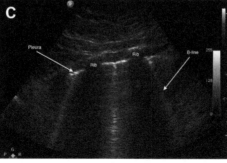

Fig. 7. (A) A lines. (B) Pleural view with labeled landmarks and showing B lines and A lines. A lines and B lines may be present on the same image but they are never present in the same place, as B lines erase or cover up A lines.

rarely an AAA may be saccular and seen only in an isolated portion of the abdominal aorta. Yet rupture of the smaller saccular aneurysms is no less deadly. Do not rule out an AAA if any segment of the aorta has not been clearly visualized.

- Ruling out rupture of an AAA with emergency POCS. Although nearly 100% sensitive and specific for the presence of an AAA, emergency POCS does not reliably detect rupture. If no AAA is seen, there is no rupture. However, when an AAA is present in a symptomatic patient, emergency POCS cannot reliably detect retroperitoneal rupture. Subtle sonographic findings of retroperitoneal hemorrhage such as anteriorly displaced kidneys are often difficult to appreciate in the critically ill or obese patient.[17]

Pearls

- Apply consistent transducer compression to displace bowel gas. Provide adequate pain control when possible. Then ask the patient to relax his abdominal walls by bending his knees and not "push back" with the abdominal muscles. Occasionally, right-flank coronal imaging may be used if excess bowel gas is still present.[17]
- Always scan the aorta in 2 anatomic planes. From the sagittal plane, a clinician may mislabel the IVC as the aorta if not being careful to identify proximal aorta branch vessels. In addition, the scanning plane may be off center of a large AAA. This anomaly may cause the busy clinician to mistakenly measure the lateral portion of the lumen as a normal-size aorta because of the cylinder tangential effect. Visualizing the vertebral body, aorta, and IVC from the axial plane avoids these errors.
- Be sure to measure the outside wall to outside wall in 2 perpendicular measurements when an AAA is present. Often the lumen of a now ovoid AAA is partially filled with echogenic clot of varying age, which may cause the clinician to underestimate the true size of the AAA.
- AAA is most frequently misdiagnosed as renal colic. In any patient with risk factors for AAA with a new diagnosis of suspected renal colic, be sure to visualize the kidneys as well as the aorta.
- Remember that an adequate emergency POCS aorta examination rules out an AAA. However, emergency POCS cannot exclude an aortic dissection. Additional imaging is needed to exclude thoracic or abdominal aortic dissection.

- The longitudinal plane is helpful in identifying a dissection flap within the aortic lumen. In addition, the longitudinal plane is useful for measuring turbulent Doppler flow within the aortic lumen surrounding the intimal. Doppler flow is best measured when the ultrasound waves are either in the same or opposite direction of blood flow. Flow is not apparent when the scanning waves are directly perpendicular to flow. Adjust the angle of the scan plane or Doppler gate to confirm the presence or absence of flow within a vessel (**Fig. 8**).

GALLBLADDER POCS

In comparison with evaluation of an AAA, emergency POCS to evaluate for cholelithiasis and related complications is often more challenging to perform and interpret. Anatomic variability of gallbladder, nearby bowel gas, and patient obesity make the examination more difficult. For several years clinicians have been able to reliably detect cholelithiasis on POCS, but until recently findings of acute cholecystitis were considered less reliable on emergency POCS in comparison with consultative ultrasonography.[18]

Pitfalls

- Bowel gas and body habitus often limit visualization of the gallbladder. Patients with symptomatic cholelithiasis are typically obese. Hyperechoic air in the stomach or duodenum immediately adjacent to the gallbladder may mimic gallstones.
- Failing to consider other causes of gallbladder wall thickening. Common causes include postprandial state, ascites, CHF, hepatitis, renal failure, and several other chronic conditions.[21]

Pearls

- Begin the examination by positioning the patient in the left lateral decubitus position. Intermittently instruct the patient to take a medium to deep breath in and hold for 5 to 10 seconds. This action causes the gallbladder to fall out from the gallbladder fossae closer to the transducer. Start with the transducer in the longitudinal scanning plane in the midclavicular line. Next, rotate the transducer as needed to visualize the long axis of the gallbladder. Alternatively, follow the main lobar fissure from the portal vein to locate the long axis view of the gallbladder.[19]
- In patients with a long or prominent rib cage, the liver and gallbladder may be identified through an intercostal approach. Select a

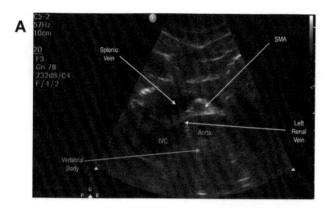

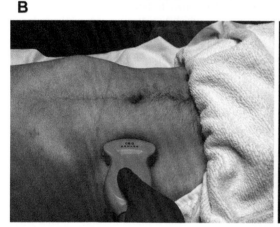
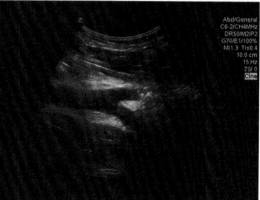

Fig. 8. Aorta in short-axis view and coronal view of aortic bifurcation. (*A*) Midabdominal aorta in the short-axis view. The left renal vein is labeled to remind the sonographer that the renal vessels serve as a landmark for finding aortic aneurysms. (*B*) Coronal view of the aortic bifurcation.

small-footprint phased-array or microconvex probe to facilitate visualization of the liver and gallbladder from in between the ribs.

- Distinguish hyperechoic gallstones from air in nearby bowel by shadow type. Hyperechoic gallstones create a clean anechoic shadow. Hyperechoic bowel gas creates a dirty echoic shadow of ring-down air artifact. In addition, close inspection will reveal peristalsis within bowel loops.
- The neck of the gallbladder should be carefully scanned to avoid overlooking impacted gallstones. Obstructive symptoms can occur when the neck of the gallbladder is obstructed by a stone, leading to cholecystitis.
- The wall echo shadow sign (WES) helps correctly identify a gallbladder nearly filled with stones. The WES consists of a curved hyperechoic line formed by the gallbladder wall, followed by a thin hypoechoic space from remaining bile, then a second hyperechoic line with clean shadowing (**Figs. 9** and **10; Fig. 22**).

UROLOGIC POCS

Nephrolithiasis is a common urologic emergency. Over the last decade, helical CT has become the standard of care, owing to its rapidity and accuracy. However, increasing concern over radiation exposure and costs of medical care has prompted renewed utilization of POCS to for nephrolithiasis. In addition, POCS is also helpful in detecting life-threatening mimics of renal colic such as AAA. Like nephrolithiasis, testicular torsion requires immediate diagnosis and management. Emergency POCS may rapidly confirm testicular torsion at the bedside, prompting immediate surgical consultation when consultative ultrasonography is not available. Despite the fact that urological imaging is relatively straight forward, several unique considerations that may aid ED physicians in their ability to detect pathology will be reviewed.

Pitfalls

- Failing to consider factors affecting the detection of hydronephrosis. In symptomatic

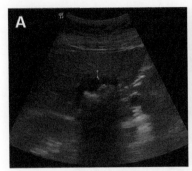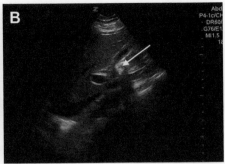

Fig. 9. Gallstones versus false-positive shadow. (*A*) Shows a gallbladder that has a thickened wall and multiple gallstone that are casting shadows. These shadows are uniformly anechoic, unlike those caused by the bowel gas in (*B*) (*arrow*). (*B*) Shows a dirty shadow that originated from a piece of hyperechoic peristalsing bowel below the gallbladder. Note the shadow originates below the gallbladder wall, which appears thickened in this patient's postprandial image.

nephrolithiasis, vomiting may result in dehydration that prevents the development of hydronephrosis. Pregnancy, polycystic kidney disease, vesicoureteral reflux, a well-hydrated patient, and an overdistended bladder may all be misinterpreted as pathologic hydronephrosis.[20,21]

- Imaging only the symptomatic testicle with suspected torsion may result in a false-negative examination. A partially torsed testicle may appear to have adequate flow if not compared with the contralateral side. Subtle asymmetries in color and pulsed Doppler flow are clues in detecting partial torsion.

Pearls

- Use the appropriate transducer and patient positioning. With thinner patients, consider the use of a small-footprint phased-array or

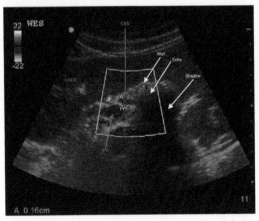

Fig. 10. Wall echo shadow (WES) sign. The labeled image demonstrates the appearance of a gallbladder full of stones. The hyperechoic wall and stones almost appear as one casting a large uniformly anechoic shadow.

microconvex probe to scan between the ribs. When scanning the long axis of the kidneys, move the transducer from the coronal scanning plane into an oblique plane by turning the transducer indicator toward the bed, thus facilitating visualization through the ribs. In addition, this slightly oblique orientation of the transducer is parallel to the true long axis of the kidney. If optimal views are not easily obtained with the patient supine, immediately reposition the patient in the decubitus or even prone position.[20,21] Examining through the psoas muscles removes bowel gas and improves visualization of the kidneys and ureters.

- Always visualize both kidneys and bladder to detect clinically significant hydronephrosis. Mild bilateral hydronephrosis may be seen in the adequately hydrated patient with a distended bladder. Prominent renal pyramids and vasculature may also be confused with mild hydronephrosis. Remember that dilated pyramids only surround the renal pelvis. Use color flow to distinguish mild hydonephrosis from vasculature. Moderate and severe hydronephrosis will be more obvious. However, bilateral comparison and bladder views are always helpful to evaluate for postrenal obstructive uropathy from unsuspected pelvic masses compressing the ureters, or bladder outlet obstruction.

- Carefully inspect common sites of stone impaction. The ureteropelvic junction and ureterovesicular junction (UVJ) can be seen on transabdominal ultrasonography. Transvaginal imaging may be helpful in detecting UVJ stones in pregnant women. Ureteropelvic junction stones are more difficult, but may be detected when scanning posterior through the psoas. Use color flow to check for twinkle artifact confirming suspected stones.

- Note that the presence of bilateral ureteral jets does not rule out nephrolithiasis. A non-obstructing stone may cause ureteral spasm and actually increase the frequency of urinary jets on the affected side.[20,21] In addition, the time required for the accurate assessment of bilateral urinary jets may not be feasible in the busy emergency department (ED).
- When performing an emergency POCS examination for testicular torsion, begin by optimizing Doppler and gain settings on the normal testicle. Use color Doppler followed by spectral Doppler to independently assess both arterial and venous flow in the normal testicle. Venous inflow is lost first, followed by arterial inflow. Then repeat the examination on the affected testicle. If flow is difficult to detect, use power Doppler. Remember that immediately after detorsion, the affected testicle may have increased flow. Recording images both before and after detorsion maneuvers will document initial findings and results, thus ensuring appropriate surgical management even after detorsion.[22] Obtain consultative ultrasonography, once available, to confirm findings (**Figs. 11** and **12**).

COMPRESSION POCS FOR DEEP VENOUS THROMBOSIS

Venous thromboembolism results in significant short-term and long-term morbidity and mortality. Early diagnosis and treatment is key to preventing complications. A decade of research has demonstrated that emergency compression POCS for deep venous thrombosis (DVT) is both rapid and accurate. In many low-risk patients, a normal examination prevents the need for additional laboratory or imaging studies. In high-risk critically ill patients, a positive examination may confirm clinical suspicion, allowing for more timely treatment.

Pitfalls

- Obtaining incomplete views and inadequate compression. Although relatively straightforward, complete coaptation of vein walls should be achieved during compression.
- Chronic thrombus may be difficult to distinguish from acute thrombus. Compare the size of the vein with that of the adjacent artery. If the vein appears distended in comparison with the adjacent artery, acute thrombus is more likely. Echogenic thrombus with collaterals is chronic.
- The absence of DVT in the symptomatic extremity does not always rule out PE. Embolization of the entire clot may result in PE with a negative ultrasonogram.
- Lymph nodes may be confused with blood clots if the operator does not take the time to view the vessel in both the short and the long axis.

Pearls

- Preparation is key to success. Elevate the head of the bed slightly to 15° to 30° of flexion at the hips. When possible, ask the patient to roll partially into the lateral decubitus position so that the affected extremity is externally rotated. Alternatively, drape the pelvis and place the lower extremities in a frog-leg position. To improve visualization of the popliteal fossa, position the patient seated or prone with the leg flexed at the knee.
- Once the vessels are visualized, apply ultrasound gel over the expected course of the vein to avoid the need to constantly reapply gel. In most patients, a high-frequency linear transducer provides optimal visualization and adequate depth. With limiting adipose

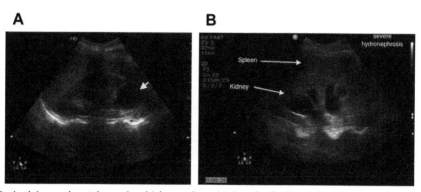

Fig. 11. (*A*) Peripelvic renal cyst (*arrow*), which may be mistaken for hydronephrosis. (*B*) Severe hydronephrosis.

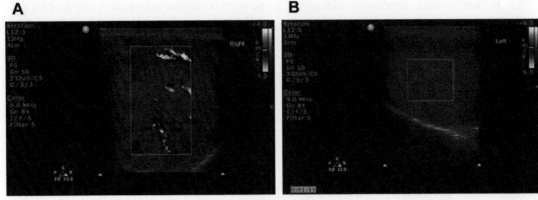

Fig. 12. Testicle, normal versus torsion. (*A*) A normal testicle with positive color Doppler flow, in sharp contrast to the absence of flow in the region of interest seen in (*B*).

tissue or edema, select a curvilinear probe to visualize deeper structures.

- If no thrombus is visualized, complete short-axis compression of a vein without significant arterial deformation rules out a DVT. In challenging cases, visualize the vein in long axis. Use color flow to identify deeper vessels. Normal venous respiratory variation in the femoral vein on spectral Doppler imaging helps to rule out a more proximal acute clot.[23,24] Normal augmentation in the femoral vein on spectral or color Doppler imaging with manual compression of the gastrocnemius helps to rule out a more distal acute clot. Because of the significant morbidity and mortality with venous thromboembolism, equivocal and positive cases require consultative ultrasonography whenever feasible (**Fig. 13**).

MUSCULOSKELETAL AND SOFT-TISSUE POCS

POCS is very helpful for the evaluation of several ED musculoskeletal (MSK) and soft-tissue complaints. The rapid identification of injury, infection, and foreign bodies by POCS often speeds appropriate management and ensures timely follow-up. Given the wide range of indications for MSK and soft-tissue POCS, there are several unique pitfalls and pearls to review.

Pitfalls

- Relying on POCS to exclude foreign bodies. Ultrasonography is not very sensitive in detecting small foreign bodies. Subcutaneous tissues with similar echogenicity can obscure foreign bodies.
- Confusing anisotropy with pathology. Tendons may have hypoechoic areas suggesting injury or inflammation if not scanning

perpendicular to the tendon fiber. Both tendons and nerves are subject to anisotropy artifact that must be accounted for when scanning (**Fig. 14**).

- Misinterpreting joint pannus as effusion. Joint pannus is hypoechoic soft tissue adjacent to the articular surfaces, which lacks compressibility and has increased flow on power Doppler.
- Failing to use POCS to help distinguish cellulitis from suspected abscess in skin or intraoral and peritonsillar areas. Pediatric patients often require procedural sedation for abscess incision and drainage. Parents are understandably unhappy when an unnecessary incision confirms cellulitis or a localized area of induration from an insect bite. The same approach should be used in the management of adult patients without clear-cut indications for incision and drainage.

Pearls

- Identify normal regional anatomy by scanning the unaffected extremity or adjacent areas in 2 planes first. This approach helps identify abnormalities even if the clinician is not familiar with normal sonographic anatomy. However, the clinician must recognize the sonographic appearance of skin, subcutaneous tissue, fascia planes, muscles, nerves, tendons, and ligaments, as well as bones in 2 orthogonal planes. When scanning the affected area, use a standoff pad or water bath to improve patient comfort and thereby image quality (**Fig. 15**).[25,26]
- Inform patients that a negative POCS does not ensure the absence of small foreign bodies. Explain to the patient the natural history of most soft-tissue foreign bodies. In

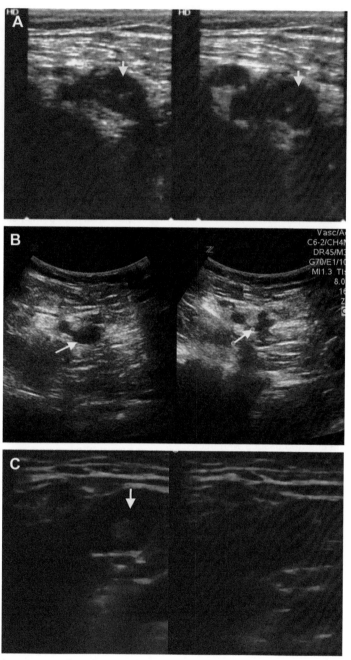

Fig. 13. (*A*) Positive deep venous thrombosis with incomplete venous compression and luminal clot (*arrows*). By contrast, (*B*) shows incomplete compression secondary to body habitus and (*C*) appears to be a luminal clot but is actually a lymph node (*arrow*).

addition, deeper soft-tissue foreign bodies are often best removed in the relative calm of the specialist's office. In either situation, provide and document adequate patient instructions and follow-up.

- Minimize anisotropy artifact by ensuring that the ultrasound beam remains perpendicular to the tendon or nerve fibers. This action typically requires gentle rocking of the probe as the entire course of the tendon is evaluated. Confirm all findings in 2 planes.
- Hypoechoic areas are also common at the insertion points of tendons into the articular cartilage of younger children. Comparison

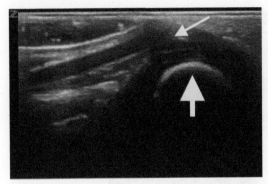

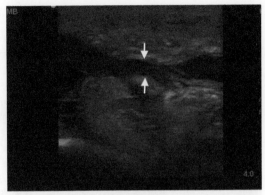

Fig. 14. False-positive rupture in the Achilles tendon showing a hypoechoic area (*small arrow*). However, it was present bilaterally and does not represent abnormality but rather an apophysis (*large arrow* represents the calcaneous).

Fig. 15. True-positive rupture of tendon with a similar hypoechoic area. It is outlined bilaterally by fluid that is secondary to the inflammatory reaction that was caused by this tendon rupture.

views of the contralateral limb or unaffected nearby joint must be obtained. Articular cartilage is found bilaterally, whereas pathology is more commonly unilateral (**Fig. 23**).[27]

- Tendon tears result in fluid visible in the inflamed tissues not only below the tendon but also above it. Isolated joint injuries causing inflammatory or traumatic effusions will be located solely underneath the tendon (**Fig. 16**).[27]
- Cellulitis typically results in relative hyperechogenicity of the affected tissues with thickening of skin and subcutaneous tissue planes. Abscess appearance may vary. A classic abscess is anechoic to hypoechoic, with posterior wall enhancement, and movement of contents of the abscess cavity with gentle probe pressure. However, MRSA abscesses associated with methicillin-resistant *Staphylococcus aureus* often have a more loculated appearance within planes of surrounding cellulitis. Determine the largest pocket of infection that is in close proximity to the skin. Mark the area with a surgical pen in 2 planes to identify

the optimal site for incision and drainage. Then use color Doppler to determine proximity of the abscess cavity to nearby lymph nodes, blood vessels, nerves, and joints.[28,29] Repeat the ultrasonography if needed to ensure adequate drainage of large abscess cavities (**Fig. 17**).

- Use POCS to both diagnose and treat peritonsillar abscess (PTA). POCS for PTA is more accurate than the physical examination, reduces the need for both CT and Ear/Nose/Throat consultation, and guides drainage. If no focal PTA is noted, unnecessary aspiration may be avoided. When necessary, POCS guidance provides direct visualization of the nearby carotid artery, reducing the likelihood of arterial injury during aspiration attempt.[30,31]

OCULAR POCS

Ophthalmologists have recognized for decades that the orbit is the perfect ultrasound medium. Over the past several years, clinicians have likewise begun to use ultrasonography for a variety of emergent disorders. Ocular POCS helps to

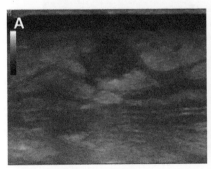
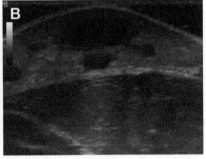

Fig. 16. Variation in appearance of abscess (*A, B*) demonstrates the heterogeneous appearance of soft-tissue abscess.

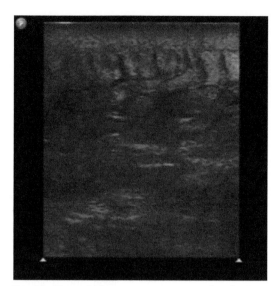

Fig. 17. The cobblestone appearance of soft tissue associated with cellulitis.

identify medical conditions such as retinal detachment and central retinal artery occlusion more accurately than the traditional ED eye examination. With careful preparation, Ocular POCS may likewise even be used for traumatic ocular disorders.

Pitfalls

- Injury to the already traumatized eye resulting from excessive probe pressure. Careful patient selection, preparation, and probe stabilization is essential to prevent unnecessary pressure on the orbit.
- Failure to distinguish between a vitreous detachment and retinal detachment. Although both require specialty consultation, retinal detachment may require emergent intervention.

Pearls

- Prevent contamination of the conjunctiva with ultrasound gel. Although the ultrasound gel is not an eye irritant, gel contamination can be bothersome to the patient. If preferred, instruct the patient to close his or her eye and gently apply a tegaderm before applying copious ultrasound gel.
- When performing ocular POCS, first stabilize the hand holding the transducer on the patient's forehead, maxillary bone, or nasal bone. As with all POCS examinations, scan the normal then the affected anatomy in 2 scanning planes. During the examination, instruct the patient to move through the cardinal positions of gaze to fully visualize all orbital structures.

- The only contraindication to ocular POCS for traumatic disorders is an obvious open globe injury. Ocular POCS is very helpful in the detection of lens dislocation, foreign bodies, and increased intracranial pressure. Apply a large quantity of gel to avoid contact between the transducer and the eyelid. Detecting a collapsed anterior chamber on POCS indicates occult globe rupture.[32–34]
- Differentiate a vitreous detachment from a retinal detachment by reducing the overall gain. Both may appear funnel-shaped and attached to the optic disk. However, as the posterior hyaloid surface of the vitreous is less dense than the retina, a vitreous detachment will fade in when the gain is reduced, in comparison with the highly reflective retinal detachment.[32–34]
- Identify vitreous hemorrhage. In comparison with retinal detachments, vitreous hemorrhage is very mobile. The resulting image shows a swaying seaweed-like mass with rapid staccato movements. Recent retinal detachment will display only a slower undulating movement.
- To assess for central retinal artery or vein occlusion, use color or power Doppler to demonstrate an absence of flow in the affected eye. Minimize the duration of the examination, especially when using Doppler, to avoid theoretical risks of injury to the eye. In addition, minimize power levels and gain to decrease image-distorting echoes caused by the closed eyelid (**Figs. 18 and 19**).[32–34]

FOCUSED CARDIAC ULTRASONOGRAPHY

According to a joint consensus statement by the American Society of Echocardiography and the American College of Emergency Physicians, focused cardiac ultrasonography (FOCUS) has now become a "fundamental tool to expedite the diagnostic evaluation of the patient bedside and to initiate emergent treatment and triage decisions." With improvements in technology and increasing POCS residency training, FOCUS is now widely used for the assessment of pericardial effusion, systolic function, ventricular enlargement, and volume status. In addition, FOCUS provides procedural guidance for pericardiocentesis and placement of transvenous pacemakers.[35,36]

Pitfalls

- Relying on the performance of only one view to determine systolic function. In the volume-

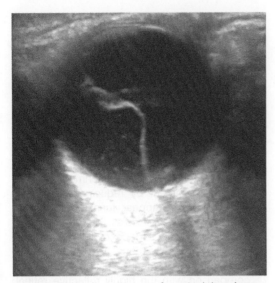

Fig. 18. A classic linear image of a retinal detachment.

depleted tachycardic patient, the rapidly beating but relatively empty heart may appear vigorous even when pump function is impaired.

- Excluding PE after a FOCUS examination. Although numerous echocardiographic findings support the diagnosis of massive PE, none has yet been demonstrated to exclude the diagnosis.
- Administering fluid boluses based only on IVC measurements. Beyond the extremes, IVC is not an accurate independent measure of the patient's need for or ability to tolerate additional fluid therapy.
- Not recognizing the limitations of FOCUS. The misuse or inappropriate interpretation of any diagnostic tests may result in adverse patient outcomes.

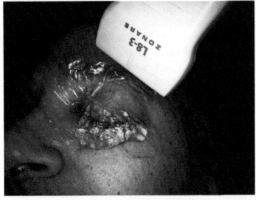

Fig. 19. This image shows how a tegaderm dressing can be applied over the eye to keep the coupling gel from irritating the patient's conjunctiva.

Pearls

- Proper patient positioning is required to obtain the optimal cardiac windows. After the subxiphoid view, elevate the head of the bed 15° to 30°. Then roll the patient into the left lateral decubitus position when possible. This positioning displaces the lung and brings the heart closer to the chest wall, improving the image quality of the parasternal and apical views.
- Parasternal views are difficult to obtain in patients with hyperinflated lungs from chronic pulmonary disease or the concurrent use of positive pressure ventilation. However, the traditional FAST examination subxiphoid view is often easily obtained in these patients. In addition, a short-axis view of the left ventricle can be obtained from the subxiphoid position. Rotate the probe into a sagittal scanning plane by turning the transducer marker toward the patient's head to visualize the posterior pericardium. From this subxiphoid long view, aim the transducer scanning plane toward the patient's left shoulder to visualize the left ventricle in short axis.
- Cardiac tamponade is primarily a clinical diagnosis in an unstable patient with a significant pericardial effusion. A pericardial effusion impairs right heart filling, then left ventricular filling, and ultimately cardiac output. The significance of the pericardial effusion depends on the rapidity of filling within the noncompliant pericardial sac. Rapid filling in the already hypovolemic trauma patient often requires emergent intervention. Do not delay appropriate life-saving treatment in the crashing patient. In the more stable medical patient with a chronic pericardial effusion, the initial FOCUS examination is often followed by specialty consultation and comprehensive echocardiography.
- Systolic function may be more difficult to assess in the volume-depleted and tachycardic patient after only one initial view. Many acute and chronic medical conditions and medications affect a patient's systolic function. After the subxiphoid view, obtain additional views and repeat the assessment to more accurately estimate systolic function and assess the individual patient's response to therapy.
- None of the echocardiographic findings of PE are sensitive enough to exclude the diagnosis. Right ventricular dilation, the McConnell sign (mid-free wall akinesia or hypokinesis with normal apical motion on the apical 4-chamber

view), right ventricular dysfunction, intraventricular septum flattening, IVC dilation without inspiratory collapse, and lower extremity DVT are moderately specific with poor sensitivity for PE.[37]

- Assessment of the IVC during FOCUS provides a good estimate of volume status at the extremes. However, ultrasonographic measurements of the IVC do not correlate reliably across the range of central venous pressure (CVP). In addition, CVP is not a reliable measure of fluid responsiveness.[38] Use ultrasonographic measurements of the IVC as one component of volume status. In addition, always perform IVC ultrasonography with the other components of FOCUS and thoracic POCS to better predict a patient's response to additional fluid therapy.
- The limitations of clinician-performed FOCUS must be recognized. Always obtain a comprehensive echocardiogram when trained clinicians are not available, findings are equivocal, or more advanced questions need to be answered (**Figs. 20** and **21**).

PELVIC POCS

Emergency Pelvic POCS accurately and safely reduces the length of stay in ED in patients presenting with first-trimester pelvic pain or bleeding suggestive of ectopic pregnancy. Over the last 2 decades, ultrasonography has significantly improved outcomes in ectopic pregnancy, although it remains a leading cause of first-trimester morbidity and mortality.[39–42] The primary role of the emergency clinician is to rule out ectopic pregnancy by ruling in an intrauterine pregnancy (IUP). When an IUP is not readily visualized, the clinician evaluates for evidence of ectopic pregnancy rupture and the ectopic pregnancy itself. In stable patients the emergency pelvic POCS may then be followed by consultative ultrasonography. In addition, there are several extended indications for emergency pelvic POCS. This section focuses on the unique pitfalls and pearls in effective use of pelvic POCS in the pregnant patient.

Pitfalls

- Failing to perform pelvic ultrasonography owing to a β–human chorionic gonadotropin (β-hCG) level below the discriminatory zone. The discriminatory zone is the β-hCG level at which early evidence of an IUP should be seen on an ultrasonogram. However, ectopic pregnancy can occur at any β-hCG value.[40]
- Relying on possible early signs of IUP during emergency pelvic POCS. Following a nondiagnostic emergency pelvic POCS examination, consultative ultrasonography may report early evidence of an IUP such as an intradecidual sac sign. However, a pseudosac from an ectopic pregnancy may have a similar appearance.
- Inadequate visualization of pregnancy location. Visualization in 2 planes is essential to determine whether the pregnancy is safely within the uterus, in an abnormal location within the uterus, or outside the uterus.
- Ending a nondiagnostic emergency pelvic POCS examination in an unstable patient before assessing for fluid in the Morison pouch. Because of pain, bowel gas, obesity, or high gain settings, free fluid in the pelvis may be missed. However, free fluid in the Morison pouch is more readily assessed and confirms the need for immediate operative intervention for ruptured ectopic pregnancy.[39–42]

Pearls

- Perform emergency pelvic POCS on any patient with suspected ectopic pregnancy without waiting for β-hCG results. The role of the emergency clinician is to detect an IUP. Then identify evidence of ectopic pregnancy. When not present, the goal of consultative ultrasonography is to then detect more subtle evidence of an IUP, ectopic pregnancy, or other pelvic abnormality. Although β-hCG levels provide a context for the interpretation of findings, obtaining images is not dependent on knowledge of the β-hCG level.
- Use the visualization of a gestational sac with a yolk sac as the earliest definitive evidence of IUP. Other earlier evidence possibly suggestive of an IUP must always be confirmed on consultative ultrasonography. In addition, always consider the possibility of an additional heterotopic ectopic pregnancy in patients receiving fertility treatments.
- Ensure that the pregnancy is symmetrically properly positioned within the uterus on 2 planes. Two types of ectopic pregnancies may initially appear intrauterine, yet result in rapid and fatal hemorrhage. An interstitial ectopic pregnancy occurs when a gestational sac implants eccentrically into the very proximal portion of the fallopian tube while still within the muscular walls of the uterus. Sonographic findings of interstitial ectopic pregnancy include a gestational sac with an endomyometrial mantle of less than 8 mm,[43] an empty uterine cavity, and the interstitial-line sign connecting the gestational sac to

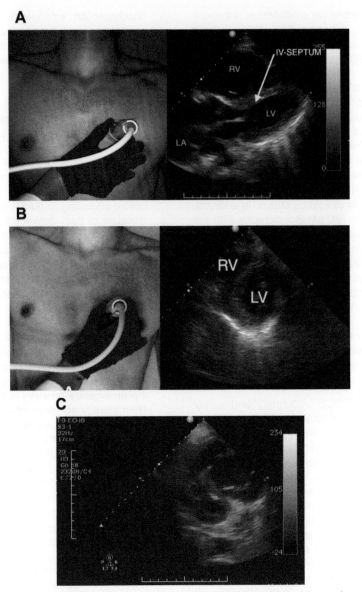

Fig. 20. PSL axis versus parasternal short (PSS) axis versus D sign. (*A*) The probe position and corresponding normal anatomy. When looking for the septal deviation that occurs secondary to right heart strain, one should rotate the probe by 90° (*B*) to the PSS axis. If the right heart strain is strong enough, the operator will obtain a positive D sign (*C*).

the endometrium. A cervical ectopic pregnancy may sometimes be confused with an impending miscarriage. Sonographic findings of cervical ectopic pregnancy include a pregnancy within the cervix, an empty uterine cavity, and an hourglass-shaped uterus in a patient with a closed cervical os (see **Fig. 22**).

POCS FOR PROCEDURAL GUIDANCE

Emergency POCS for procedural guidance improves the safety and efficiency of numerous common and infrequently performed emergency medicine procedures.[25,26] As early as 2001, the Agency for Healthcare Research and Quality (AHRQ) endorsed POCS for procedural guidance during central-line insertion as 1 of the top 11 methods to improve patient safety in the United States (American College of Emergency Physicians [ACEP] 2009 Ultrasound Guidelines). Indications for POCS procedural guidance now include several diverse procedures ranging from arthrocentesis to pericardiocentesis, and even cricothyrotomy. This section reviews pitfalls and

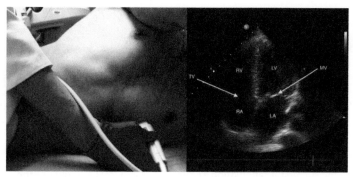

Fig. 21. Apical 4-chamber split screen. This image demonstrates the correct patient position and expected image an apical 4-chamber view.

pearls of POCS for central venous line guidance that apply to numerous other procedural applications.

Pitfalls

- Failing to use POCS procedural guidance for patients with difficult central venous access. The use of ultrasonography for this application is widely endorsed by both ACEP and the AHRQ. Emergency POCS is part of the core curriculum in emergency medicine residency education, and is quickly becoming part of the standard of care in EDs where POCS is readily available.
- Repositioning the patient after marking the skin when only using POCS for static guidance. Movement of the patient may change the relationship of the skin to relevant deeper structures in numerous procedures including central lines, abscess drainage, lumbar puncture, and pericardiocentesis.[25,26]

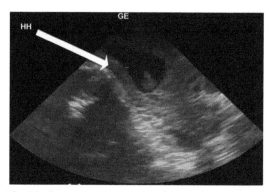

Fig. 22. Correct measurement of an endomyometrial mantle (EMM), which is necessary in early pregnancy to avoid missing a cornual pregnancy. The image shows a positive cornual pregnancy with an EMM of less than 8 mm.

Pearls

- Practice emergency POCS for procedural guidance before the next patient with difficult central venous access. Trained clinicians are already competent in traditional blind approaches to emergent procedures. Given this experience, the number of procedures required for proficiency in the additional steps of POCS procedural guidance is less than that required for diagnostic applications (ACEP Ultrasound Policy Statement). Adhering to specialty-specific training guidelines ensures appropriate utilization and credentialing. Learn scanning protocols on normal models. Perform practice procedures on phantoms and simulators. Begin with static guidance when needed. Progress to 2-person dynamic guidance and ultimately 1-person dynamic guidance as proficiency develops.
- Visualize proper guide-wire placement in the long axis of the central vein before dilation. When visualized in the short axis, inadvertent loss of the needle tip may result in puncture of the carotid artery. Before dilation of the vessel, obtain long-axis visualization of the guide wire only within the lumen of the vein to prevent arterial cannulation.[44–46] Dynamic in-plane visualization of the location of needle or guide wire provides the best confirmation of appropriate location (see **Fig. 23**).
- Confirm proper placement by visualizing routine saline flush. For central lines above the waist, visualizing opacification of the right heart during routine saline flush helps confirm central venous location. Likewise, confirm placement by visualizing small amounts of saline flush proximal to peripheral venous cannulation. This technique is also helpful in identifying needle-tip location during POCS

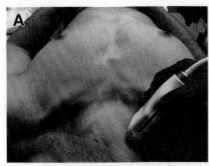
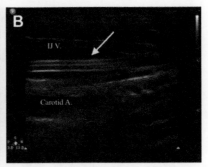

Fig. 23. View of IJ showing successful cannulation and in vein. These images highlight the relationship between the guide wire/triple lumen catheter and the ultrasound probe (*A*) and the resulting image proves successful cannulation (*B*) (*arrow* points to triple lumen catheter in in internal jugular vein).

guidance for pericardiocentesis, and when injecting small amounts of anesthetic in POCS-guided nerve blocks.

SUMMARY

Emergency POCS is a versatile diagnostic and procedural tool that has improved patient care in the fast-paced world of the ED for nearly 2 decades. As utilization further increases, so will the risk of liability. However, a recent study evaluated a large legal database and found no recorded cases brought against emergency physicians for using ultrasonography to aid in their evaluation of patients. Conversely, their search did uncover a single case whereby the emergency physician had been subjected to legal scrutiny for not using POCS.[47] Emergency POCS programs must be developed according to specialty-specific training, documentation, and quality assurance guidelines. Recognizing the unique role and limitations of POCS by recalling the pitfalls and pearls discussed will help the emergency physician use POCS safely and efficiently.

REFERENCES

1. Rozcyki GS, Ballard RB, Feliciano DV, et al. Surgeon-performed ultrasound for the assessment of truncal injuries. Ann Surg 1998;228(4):557–67.
2. Mandavia DP, Joseph A. Bedside echocardiography in chest trauma. Emerg Med Clin North Am 2004; 22(3):601–19.
3. Sierzenski PR, Schofer JM, Bauman MJ, et al. The double-line sign: a false positive finding on the Focused Assessment with Sonography for Trauma (FAST) examination. J Emerg Med 2011;40(2):188–9.
4. Daignault MC, Saul T, Lewiss RE. Right flank pain: a case report of an interesting sonographic finding. J Emerg Med 2012;43(6):1059–62.
5. Blaivas M, DeBehnke D, Phelan MB. Potential errors in the diagnosis of pericardial effusion on trauma ultrasound for penetrating injuries. Acad Emerg Med 2000;7(11):1261–6.
6. Ferrada P, Vanguri P, Anand RJ. Flat inferior vena cava: indicator of poor prognosis in trauma and acute care surgery patients. Am Surg 2012;78(12):1396–8.
7. McGahan JP, Richards J, Gillen M. The focused abdominal sonography for trauma scan: pearls and pitfalls. J Ultrasound Med 2002;21(7):789–800.
8. Perera P, Mailhot T, Riley D, et al. The RUSH exam: rapid ultrasound in shock in the evaluation of the critically ill. Emerg Med Clin North Am 2010;28(1):29–56.
9. McGahan JP, Richards J, Fogata ML. Emergency ultrasound in trauma patients. Radiol Clin North Am 2004;42(2):417–25.
10. Rose JS. Ultrasound in abdominal trauma. Emerg Med Clin North Am 2004;22(3):581–99.
11. Gillman LM, Ball CG, Panebianco N, et al. Clinician performed resuscitative ultrasonography for the initial evaluation and resuscitation of trauma. Scand J Trauma Resusc Emerg Med 2009;17:34.
12. Chan SS. Emergency bedside ultrasound to detect pneumothorax. Acad Emerg Med 2003;10(1):91–4.
13. Lichtenstein DA. Ultrasound in the management of thoracic disease. Crit Care Med 2007;35(Suppl 5):S250–61.
14. Ding W, Shen Y, Yang J, et al. Diagnosis of pneumothorax by radiography and ultrasonography: a meta-analysis. Chest 2011;140(4):859–66.
15. Kennedy S, Simon B, Alter HJ, et al. Ability of physicians to diagnose congestive heart failure based on chest x-ray. J Emerg Med 2011;40(1):47–52.
16. Kataoka H. Ultrasound pleural effusion sign as useful marker for identifying heart failure worsening in established heart failure patients during follow up. Congest Heart Fail 2012;18(5):272–7.
17. Barkin AZ, Rosen CL. Ultrasound detection of abdominal aortic aneurysm. Emerg Med Clin North Am 2004;22(3):675–82.

18. Shah K, Wolfe RE. Hepatobiliary ultrasound. Emerg Med Clin North Am 2004;22(3):661–73.

19. Summers SM, Scruggs W, Menchine MD, et al. A prospective evaluation of emergency department bedside ultrasonography for the detection of acute cholecystitis. Ann Emerg Med 2010;56(2):114–22.

20. Noble VE, Brown DF. Renal ultrasound. Emerg Med Clin North Am 2004;22(3):641–59.

21. Vallurupalli K, Atwell TD, Krambeck AE, et al. Pearls and pitfalls in sonographic imaging of symptomatic urolithiasis in pregnancy. Ultrasound Q 2013;29(1):51–9.

22. Blaivas M, Brannam L. Testicular ultrasound. Emerg Med Clin North Am 2004;22(3):723–48.

23. Bramante RM, Raio CC. Near-miss in focused lower-extremity ultrasound for deep venous thrombosis. J Emerg Med 2013;45(2):236–9.

24. Tracy JA, Edlow JA. Ultrasound diagnosis of deep venous thrombosis. Emerg Med Clin North Am 2004;22(3):775–96.

25. Tibbles CD, Porcaro W. Procedural applications of ultrasound. Emerg Med Clin North Am 2004;22(3):797–815.

26. Tirado A, Wu T, Noble VE, et al. Ultrasound-guided procedures in the emergency department-diagnostic and therapeutic asset. Emerg Med Clin North Am 2013;31(1):117–49.

27. Valley VT, Stahmer SA. Targeted musculoarticular sonography in the detection of joint effusions. Acad Emerg Med 2001;8(4):361–7.

28. Tayal VS, Hasan N, Norton HJ, et al. The effect of soft-tissue ultrasound on the management of cellulitis in the emergency department. Acad Emerg Med 2006;13(4):384–8.

29. Gaspari RJ, Resop D, Mendoza M, et al. A randomized controlled trial of incision and drainage versus ultrasonographically guided needle aspiration for skin abscesses and the effect of methicillin-resistant Staphylococcus aureus. Ann Emerg Med 2011;57(5):483–91.

30. Costantino TG, Satz WA, Dehnkamp W, et al. Randomized trial comparing intraoral ultrasound to landmark-based needle aspiration in patients with suspected peritonsillar abscess. Acad Emerg Med 2012;19(6):626–31.

31. Lyon M, Blaivas M. Intraoral ultrasound in the diagnosis and treatment of suspected peritonsillar abscess in the emergency department. Acad Emerg Med 2005;12(1):85–8.

32. Schott ML, Pierog JE, Williams SR. Pitfalls in the use of ocular ultrasound for evaluation of acute vision loss. J Emerg Med 2013;44(6):1136–9.

33. Borloz MP, Frohna WJ, Phillips CA, et al. Emergency department focused bedside echocardiography in massive pulmonary embolism. J Emerg Med 2011;41(6):658–60.

34. Blaivas M, Theodoro D, Sierzenski PR. A study of bedside ocular ultrasonography in the emergency department. Acad Emerg Med 2002;9(8):791–9.

35. American College of Emergency Physicians. Emergency ultrasound imaging criteria compendium. American College of Emergency Physicians. Ann Emerg Med 2006;48(4):487–510.

36. Labovitz AJ, Noble VE, Bierig M. Focused cardiac ultrasound in the emergent setting: a consensus statement of the American Society of Echocardiography and American College of Emergency Physicians. J Am Soc Echocardiogr 2010;23(12):1225–30.

37. Borloz MP, Frohna WJ, Phillips CA, et al. Emergency department focused bedside echocardiography in massive pulmonary embolism. J Emerg Med 2011;41(6):658–60.

38. Corl K, Napoli AM, Gardiner F. Bedside sonographic measurement of the inferior vena cava caval index is a poor predictor of fluid responsiveness in emergency department patients. Emerg Med Australas 2012;24(5):534–9.

39. Moore C, Promes SB. Ultrasound in pregnancy. Emerg Med Clin North Am 2004;22(3):697–722.

40. Wang R, Reynolds TA, West HH, et al. Use of a β-hCG discriminatory zone with bedside pelvic ultrasonography. Ann Emerg Med 2011;58(1):12–20.

41. Lambert MJ, Villa M. Gynecologic ultrasound in emergency medicine. Emerg Med Clin North Am 2004;22(3):683–96.

42. Ong CL. Pitfalls of gynaecological ultrasonography. Singapore Med J 2004;45(6):289–94.

43. Moore C, Todd WM, O'Brien E, et al. Free fluid in Morison's pouch on bedside ultrasound predicts need for operative intervention in suspected ectopic pregnancy. Acad Emerg Med 2007;14(8):755–8.

44. Blaivas M. Video analysis of accidental arterial cannulation with dynamic ultrasound guidance for central venous access. J Ultrasound Med 2009;28(9):1239–44.

45. Stone MB, Nagdev A, Murphy MC, et al. Ultrasound detection of guidewire position during central venous catheterization. Am J Emerg Med 2010;28(1):82–4.

46. Phelan M, Hagerty D. The oblique view: an alternative approach for ultrasound-guided central line placement. J Emerg Med 2009;37(4):403–8.

47. Blaivas M, Pawl R. Analysis of lawsuits filed against emergency physicians for point-of-care emergency ultrasound examination performance and interpretation over a 20-year period. Am J Emerg Med 2012;30:338–41.

Focused Cardiac Ultrasonography in the Emergent Patient

Anthony J. Weekes, MD[a],*, James Hwang, MD, MPH[b],
Sama Ghali, MD[a]

KEYWORDS

- Focused cardiac ultrasonography • Emergency medicine • Critical care • Resuscitation • Echo

KEY POINTS

- Focused cardiac ultrasonography requires skill and knowledge for image acquisition, detection of key findings, and appropriate clinical interpretation. The goal of the treating physician using cardiac ultrasonography is to answer focused clinical questions within each individual patient's clinical context.
- Basic global systolic function evaluation includes qualitative distinction of the spectrum from left ventricular contractions (absent to hyperdynamic). Advanced focused cardiac ultrasonography involves quantitative evaluations of cardiac function.
- Pericardial effusion assessment and detection of tamponade physiology are best assessed with cardiac ultrasonography.
- Right ventricle dysfunction is not diagnostic of pulmonary embolism (PE) but serves as an important risk stratification tool in suspected or confirmed PE.
- A plethora of emergency medicine and critical care research has increased the breadth and depth of focused cardiac ultrasonography. Two-dimensional transthoracic ultrasonography is the main modality used but M-mode, Doppler technology, and transesophageal technology are being used by emergency medicine and critical care specialists.
- Emerging advanced applications include diastolic function; hemodynamic measurements and monitoring; valve assessment; and volume status assessment.

 Videos of abnormal chambers, pericardial disease, myocardial and valve dysfunction, dissection, and other interesting findings accompany this article at http://www.ultrasound.theclinics.com/

Focused cardiac ultrasonography is one of the most important and frequently used applications in clinical ultrasonography. The treating physician performs and interprets the focused cardiac ultrasonography within the clinical context of that individual patient. The ultrasonographic findings do not make the diagnosis by themselves. Emergency medicine and critical care physicians often

The authors have nothing to disclose.
[a] Department of Emergency Medicine, Carolinas Medical Center, 1000 Blythe Boulevard, Charlotte, NC 28230, USA; [b] Emergency Ultrasound, Scripps Memorial Hospital, La Jolla, CA, USA
* Corresponding author.
E-mail address: anthony.weekes@carolinashealthcare.org

ultrasound.theclinics.com

require time-sensitive information and evaluations on heart structure and function in symptomatic, critically ill patients.

The *Emergency Ultrasound Guidelines*[1] from the American College of Emergency Physicians list the primary indications of basic focused cardiac ultrasonography as:

- Understand basic transthoracic cardiac windows (parasternal, subcostal, and apical) and planes (4 chamber, long and short axes)
- Recognition of relevant cardiac anatomy (chambers, pericardium, valves, and aorta)
- Qualitative global cardiac function
- Pericardial effusion detection and features of tamponade
- Inferior vena cava (IVC) assessment and its relationship with volume and central venous pressure (CVP)
- Recognition of a dilated aortic root and descending aorta

Focused cardiac ultrasonography exemplifies clinical ultrasonographic application with its wide scope of practice, which can be classified into the following clinical functions:

- Resuscitative
- Diagnostic
- Symptom or sign based
- Procedural guidance
- Therapeutic and monitoring

There is significant overlap in the practice of emergency medicine and critical care medicine. The increase in emergency ultrasonography fellowships, collaborative efforts between the specialties of emergency and critical care, and progression of focused cardiac ultrasonography research from basic to more advanced cardiac assessments have expanded and advanced the scope of focused cardiac ultrasonography applications, increased the depth of knowledge, and broadened the use of technology modalities.[2–5]

Two-dimensional transthoracic echocardiography (TTE) remains the primary modality and approach of focused cardiac ultrasonography. However, more and more emergency and critical care practitioners are showing increased proficiency in echocardiography and are now performing the focused application of M-mode and Doppler (pulsed wave, continuous wave, and tissue Doppler) when applicable.

The limitations and challenges of TTE include:

- Multiple views are often required
- Each window has its benefits and limitations
- Patient repositioning is often required

- Patient characteristics that challenge image acquisition include:
  - Lung interference (eg, chronic obstructive pulmonary disease, mechanical ventilation)
  - Crepitus
  - Narrow intercostal spaces
  - Obesity
  - Chest wall tenderness
  - Muscular chest
- Interference with cardiac monitoring device
- Ongoing chest compressions and defibrillation in periarrest and resuscitation scenarios

CASE

A 56-year-old man with hypertension reported fatigue and dyspnea. His blood pressure was 90/50 mm Hg.

The physician had to quickly determine the causes of unexplained dyspnea and hypotension. This patient may have had significant cardiac dysfunction. Echocardiography provided an immediate and readily accessible diagnostic assessment of overall cardiac function. Ruling in and ruling out systolic dysfunction can strongly influence both the differential diagnosis and clinical management.

CARDIAC FUNCTION ASSESSMENT

Cardiac function affects the hemodynamic profile of any patient and influences both respiratory status and exercise tolerance. Basic and intermediate level focused cardiac ultrasonography evaluates qualitative and quantitative left ventricular (LV) systolic function, respectively. More advanced focused cardiac ultrasonography involves advanced views, cardiac output (CO) measurements, and evaluation of LV diastolic function.

The clinical indications for assessing overall LV systolic function include, but are not limited to, the following:

- Periarrest
- Unexplained hypotension
- Shock states
- Dyspnea
- Syncope
- Chest pain
- Signs suggestive of increased CVP
- Suspicion of cardiomyopathy or cardiac failure

The primary emphasis of focused cardiac ultrasonography is contractility. However, contractility is just one of the key factors that influence overall cardiac function. Preload, afterload, and cardiac chamber shape all influence the function of the heart and its ability to eject a volume of blood to vital organs. Physicians performing focused cardiac ultrasonography must be aware of its limitations and know the indications for more detailed evaluation by comprehensive echocardiography.

Global Cardiac Contractility/Systolic Function

Normal heart mechanics involves a complex twisting action, with circumferential, radial, and longitudinal contractions. Visual estimation comes after viewing numerous cardiac ultrasonographic images of patients with varying degrees of LV function (LVF). Visual and measured evaluations of the contractility of the heart concentrate on the following parameters:

- Diastolic and systolic changes in chamber dimensions: the ventricle volume, area, and diameter decrease from the diastole phase to the systole phase; reference ranges are provided
- Thickening of myocardium with systole
- Motion of endocardium and valves: endocardial surfaces move radially inward but do not touch; severely depressed with barely any movement to hyperdynamic where near obliteration of the chamber during systole
- Longitudinal movement of annulus of valves along the long axis of the heart

Comprehensive echocardiography includes regional wall motion analysis, tissue Doppler, and use of pulsed wave Doppler to determine the Tei index of myocardial performance.

Basic: detection of asystole (ventricular standstill).

CHAMBER SHAPE AND SIZE

An appreciation of normal and relative chamber sizes and wall thicknesses allows physicians to assess for underlying cardiac disease caused by chamber enlargement, wall thickening and thinning, and abnormal dynamics when they appear (**Table 1**, Videos 1–3).

Qualitative Assessment of Global LV Systolic Function

Absolute dimensions and relative dimensions are important (**Table 2**). Visual estimates are helpful. A useful pearl is to look at the parasternal long axis (PSLA) view; the normal aortic root diameter should be similar in size to both normal left atrium (LA) and right ventricle (RV) diameters.

Ideally 1:1:1. This simple eyeball screen can detect chamber enlargement, LA size can still be underestimated. View dimensions in different windows, especially the apical 4-chamber window.

Categorization of LV systolic function:

- Severely depressed
- Moderately depressed
- Mildly depressed
- Normal
- Hyperdynamic

Quantitative Assessments of LV Systolic Function

Measurements

- Ejection fraction (EF) (**Table 3**)
  - Calculation assumes that maximum inward and outward movement of LV walls occur at the same time
  - Volumetric change of LV from diastole to systole expressed as a ratio or percentage.
  - Requires LV diastolic and systolic internal area measurements in apical 4-chamber and apical 2-chamber views
  - Generally represents systolic function
  - May overestimate cardiac function
- Limitations:
  - EF may not represent overall CO if with:
    - Significant valve abnormalities such as severe mitral insufficiency (pump leakage); reduced afterload and reduced outflow despite chamber size change and normal to increased EF calculation
    - LV hypertrophy (LVH) or hypertrophic cardiomyopathy (HCM) may lead to normal/hyperkinesis by EF values but less than normal stroke volume (SV) or CO caused by small chamber size
    - Dyssynchrony (eg, left bundle branch block [LBBB]) inward and outward motion of all LV walls do not occur at the same time. This situation makes EF measurements and interpretation of LV systolic function with LBBB unreliable
- Fractional shortening (FS):
  - The percentage decrease in either the area or the diameter of the ventricle from diastole to systole is measured. Normal LV contractility yields FS measurement approximately 45%. Fractional diameter measurements are taken at the basal aspect of the LV (**Fig. 1**).
    - Not reliable in conditions such as dyssynchrony (eg, LBBB) or septal shift

Table 1
Reference values for cardiac chamber dimensions with echocardiography

Chamber Measurement	Normal Range	Severe Increase
LV		
Ventricle diastolic diameter (cm)	4.2–5.9 (men)	>6.9
	3.9–5.3 (women)	>6.2
Posterior or septal wall thickness (cm)	0.6–1.0 (men)	≥1.7
	0.6–0.9 (women)	≥1.6
LA		
Diameter minor axis (cm)	3.0–4.0 (men)	>5.2
	2.7–3.8 (women)	>4.7
Length major axis (cm)	≤5.0	>7.0
Area (cm²)	≤20	>40
RV		
Basal diameter (cm)	2.0–2.8	>3.9
Mid diameter (cm)	2.7–3.3	>4.2
Base to apex length (cm)	7.1–7.9	>9.2
RV diastolic area (cm²)	11–28	>38
RV systolic area (cm²)	7.5–16	>23
RVOT diameter above aortic valve (cm) (parasternal short axis window)	≤2.9	≥3.6
RV free wall thickness (cm)	<0.5	
RA		
RA minor axis (cm)	2.9–4.5	>5.5
Aortic Dimensions		
LVOT diameter (systole) (cm)	1.2–2.2	
Proximal ascending aorta (cm)	3.0 ± 0.4 (men)	≥4.0
	2.7 ± 0.4 (women)	
Descending aorta (cm)	2.0–3.0	
Chamber Comparison Pearls		
Ratio RV/LV diameter	0.4–0.6	≥1.0
Ratio RV/proximal aorta: LA diameters in PSLA	1.0:1.0:1.0	

Minor axis refers to anteroposterior diameter of the chamber in the long axis view. Base to apex (major axis) length is perpendicular to minor axis measurement.
Abbreviations: LA, left atrium; RA, right atrium; RV, right ventricle; RVOT, RV outflow tract.
Data from Refs.[6–8]

- Isolated regional wall motion abnormalities
  - Measurement within a region of wall hypokinesis can underestimate overall systolic function
  - Measurement outside a region of wall hypokinesis can overestimate overall systolic function

CARDIAC OUTPUT

Cardiac output refers to the volume of blood pumped out of the heart per minute. Although EF measures the change in LV chamber dimensions between diastole and systole, the SV is the volume of blood passing through the outflow tract into the proximal aorta with each systolic contraction of the LV. Typically, CO is measured through the LV outflow tract (LVOT). The velocity time integral measures the distance traversed by most of the blood (integral of the velocities over the single systolic output through the LVOT) (**Fig. 2**).

SV = π (LVOT diameter/2)^2 × velocity time integral (VTI). It is total volume of blood ejected over the course of 1 minute of cardiac contractions (heart rate [beats/min] × SV).

The following features of LV systolic function may be useful in focused cardiac ultrasonography to recognize abnormal function and lead to more definitive assessments of LVF.

Longitudinal shortening: the mitral annulus of the LV is the reference point.

Table 2
Focused cardiac ultrasonography assessments of cardiac function

Measures of Ventricle Function	Reference Range	Severe Dysfunction
LV Systolic Function		
Ejection fraction (%)	>55	<30
FS: chamber diameter change (%)	25–43 (men)	≤14
	27–45 (women)	≤16
FS: wall thickness change (%)	14–22 (men)	≤10
Aortic VTI (cm)	18–25	
Stroke volume (mL)	70–110 (rest)	
	80–130 (exercise)	
CO (L/min)	5–8.5 (rest)	
	10–17 (exercise)	
Other Screens of LV Systolic Function		
EPSS (mm)	<5	>8
Aortic root excursion (cm)	1.16 ± 0.15	
Mitral annulus long axis movement (mm)	>12	<8
LV Diastolic Function		
E/A ratio (pulsed wave Doppler)	E>A	≥2.0 (restrictive) See **Fig. 1B**
RV Systolic Function		
RV fractional change (%)	32–60	≤17
TAPSE (cm)	1.5–2.0	<1.0

E/A ratio: transmitral flow velocity during early diastole to atrial systole.
   Abbreviations: EPSS, E-point septal separation; FS, fractional shortening; LA, left atrium; RA, right atrium; RV, right ventricle; TAPSE, tricuspid annular plane systolic excursion; VTI, velocity time integral.
   Data from Refs.[6,9–12]

- Good systolic motion moves the annulus along the long axis toward the apex. This is subtle movement. Poor systolic function barely moves the annulus
- Apical movement less than 8 mm suggests EF less than 50%
- Can be visually assessed
- Tissue Doppler used in comprehensive echocardiography

Table 3
Classification of LV systolic function by visual estimation and measurements methods

Visual Estimation/ Categorization	EF Simpson's Method (%)	Fractional Shortening LV Diameter (%)
Hyperdynamic	>65	>55
Normal	>55	25–45
Mild decrease	45–54	20–24
Moderate decrease	30–44	15–19
Severe decrease	<30	<14

E-Point Septal Separation

- Semiquantitative (**Fig. 3**)
- Looks at closest distance between the anterior mitral leaflet tip and basal LV septum during diastole
- Better at binary categorization of LV systolic function into severely depressed versus not severely depressed
- E-point septal separation (EPSS) ≥7 mm is very sensitive for severe dysfunction, but with poor specificity
- Best evaluated in PSLA; allows confident M line placement at leaflet tip; parasternal short axis (PSSA) at mitral valve level may not be at leaflet tip (falsely increased EPSS measurement)
- EPSS does not provide further distinctons of LVF along spectrum of values
- EPSS is increased by aortic regurgitation, mitral stenosis, LV dilation
- EPSS may be decreased by LVH, sigmoid septum
- Unreliable in conditions such as atrial fibrillation and LBBB

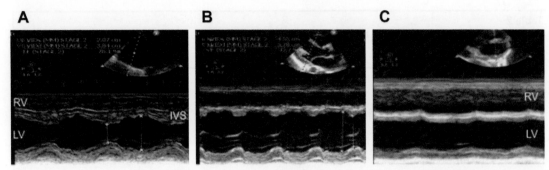

A   **B**   **C**

RV

LV   IVS

RV

LV

Fig. 1. FS comparison. Parasternal views with M-mode placed mid-LV. The M line is applied through a region of middle to basal aspect of the LV. M-mode tracings show measurements of LV internal diameter during diastole and systole. FS is a global assessment of LVF but is a regional sampling of LV dynamics. If significant regional wall motion abnormalities exist, the FS assessment can either underestimate or overestimate overall LV systolic function. (*A*) Hyperdynamic LV. (*B*) Normal LV systolic function. (*C*) Poor LV systolic function is shown using the parasternal short axis window.

Aortic Root Displacement

- Sinusoidal movement of the aortic root, as displayed on M-mode tracing, suggests normal LV systolic function (**Figs. 4** and **5**)
- Normal LV systolic function associated with normal LA filling and emptying leads to antero-posterior (AP) displacement of the aortic root
- Diminished root excursions (<0.6 cm) occur with diminished LA filling and emptying caused by poor LV systolic function[13]
- Aortic root displacement may also increase with severe mitral regurgitation (MR)
- Emergency physician performed measurement of aortic root displacement study shown to correlate well with EF[13]

Visual eyeball estimates of EF:

- Accurately distinguishes clinically significant LV systolic categories

- Less so for moderately decreased and normal
- Strong interrater agreement by emergency physician
- Useful criteria for visual estimation include:
- Motion of LV endocardial surfaces toward center (along LV minor axis)
- Movement of mitral annulus (along long axis of LV)
- Proximity of mitral leaflet tip to septal wall at early diastole

Videos 4–9 show examples of different degrees and measurements of cardiac contractility with chamber size abnormality.

LV systolic function (at the time of your evaluation of the patient) must be carefully interpreted within the context of the patient's symptoms and signs, including previous cardiac function studies if available (**Table 4**). LV systolic function is 1 component of the focused cardiac

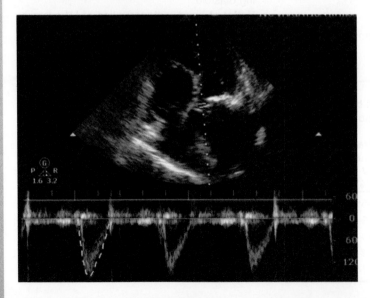

Fig. 2. CO velocity time integral (VTI). Doppler analysis of the aortic outflow tract produces a velocity profile during systole. The pulse wave sample gate is positioned within the outflow tract in the apical 5-chamber window. A tracing of the crescendo and decrescendo of blood velocities is the VTI. This information is used with the diameter of the LVOT and the heart rate to calculate the volume of blood pumped out into the aorta each minute (CO).

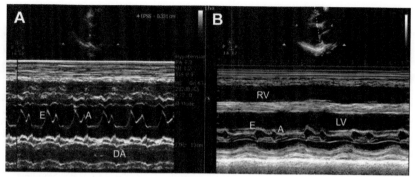

Fig. 3. E-Point septal separation (EPSS). M line applied to the mitral leaflet tip in PSLA window. (*A*) This patient has normal systolic function and normal LV and RV dimensions. The first and main movement of the mitral leaflet (E wave) comes close (0.3 cm) to the septum. An EPSS of 0 to 5 mm is associated with normal LV contractility. The second phase of diastole (E wave) is caused by atrial contraction. The relative size of the E and A waves also reflects on diastolic function. The descending aorta is noted posterior to the LV wall. It was interrogated by the M line. The echolucent region behind the posterior LV wall is the descending aorta. This region can be mistaken for a pericardial effusion if only the M tracing is looked at. Refer to the two-dimensional image and note the position and path of the M line. (*B*) Poor systolic function is shown here. The LV is mildly dilated and the tip of the E wave is 3.3 cm from the septum. At this M line position, the LV wall motion is not well depicted.

ultrasonography evaluation. Cardiac dysfunction signs may be caused by primary myocardial disorder. The 3 most common myocardial disorders are shown in **Table 5**. Clinical interpretation of overall cardiac function also includes an appreciation of the influences of preload, afterload, and valve function on the size, shape of ventricles and atria, and the appearance of their walls.

CASE

A patient arrived with dyspnea. He had increased heart rate and a blood pressure 240/130 mm Hg. His neck veins were distended and you heard rales throughout his lungs. A bedside focused cardiac ultrasonography showed thickened LV walls and his EF was clearly more than 65%. Before the echo, congestive heart failure (CHF) was

highest on the differential list. How was that list affected?

CHF is a common syndrome that involves dyspnea and fatigue with underlying cardiac dysfunction. Most patients with heart failure have both systolic and diastolic dysfunction. About half of patients with systolic dysfunction also have diastolic dysfunction. Effective CO requires good contractility after adequate filling of the LV. Ineffective filling (diastolic dysfunction) is caused by increased filling pressures. Increased LV filling pressures are caused by impaired relaxation and decreased compliance of the LV walls. Other causes of increased LV filling pressures include increased systemic vascular resistance (eg, hypertension).

Diastolic heart failure is the diagnosis assigned to patients with CHF symptoms and signs with LV systolic function that is considered

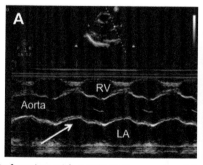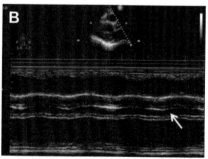

Fig. 4. Systolic function with aortic root excursion. M-mode of the aortic root and LA shows: (*A*) the sinusoidal undulations (*long arrow*) of the parallel aortic root walls in response to normal systolic movement of the LV and LA filling and emptying; (*B*) in contrast, these aortic root walls barely show any undulations (*short arrow*), with poor LV systolic function.

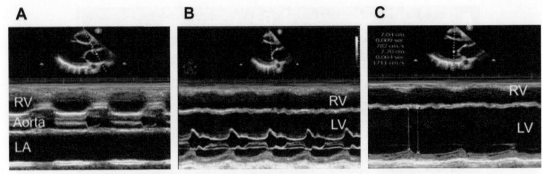

Fig. 5. Dilated heart with poor systolic function. Different placements of the M line on this PSLA view provide semiquantitative assessments of systolic function. This patient has severely depressed systolic function. The M tracings show the following: (*A*) slight aortic root undulations. The LA is dilated (LA is larger than the aortic root). (*B*) Dilated LV with large EPSS (3.0 cm). (*C*) Dilated LV (7.7 cm) with little variation between systolic and diastolic LV diameters. FS was 9%.

preserved or not severely depressed (mildly deceased to normal EF, ie, >40%). Diastolic dysfunction was previously underappreciated. It is now recognized as a significant cause of CHF. A focused cardiac ultrasonography assessment that rules out severely depressed LVF does not rule out CHF.

Table 4 Classification of LV systolic function and potential clinical interpretations	
Myocardial Contractility Findings	Associated Clinical Considerations[a]
Severely depressed	Acute vs chronic; myocarditis, sepsis, ischemic cardiomyopathy, non ischemic cardiomyopathy; acute myocardial infarction, myocardial stunning, cardiac standstill
Moderately depressed	Acute vs chronic, if CHF, consider diastolic failure
Normal	Baseline normal vs acute change; if CHF suspected, consider diastolic heart failure
Hyperdynamic	Acute; compensatory; hypovolemia; adrenergic medications, acute or chronic valve dysfunction (severe MR, severe aortic regurgitation), massive PE (assess and compare chamber size), anaphylaxis

Abbreviation: CHF, congestive heart failure.
[a] Includes, but is not limited to, these considerations or may warrant comprehensive echocardiography evaluation.

DIASTOLIC FUNCTION

Normal LV filling involves 2 stages:

- Initial isovolumetric relaxation of the left ventricle with rapid passive filling
- Second phase is supplemental filling from LA contraction
- Isovolumetric LV relaxation is the main component of diastole filling
- Focused cardiac ultrasonography evaluating mitral tip movement also provides information on diastolic function

Assessment Methods

M-mode

- Assess mitral valve leaflet tip motion during diastole
- M line applied to perpendicular to long axis of heart (parasternal long view)
- Movement of anterior mitral leaflet tip toward and away from LV septum
- Early diastole
  - E wave depicts leaflet opening during isovolumetric relaxation phase
- Late diastole
  - A wave depicts leaflet opening caused by LA contraction

Pulsed wave Doppler

- Assess transmitral blood flow velocity during diastole
- Use apical window (2 chamber or 4 chamber)
- Sample gate positioned at apical side of mitral leaflet tips
- Parallel (0°–20°) to blood flow

Table 5
Distinguishing features of cardiomyopathies

Parameter Assessed	Type of Cardiomyopathy		
	Hypertrophic	Dilated	Restrictive
LV wall thickness	Asymmetric hypertrophy	Normal or thin	Concentric hypertrophy
Ventricle size	Normal or decreased	Dilated	Normal or decreased
Atrial size	Dilated if MR present	Dilated	RA and LA dilated
LV systolic function	Normal	Depressed: moderate to severe	Normal (decreased in late stages)
LV diastolic function	Abnormal	Abnormal	Predominant abnormal

Tissue Doppler used by comprehensive echocardiography

- Assess mitral annulus muscle movement during diastole
- Diastolic function patterns used in comprehensive echocardiography

Normal diastolic LVF profile

- E wave is larger than the A wave
- E/A ratio greater than 1

There are 3 patterns of diastolic dysfunction severity (**Fig. 6**, Video 10).

Abnormal Diastolic Function Profiles

Impaired relaxation

- Reversal of E/A ratio; E/A less than 1
- Diminished E wave size; similar to normal A wave
- Sharply spiked and taller A wave
  - Increased resistance to passive inflow (impaired isovolumetric relaxation)
  - Increased A wave indicates greater contribution of atrial contraction to diastolic filling

Pseudonormalization

- E wave greater than A wave

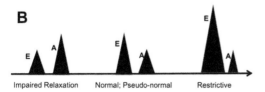

Fig. 6. Diastolic dysfunction severity patterns. Pulsed wave Doppler evaluation of blood flow across the mitral valve can provide information on diastolic functioning. The normal diastolic flow during the isovolumetric relaxation phase of the LV produces the E wave followed by a smaller A wave (atrial contraction). (*A*) Impaired relaxation is the first stage of diastolic dysfunction. The A wave is now larger than the E wave. (*B*) Worsening severity produces a restrictive pattern. The E and A wave patterns from tissue Doppler analysis are different. Other important aspects of Doppler analysis not depicted here include isovolumetric relaxation time (IRT) and deceleration of the E wave. Tissue Doppler and analysis of IRT and decelerations can distinguish normal diastolic function from the pseudonormal pattern associated with moderate severity of diastolic dysfunction.

This second pattern looks similar to normal diastolic function profile (hence its name pseudo-normal), but has a deceleration of E wave greater than 130 m/s. The differentiation of normal diastolic profile from pseudonormal pattern of diastolic dysfunction is considered beyond the scope of this discussion of focused cardiac ultrasonography.

Restrictive pattern

- Most severe form of dysfunction
- E/A ratio greater than 2
- Sharply spiked E wave
- Rapid deceleration time of early transmitral velocity less than 130 m/s

Two emergency medicine research studies performed pulsed wave Doppler mitral valve evaluations on suspected patients with CHF in the emergency department (ED). Both studies used the restrictive pattern findings on Doppler flow analysis to define diastolic dysfunction. The diastolic restrictive pattern was 82% to 89% sensitive and 80% to 90% specific in both studies.[13,14] In 1 study, the Doppler restrictive pattern was better than the FS determination of systolic dysfunction for the diagnosis of LV heart failure causing acute dyspnea.[14] Diastolic dysfunction management goals include increasing relaxation time by decreasing tachycardia; controlling dysrhythmias and maintaining sinus rhythm; reducing hypertension and afterload; prevention of myocardial ischemia.

LA chamber size assessment is an important part of the assessment of diastolic and cardiac function. The LA volume can accurately reflect the degree of diastolic function. Normal LA dimensions occur with normal diastolic function (Video 11)

- LA enlargement reflects the duration and severity of increased LV filling pressures
- Can be caused by valve stenosis and regurgitation
- LA dilation usually is not symmetric
  - Length increases more than AP diameter
  - Underestimates volume of enlarged LA if only AP diameter assessed
  - Evaluate length in apical window

Bottom line: focused cardiac ultrasonography evaluation of both systolic and diastolic function can help with the diagnosis of CHF in symptomatic patients with acute dyspnea. Maintain a concern of diastolic failure in patients with dyspnea with preserved LVF, especially those with hypertension, LVH, and tachycardia.

In patients with acute symptomatic hypotension and cardiac arrest, the focus is on ruling in or ruling out severe LV systolic dysfunction.

CASE

A 45-year-old with end-stage renal disease had increased shortness of breath and hypotension. He was lethargic and could not provide details of his symptoms. A bedside echocardiogram was performed by the sonologist and showed that his heart function was moderately depressed and there was fluid around his heart. Next, the provider confirmed that the fluid was pericardial (not pleural or peritoneal fluid) and estimated that it was a moderate to large size with signs of tamponade. Cardiology was emergently consulted. The patient remained stable, and pericardial window drainage of 2 L of fluid led to clinical improvement.

PERICARDIAL EFFUSION ASSESSMENT

Echocardiography is the ideal modality for rapidly and accurately ruling in and ruling out the presence of a pericardial effusion. Emergency medicine performed focused cardiac ultrasonography has a high sensitivity and specificity for the detection of pericardial effusion.[15] In penetrating and blunt trauma, there is a high sensitivity and specificity with subcostal parasternal cardiac evaluation within the FAST (Focus Assessment of Sonography in Trauma) protocol.[16,17] There are many clinical indications for suspecting pericardial effusion in the non-trauma patient.

PERICARDIAL EFFUSION

- Allows heart movement within a protective casing
- Cushions the heart
- Fluid accumulation limited by fibrous pericardial sac
- Pericardial sac surround heart tapers at atrioventricular sulcus
  - Near coronary sinus
  - Near descending thoracic aorta

Symptoms caused by:

- Mechanical compression of adjacent structures
- Intrapericardial pressure increase
- Decrease in CO

Ultrasonography appearance:

- Pericardial effusion is usually echolucent
- The fibrous pericardium is echogenic
- Pericardial fluid detected between outer myocardium and pericardium
- Pericardial fluid accumulations taper toward the base of the heart and do not extend posterior to the descending aorta, as shown on parasternal views (Video 12)

Volume estimate: not precise

- Size estimate by width in diastole
- Small: confined to posterior space, less than 0.5 cm
- Moderate: circumferential, less than 1 cm at widest point
- Large: greater than 1 cm at any point
- Fluid accumulation may be clinically silent

Clinical Considerations

A single view can confirm the presence of an effusion. The appearance and size of an effusion can vary from 1 cardiac window to another. When a pericardial effusion is present, signs of cardiac tamponade should be sought in as many views as possible.

RATE OF ACCUMULATION

Rapid pericardial fluid accumulation leads to rapid increases of intrapericardial pressure. Classic conditions in which tamponade physiology develops quickly include proximal aortic dissection and penetrating trauma injuries to the heart (Video 13).

Gradual accumulations of fluid may allow gradual stretch of the pericardium. Large fluid accumulation may be tolerated before intrapericardial pressure increase can provoke tamponade (Videos 14–16).

Chronic Pericardial Effusions

- Often well tolerated
- Previous pericarditis, end-stage renal disease, hypothyroidism and neoplasm, connective tissue or autoimmune disease, infection, heart failure, nephrotic syndrome, cirrhosis, pulmonary hypertension

If stable and idiopathic: no immediate treatment.

False-Positive Results

- Epicardial fat (Video 17)
- Pleural effusion

False-Negative Results

- Penetrating pericardial injuries can prevent pericardial fluid accumulations as leakage into the pleural space[18]
- Most pericardial fluid accumulations are unloculated. However, postcardiac surgery patients or those with previous history of pericardial effusion drainage can develop loculated or localized pericardial effusion. In this special patient population, TTE may miss up to 50% localized effusions.

In this special patient population, try many different windows or seek comprehensive echocardiography. If the patient is critically ill and an effusion is detected, then strongly consider the presence of tamponade.

Penetrating trauma: unclear path and depth of penetrating object can lead to significant intrathoracic injuries including to the heart.

Blunt trauma:

- Look for disorganized cardiac activity caused by cardiac contusion
- False-positive result: preexisting pericardial effusion and not caused by acute trauma

Pericarditis can occur without a pericardial effusion. Pericardial effusions may occur with pericarditis and may accompany myocarditis. Myocardial dysfunction is the main echocardiographic finding with myocarditis.

DETECTION OF TAMPONADE

- Two-dimensional (2D) real-time evaluation for RV and right atrial (RA) wall motion (**Table 6**)[19,20]
  - Distinguish systole from diastole
  - Frame-by-frame review of cine loop or recorded digital video
    - Diastole: mitral opening to mitral closure
    - Systole: as aortic valve opening to closure
  - RA collapse
    - Earliest sign of tamponade
    - Nonspecific
    - Can also occur with large pleural effusion and hypovolemia
  - RV wall collapse during diastole
    - Key finding
    - May not occur with high right-sided pressure and RV hypertrophy
      - Example: pulmonary hypertension
  - Both may be subtle or obvious
  - Tachycardia can make this tamponade feature difficult to discern

Table 6
Level of pericardial effusion assessment with echocardiography

Pericardial Effusion	Basic Focused Cardiac Ultrasonography	Advanced Focused Cardiac Ultrasonography	Comprehensive Echocardiography
Presence or absence	+ Distinguishes pleural and peritoneal fluids from pericardial fluid	+ Identifies heterogeneous pericardial effusion and pericardial constriction	+ Multiple views for loculated effusions
Size estimation (cm)	Qualitative	Small (<0.5); moderate (0.5–2.0); large (>2.0)	Qualitative and quantitative
Tamponade features	Collapse of RV free wall; includes IVC plethora	Right atrial collapse; RV diastolic collapse M-mode evaluation in subcostal or parasternal window (diastole depicted by mitral E-A waves)	Inspiratory variation Doppler inflow across mitral and tricuspid valve in apical views; RV and RA wall motion correlated with real-time electrocardiographic monitoring in any window

- M-mode evaluation
  - Subcostal or parasternal views
  - More detailed show of diastolic RV collapse
- Doppler evaluation
  - During spontaneous breathing
    - Mitral valve flow decrease greater than 25%
    - Tricuspid valve flow increase greater than 40%
  - Mechanical ventilation/adrenergic medications/severe hypotension can limit/alter this feature

CASE

A healthy 71-year-old woman had new dyspnea for 2 weeks and it had got worse today. She had labored breathing, jugular venous distension, and clear lung sounds. Her abdomen was nontender and her extremities not tender or swollen. The patient's electrocardiogram showed inverted T waves, no ST segment increase, and right bundle branch pattern. Laboratory tests: normal hemoglobin level, troponin: 0.02, brain natriuretic peptide: 2800. Her pulse oximetry reading decreased to 89% despite 7 L/min of oxygen. Chest radiography was normal. PE was the leading cause on the differential in this patient with unexplained respiratory insufficiency.

RV SIZE AND FUNCTION ASSESSMENT

Contrast-enhanced computed axial tomography of the thorax and a ventilation perfusion test are better diagnostic imaging tests for the detection of suspected PE. The risks include radiation exposure and contrast nephropathy but, most importantly, transportation of an unstable patient away from close physician and nurse monitoring.

NORMAL ANATOMY

The normal RV is a thin-walled, compliant low-pressure chamber, the size and function of which can be strongly influenced by several factors. The size and function of the RV is related to the severity and duration of pulmonary hypertension and is associated with worsening symptoms and reduced survival.

The RV free wall and septal wall contractions contribute equally to RV SV. There is significant ventricular interdependence. The RV may be enlarged primarily or secondary to LV disease. Furthermore, RV compromise can then affect LVF. The RV should be direct assessed and then compared with the LV.

The normal LV chamber is larger, with more muscular walls than the RV. The LV apex occupies two-thirds of the overall apex of the heart. The interventricular septum is curved toward the right heart because of the pressure difference between both ventricles. This feature can be seen on the any of the basic cardiac windows (Video 18).

There are several important and common causes for RV enlargement and dysfunction (**Box 1**). Obstruction to RV outflow is a common cause.

Pulmonary pressure increases because of acute respiratory distress syndrome, mechanical ventilation with increased positive end expiratory pressure settings, disease such as severe asthma and chronic obstructive pulmonary disease, and primary and secondary pulmonary hypertension. A common cause of pulmonary vascular congestion and an increased right outflow resistance is LV myocardial or valve failure.

PE is an important cause of acute RV enlargement and dysfunction. However, not all pulmonary artery occlusions compromise cardiac and respiratory function. The physiologic cycle of massive and submassive PE can fully explain key echocardiographic findings. A primary insult of pulmonary arterial obstruction may lead to pressure load. Increased RV wall tension and oxygen demand can lead to RV ischemia and decreased RV systolic function. In addition, the RV wall stretches and the RV chamber enlarges. The expansion of

RV volume is limited by the pericardium, so further increases in RV volume and pressure lead to a shift of the intraventricular septal wall toward, or even into, the LV chamber. The LV now has restricted filling (by the pericardium and inward bulge of septal wall) and decreased CO. This situation results in decreased RV preload and worsening of conditions of hypotension and respiratory distress and hypoxemia.

Acute PE has a clinical spectrum and is categorized by the level of hemodynamic compromise. Massive and submassive categories require more than heparin and oral anticoagulant therapy. These patients are better served with fibrinolytic treatments or direct administration of fibrinolytic agents within the pulmonary artery at the embolism site or surgical embolectomy. Patients with compromised right heart function (submassive PE) treated only with heparin and oral anticoagulants suffer long-term exercise intolerance dysfunction caused by persistently increased and uncorrected RV pressures.[21]

Echocardiography is not specific or sensitive enough to rule out or rule in all cases of PE.[22] A recent study[23] showed that RV dilatation and dysfunction seen on bedside cardiac ultrasonography performed by emergency physicians was 50% sensitive and 98% specific for PE. However, it has a definite role in risk stratifying patients with suspected or confirmed PE.[24] Patients with high acuity symptoms and signs with PE and RV strain are at increased risk for death shock and intubation, but even submassive PE survivors receiving heparin and oral anticoagulant (not fibrinolytics) have increased long-term risk for persistent RV dysfunction on echocardiogram with poor 6-minute walk test distance and dyspnea at rest (New York Heart Association score >2).[21] The American Heart Association's current evidence-based risk stratification and clinical management guidelines for PE use clinical acuity, RV dysfunction signs on computed tomography images and echocardiograms, electrocardiographic markers, and serum biomarkers for cardiac dilation and ischemia.[25]

Key focused cardiac ultrasonography features used for risk stratification of massive or submassive PE cases include:

- RV enlargement (Videos 19 and 20):
  - Not definitely defined
  - RV end diastolic (RVED) diameter: LV end diastolic (LVED) diameter ratio
  - Measured at base in apical 4 window
  - RV apex changes in apical 4-chamber view
    - Widens
    - Less sharp; may appear blunt (like LV apex)

Box 1
Common causes of RV enlargement

Volume Overload

- Severe tricuspid regurgitation
- Right to left shunt
- LV failure

Pressure Overload

- Pulmonary valve stenosis
- Chronic pulmonary hypertension
- Primary pulmonary parenchymal disease (chronic obstructive pulmonary disease)

Acute RV Failure

- Sepsis-induced
- Massive PE
- RV infarction
  - LV inferior wall
- Acute respiratory distress syndrome
  - Mechanical ventilation
    - Increased positive end expiratory pressure, tidal volume
  - Pulmonary vascular bed constriction/occlusion
    - Hypoxia, acidosis, thrombi, edema, and so forth

- Extends to the same level of the LV apex
  - RVED area: LVED area
    - Normal (0.4–0.6)
    - Moderate dilation (0.7–0.9)
    - Severe (≥1)
  - Some studies used RV/LV ratio as greater than 0.6, 0.7, 0.9 and greater than 1.0
- RV hypomotility (mild, moderate, severe)
- McConnel sign (RV free wall hypokinesis with active movements of RV apex [apical sparing])
- Septal shift (toward LV)
- Eccentricity of LV in PSSA view; the LV is not circular but has a flattened septal wall
- Thrombus in transit within RA, RV, or proximal pulmonary artery
  - Rarely obtained view (Video 21)
- Increased RV pressure
  - Tricuspid regurgitation velocity
  - IVC plethora:
    - Increased diameter
    - Decreased respiratory variation

The presence of 2 or more of these findings is suggestive of RV dysfunction. One of the best views for noting RV enlargement and septal shift is the PSSA view at the mitral level. The RV free wall evaluation is better in the subcostal 4-chamber and PSSA views, in which the RV wall is perpendicular to the ultrasound axis. The apical 4-chamber window is better for both RV and LV diameter measurements and tricuspid valve regurgitation Doppler evaluation and quantification.

Patients assigned as massive PE or submassive PE receive, or are strongly considered for, aggressive treatment with fibrinolytic therapy, unless contraindicated.

RV FUNCTION ASSESSMENT

Visual estimate of RV systolic movement is often used, but unlike the LV, the main component of RV systolic movement is along its long axis. Systolic function of the RV can be assessed using tricuspid annular plane systolic excursion (TAPSE) as a qualitative or quantitative guide. This assessment uses M-mode to evaluate movement of the lateral (free wall) tricuspid annulus along the RV long axis. Movements of the annulus show as undulations on the M-mode tracing (**Fig. 7**). The amplitude of the undulations is the TAPSE and correlates with RV systolic function. TAPSE measurements less than 1.6 cm are associated with abnormal RV systolic function.[26]

Conclusion of Case

Your bedside cardiac ultrasonography demonstrated signs of right heart strain and compromised LV filling and ruled out LV systolic dysfunction and pericardial effusion. She was given heparin and tenecteplase and admitted to the intensive care unit. Within 2 hours, she had normal breathing, and normal pulse oximetry readings on room air. Her comprehensive echocardiogram on the second hospital day showed normal size and function of the LV and RV. She was discharged from the hospital after 3 days with good exercise tolerance on a regimen of oral anticoagulants.

Case

A 55-year-old man with a history of hypertension presented with sudden severe chest pain

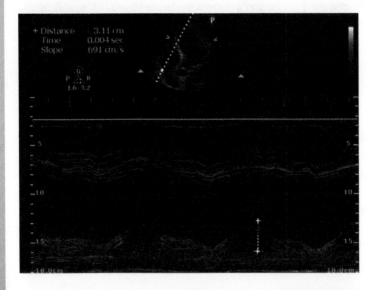

Fig. 7. RV systolic function. TAPSE: the apical 4-chamber window is used. The M line is placed through the tricuspid annulus of the RV free wall. Observe the undulating movement of the tricuspid annulus along the long axis of the RV. The measured amplitude of the tricuspid annulus movement on the M tracing (*caliper*) is called TAPSE. Measurement variations can occur because of differing angles of interrogation, patient movement, and respirations. If possible, request a brief pause in the patient's respirations, then perform TAPSE measurement.

radiating to his back. The patient denied any known history of diabetes mellitus or hyperlipidemia but admitted to recent cocaine and methamphetamine abuse. On arrival to the ED, the patient was noted to have a blood pressure of 210/120 mm Hg, heart rate of 122 beats per minute, respiratory rate of 24, and SaO_2 of 92%. On examination, the patient was clearly uncomfortable and was diaphoretic. Auscultation of the patient's heart showed a diastolic murmur over the base of the heart and faint rales over the bases. The patient had trace to 1+ bilateral lower extremity edema.

THORACIC AORTIC DISEASE

Evaluation of the aorta for acute aortic syndromes is an integral component of focused cardiac ultrasonography in the emergent patient. The aorta is divided up into segments: aortic root, ascending aorta, aortic arch, and descending aorta. Focused cardiac ultrasonography can assess parts of each of the aortic segments, particularly the aortic root and the proximal ascending aorta. Although transesophageal echocardiography (TEE) is the more optimal method for assessing for aortic emergencies, focused cardiac ultrasonography is often used as the initial modality in emergent scenarios.[27] Focused cardiac ultrasonography can provide important initial information and can also assess for some of the complications associated with aortic dissection, specifically, aortic regurgitation (discussed later) and pericardial effusion (discussed later). However, it is important to recognize the limits of focused cardiac ultrasonography (the aorta in these views lies further from the transducer, yielding suboptimal, less accurate views) and that a negative focused cardiac ultrasonography result does not rule out aortic dissection. Further imaging should always be considered (ie, TEE, computed tomography, or magnetic resonance imaging). The sensitivity of TTE in the diagnosis of ascending aorta dissection is 78% to 90%, and 31% to 55% in descending aortic dissection. The specificity for type A aortic dissection is 87% to 96%, and 60% to 83% for type B dissection.[28] Although the sensitivity and specificity for descending aortic dissection is less than ideal, this is more tenable because the management of descending aortic dissection is often more medical than surgical. Focused cardiac ultrasonography may provide earlier detection of acute ascending aortic dissection, in which mortality is as high as 1% to 2% per hour for the first 48 hours.[29]

The thoracic aorta is interrogated from multiple, composite cardiac views (**Box 2, Figs. 8–10**).

Box 2 Thoracic aorta segments shown by transthoracic cardiac ultrasonography	
Thoracic aorta segment	TTE window
Aortic root	PSLA
Ascending aorta	Right parasternal view, A3C
Aortic arch	Suprasternal notch view
Descending aorta	PSLA, A4C, A2C

Abbreviations: A2C, apical 2-chamber view; A3C, apical 3-chamber view; A4C, apical 4-chamber view.

The diagnosis of classic aortic dissection is based on showing an undulating intimal flap, which divides the aorta into 2 lumens (true and false lumens).[30] It is important to confirm the presence of an intimal flap on multiple cardiac views. The intimal flap should have a defined motion that is not parallel to the motion of any other cardiac or aortic structure. False-positive results may be caused by reverberations from atherosclerosis, sclerotic aortic root, or calcified aortic disease. Intramural hematoma is characterized by circular or crescentic thickening of the aortic wall

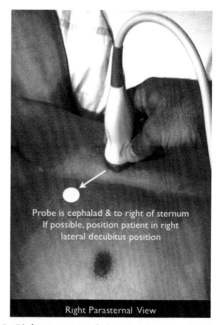

Fig. 8. Right parasternal view to assess proximal aorta and aortic valve. The probe is placed cephalad and to the right of the sternum. If possible, position the patient in the right lateral decubitus position.

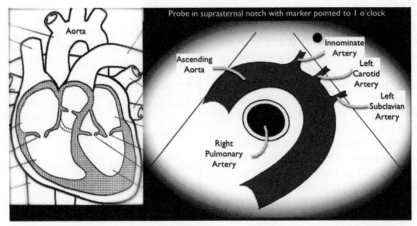

Fig. 9. Suprasternal view to assess the aortic arch. The probe is placed in the suprasternal notch, with the marker pointed toward 1 o'clock. On this view, the ascending aorta, innominate artery, left carotid artery, and left subclavian artery may be visualized.

greater than 5 mm without flow within this area of thickening. The presence of pericardial effusion in an ascending aortic dissection is an ominous sign, because it represents rupture of the false lumen into the pericardium. Aortic insufficiency can be assessed for with color flow Doppler and occurs in between 40% and 76% of patients. Aortic insufficiency may lead to volume overload and result in LV dilatation and cardiac failure. Involvement of the main coronary arteries in dissection is believed to occur in approximately 10% to 15% of patients, and the right main coronary artery is most frequently affected. Assessment for right ventricular dysfunction or regional wall motion abnormalities may raise concern for this complication. The diagnosis of thoracic aortic dilatation or aneurysm is made when the measured aortic diameter exceeds normal values (**Table 7**).[31] The standard diameter measurements are at the aortic annulus, the level of the sinuses of Valsalva, and the sinotubular junction (**Figs. 11–13**).

Case

This 72-year-old woman with a history of dementia, coronary artery disease, and chronic obstructive pulmonary disease was transported to the ED. Paramedics found her on the floor of her skilled nursing facility. As per report, the patient was usually alert and oriented x1 at baseline but her mental status was altered and responded minimally to

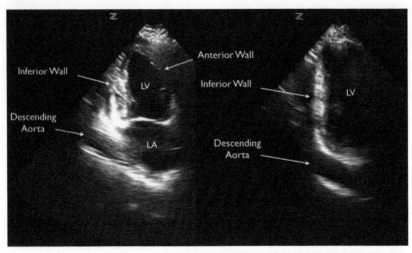

Fig. 10. Apical 2-chamber view to assess the descending aorta. The probe is placed in the apical position, and the transducer is rotated 60° counterclockwise from the apical 4-chamber view. On this view, the descending aorta is visualized deep to the LV and LA.

Table 7 Reference values for segment of the proximal thoracic aorta	
	Normal Size (cm)
Aortic annulus	2.0–3.1
Sinuses of Valsalva	2.9–4.5
Sinotubular junction	2.2–3.6
Ascending aorta	2.2–3.6
Descending aorta	2.0–3.0

verbal stimuli. Review of transfer paperwork showed that the patient had had voluminous loose stools over the last 1 to 2 days and was started on empirical treatment of possible antibiotic-associated diarrhea. Her vitals signs were 82/48 mm Hg, 128 beats per minute, 36 breaths per minute, and pulse oximetry reading of 94%. On examination, the patient had distant heart and lung sounds, very dry mucous membranes, and totally body fluid overload with 1 to 2+ pitting lower extremity edema.

Her hypotension and lethargy strongly suggested early shock. The provider was not certain about her current and underlying heart function or her volume status. Bedside cardiac ultrasonography could assist in evaluating her volume status and tolerance of fluid resuscitation.

VOLUME STATUS ASSESSMENT

Accurate assessment of a patient's intravascular volume status is often a challenge, particularly in critically ill patients with multiple comorbidities.

For patients with undifferentiated shock, volume loading and expansion is often the first-line therapy used to improve their hemodynamic status.[32] Between 40% and 70% of patients respond to a fluid challenge.[33] However, volume resuscitation is not without its risks and can have deleterious effects in patients with right heart failure, cardiogenic shock, or volume overload. Too much volume can precipitate respiratory failure and can prolong ventilation times. However, too little volume can likewise be harmful and may lead to underresuscitation and to the initiation of vasopressors before adequate volume expansion.

Evaluation of the IVC with ultrasonography (IVC-US) is an integral component of focused cardiac ultrasonography in the emergent patient. It has been proposed that IVC-US is a readily available, noninvasive estimate of a patient's intravascular volume status.[34] IVC-US examines the proximal IVC diameter as well as its change in diameter during a respiratory cycle, known as the caval index (IVC-CI) or IVC collapsibility. Tables estimating RA pressures from static and dynamic IVC measurements have been created (**Table 8**).[6] However, the data supporting such a clearly defined relationship are limited. Cutoff values for IVC diameter and collapse have since been reevaluated given the realization that the previous values performed well when estimating low or high CVP and less well with intermediate values.[26] Significant variation in baseline IVC diameter exists between individuals,[35] and a plethoric IVC may be observed in conditions not caused by intravascular volume overload (ie, pulmonary embolus, cardiac tamponade, or tension pneumothorax).

In spontaneously breathing patients, negative thoracic pressure is generated during inspiration. This process draws blood from the extrathoracic IVC up into the chest and results in a decrease

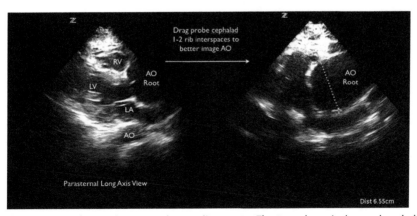

Fig. 11. PSLA view to assess the aortic root and ascending aorta. The transducer is dragged cephalad 1 to 2 rib interspaces to visualize more of the aortic root and more of the ascending aorta.

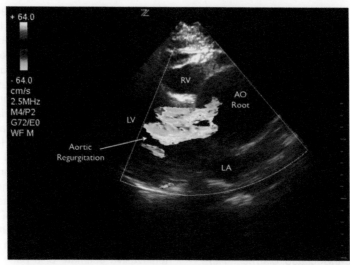

Fig. 12. PSLA view showing aortic insufficiency and aortic regurgitation caused by aortic dilatation and aortic dissection.

or collapse in the size of the IVC. During expiration, intrathoracic pressures increase and the IVC increases in size. In spontaneously breathing patients, the IVC is greatest during expiration and smallest during inspiration.

For mechanically ventilated patients, the opposite holds true. Positive pressure ventilation increases intrathoracic pressures, resulting in an increase in size of the IVC when gas flows into the lungs and a decrease in size of the IVC when gas flows out of the lungs. In mechanically ventilated patients, the IVC is greatest during inspiration and smallest during expiration (**Tables 9** and **10**).

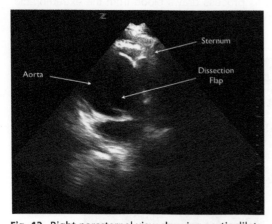

Fig. 13. Right parasternal view showing aortic dilatation and aortic dissection. The diagnosis of aortic dissection is based on showing an undulating intimal flap with a defined motion that is not parallel to the motion of any other cardiac or aortic structure.

Numerous studies have been performed to determine the usefulness of IVC-US as a reflection of CVP.[34,39] The literature is divided regarding its ability to do so. Although many studies purport a strong association,[34,39] an equal number of studies caution that IVC size is not predictable[40] based on age, sex, or body surface area and that the degree of IVC change with graded volume loading is not predictably proportional.[41] The value of these studies is called further into question by the inherent limitations of CVP as an accurate reflection of volume status. Although monitoring CVP has been shown to drive fluid resuscitation and to improve patient outcomes, it does not accurately reflect LV preload. This situation is particularly true in patients with decreased ventricular compliance, pulmonary disease, or valvular dysfunction. CVP alone can be misleading. Patients with increased CVP readings may still need

Table 8		
Correlation of IVC variables with measured RA pressures in spontaneously breathing patients		
Spontaneous Ventilation		
IVC Diameter (cm)	% Collapse	RA Pressure (mm Hg)
<1.7	Spontaneous collapse	Volume depletion
1.7	50	0–5
>1.7	>50	6–10
>1.7	<50	11–15
Dilated IVC	No collapse	>15

Table 9
Correlation of IVC variables with measured RA pressures in mechanically ventilated patients

Mechanical Ventilation		
IVC Diameter (cm)	% IVC Collapse	RA Pressure (mm Hg)
<1.2	Not reliable	<10
>2.5	<10	>15

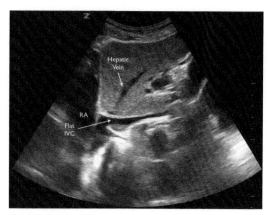

Fig. 14. Subcostal long axis view of the IVC showing a flat IVC. This IVC is small and collapses spontaneously, indicating volume depletion.

further volume resuscitation. Interpretation of IVC findings should always occur in the context of the patient's past medical history and in the context of the remainder of the patient's focused cardiac ultrasonography (ie, cardiac function, chamber shape and size, diastolic function, and CO).

The subcostal view is used to image the IVC. The IVC may be viewed in either its long or short axis. The IVC is typically measured just proximal to the junction of the hepatic veins, which lie approximately 0.5 to 3.0 cm from the junction of the IVC with the RA. When measuring percent collapse, it is important to minimize respiratory translation of the IVC into another plane (**Figs. 14** and **15**).

Case

An 84-year-old man with a history of ischemic cardiomyopathy and recent middle cerebral artery stroke presented from his rehabilitation facility with fever, respiratory distress, and

Table 10
Comparison of studies of IVC parameters and fluid responsiveness

	IVC Parameter Used (%)	FR
Spontaneously Breathing		
Muller et al	IVC-CI >40	Associated with FR
Lanspa et al,[36] 2013	IVC-CI <15	Rules out FR
Mechanical Ventilation		
Barbier et al,[37] 2004	Distensibility Index >18	Predicts FR
Feissel et al	DeltaD (IVC) >12	Identifies FR
Moretti et al,[38] 2010	Distensibility Index >16	Predicts FR

Abbreviation: FR, fluid responsiveness.

hypoxia. The patient's presentation and initial workup (leukocytosis and focal infiltrate on chest radiography) were concerning for aspiration versus health care–associated pneumonia. The patient's initial vital signs showed a blood pressure of 86/50, heart rate of 130 beats per minute, respiratory rate of 32, and an oxygen saturation of 91%. The patient was administered an intravenous fluid bolus of 1.5 L with some improvement in his heart rate but he remained hypotensive at 90/56.

Volume status assessment is performed to try and answer the more paramount question of whether a patient is fluid responsive. In general, fluid responders are those whose CO/index increases

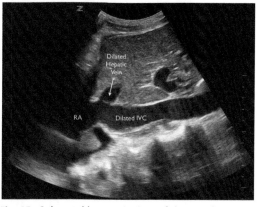

Fig. 15. Subcostal long axis view of the IVC showing a plethoric IVC. This IVC is dilated and has little respiratory collapse. Interpretation of a dilated IVC should occur in the context of the patient's medical history and in the context of the remainder of the focused cardiac ultrasonography.

by more than 15% after a fluid bolus. For patients with circulatory insufficiency, volume loading and expansion may result in an increase in IVC diameter and a decrease in IVC respiratory variation. The resultant changes tend to differ between spontaneously breathing patients and those receiving mechanical ventilation. Although threshold values may differ, the overall response of these patients to fluid challenges can be assessed with serial ultrasonography and may guide further resuscitation decisions (**Fig. 16**).

In a study on spontaneously breathing patients with circulatory failure, Muller and colleagues[42] found that IVC collapsibility cannot reliably predict fluid responsiveness, with a positive predictive value of only 72%. These investigators concluded that an IVC-CI of greater than 40% is usually associated with fluid responsiveness and that low values lower than 40% do not exclude fluid responsiveness. In a more recent but smaller study of spontaneously breathing patients with septic shock, Lanspa and colleagues[36] found that a vena cava collapsibility of less than 15% essentially rules out fluid responsiveness. More specifically, they found that a vena cava collapsibility of greater than 15% predicts a hemodynamic response, with a positive predictive value of only 62% but a negative predictive value of 100%.

In a study of mechanically ventilated septic patients, Barbier and colleagues[37] found that an IVC Distensibility Index greater than 18% predicted fluid responsiveness with a sensitivity of 90% and a specificity of 90%. A similar study by Feissel and colleagues[43] found that a DeltaD(IVC) of 12% can be used to identify fluid responders with a positive predictive value of 93% and a negative predictive value of 92%. In a more recent study of mechanically ventilated patients with subarachnoid hemorrhage, Moretti and Pizzi[38] found that an IVC Distensibility Index of greater than 16% predicted fluid responsiveness, with a sensitivity of only 70% but a specificity of 100%.

Assessing change in IVC size and dynamics is a reasonable approach; however, perhaps a more effective method of determining fluid responsiveness is to calculate the change in subaortic VTI or SV or to calculate the change in CO/cardiac index (CI) directly.[44,45] Several studies have been performed to determine the usefulness of changes in VTI or SV to dichotomize patients into fluid responders or fluid nonresponders.[46,47] Again, fluid responders are those whose CO/CI increases by more than 15% after a fluid bolus.

Calculations of VTI, SV, and CO/CI are a more advanced, but still important, component of focused cardiac ultrasonography in the emergent patient. The apical 5-chamber view is used to obtain the subaortic VTI over the LVOT. Although emergency providers have reported good image quality and measurements of VTI, VTI can be challenging in terms of interobserver and intraobserver agreement and may have fluctuations of up to 15% not related to fluid volume (**Fig. 17**).

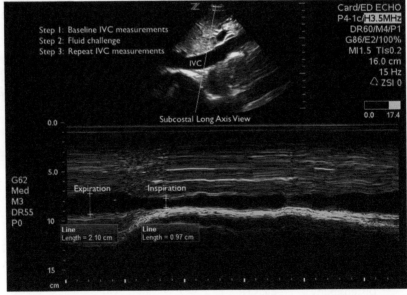

Fig. 16. Subcostal long axis view of the IVC showing IVC diameter and collapsibility. Baseline IVC diameter/collapsibility is measured, a fluid challenge is administered, and then postintervention IVC diameter/collapsibility is measured.

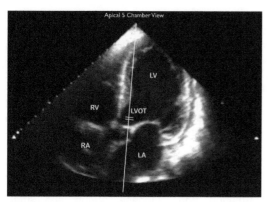

Fig. 17. The apical 5-chamber view is used to measure the subaortic VTI, which is then used to calculate the SV and CO/CI.

Passive straight leg raise is a simple, noninvasive, and reversible maneuver that redistributes blood from the lower extremities back to the central circulation.[48,49] In a study by Thiel and colleagues, a broad group of patients in a medical intensive care unit underwent passive leg raise, in which they were positioned supine with their legs straight and elevated at 45° for 2 minutes. Thiel and colleagues[48] found that an SV increase induced by passive leg raise greater than 15% predicted volume responsiveness with a sensitivity of 81%, specificity of 93%, positive predictive value of 91%, and a negative predictive value of 85%.

CASE

A 67-year-old woman with dyspnea had dilated LA and LV. Her LV systolic function was moderately poor with moderate RV enlargement. Color Doppler interrogation of her mitral region showed prominent MR jet. Comprehensive echocardiography confirmed severe mitral valve dysfunction. Her CHF was managed with afterload reduction and cardiology consults discussions about mitral valve repair.

VALVULAR ASSESSMENT

Comprehensive echocardiography provides thorough quantitative assessments of valve structure and function. This subject is considered beyond the scope of focused cardiac ultrasonography. There are suggestions that Doppler assessments for valve dysfunction may be warranted. Mild or trace MR and mild tricuspid regurgitation are common (60%–70%) among patients, especially with

aging. Emergency and critical care physicians are concerned with detection of severe valve abnormalities.

Severe valve diseases that provoke hemodynamic instability in patients are:

- Severe/critical aortic stenosis
- Severe MR (**Fig. 18**, Videos 22 and 23)
- Aortic regurgitation (Video 24)
- Severe mitral stenosis (Videos 25 and 26)

2D ultrasonography clues to valve pathology

- Calcifications
- Restricted leaflet movement
- Abnormal leaflet coaptation
- Proximal chamber dilation
- Chamber hypertrophy

SEVERE MITRAL REGURGITATION

Mitral Regurgitation (MR) creates 2 paths for blood flow with LV systole.

There is pump leakage and reduced afterload. The compensation response is typically an increased LV contractility in an attempt to create an adequate CO.

Indirect signs of significant MR:

- Dilated LV
- Hyperdynamic LV:
  - If severe MR is confirmed, cardiothoracic consultation or intervention is indicated, even with LV normal and, especially with, poor LVF

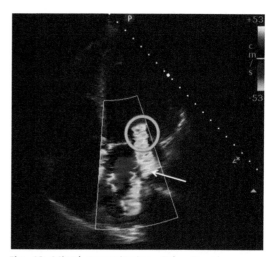

Fig. 18. Mitral regurgitation. Color Doppler assessment of the mitral valve shows regurgitant flow back into the atrium (*arrow*). The vena contracta (*circle*) shows the increased turbulence of blood flow toward the orifice. The 2-cm plus size of the vena contracta suggests moderate to severe MR.

- LA enlargement
- Interatrial septal bowing/shift to right

Direct color Doppler quantification of severe MR:

- Vena contracta greater than 0.7 cm
  - The vena contracta is a zone of maximal blood velocity as the blood drains toward the orifice causing the mitral leak. Considered akin to spiraling water draining down an unplugged bathtub. The measurement is of the narrowest color flow region between the prevalve acceleration zone and the expansion of the jets as it enters the LA.
- Area of regurgitant jet (>40% LA area) (see **Fig. 18**, Videos 22 and 23).

Mitral Stenosis

Severe mitral stenosis is commonly caused by rheumatic heart disease. Abnormal mitral opening leads to increased LA pressure and LA enlargement. The resulting pulmonary vascular congestion can lead to right heart failure. LA enlargement usually portends significant heart disease. A simple comparison of LA diameter with aortic root diameter in diastole is that LA diameter/aortic root diameter greater than 1 is a good visual marker of LA enlargement.[50] The cause can be identified with comprehensive echocardiography (see Video 25 and 26).

Aortic Regurgitation

Color Doppler in either of the parasternal views may show regurgitation but the optimal views include the apical 5-chamber and the apical long view (also called the apical 3-chamber view). Severity of aortic regurgitation is usually determined by comprehensive echocardiography. Some features of severe aortic regurgitation that can be appreciated by focused cardiac ultrasonography include: vena contracta size greater than 0.6 cm; regurgitant jet width greater than 65% of LVOT; and LV dilation (see **Fig. 12**, Video 24).

Tricuspid regurgitation, if severe, requires use of continuous wave Doppler instead of pulsed wave Doppler to quantify. Mild tricuspid regurgitation is present in many healthy asymptomatic patients. Significant tricuspid regurgitation may be secondary to acute or chronic RV pressure or size increases. Causes include pulmonary hypertension left heart failure, submassive to massive PE.

Aortic Stenosis

Aortic stenosis is a common disease that may be a consequence of aging, rheumatic heart disease, or congenital valve abnormalities. Increased afterload, compensatory LVH, and heart failure are the causes of symptoms of syncope, chest pain (angina), and heart failure in these patients. Comprehensive echocardiography can measure the critical aortic area to suggest operative intervention. Suspect aortic stenosis when these symptoms develop and when the LVH is present with or without hypertension.

PROCEDURAL GUIDANCE

Focused cardiac ultrasonography can provide information and guidance during and after procedures such as pericardiocentesis, central line placement, and transvenous pacer lead placement.

Pericardiocentesis

- Complications
  - Missed
  - Heart puncture/s
  - Coronary artery puncture/s
  - Pneumothorax
- Compounded by inexperience and haste
- Traumatic pericardial tamponade
  - Thoracotomy
  - Pericardial window
- Medical/atraumatic tamponade
  - Needle pericardiocentesis
  - Pericardial window
  - Cardiothoracic surgery (dissection)
- Dynamic/real-time guidance to observe
  - Needle enters pericardial fluid collection
  - Guidewire and pigtail catheter insertion (Seldinger technique)
  - Fluid volume decrease
  - Postprocedure heart dynamics
- Choice to sites of needle puncture and catheter insertion
  - Subcostal
  - Parasternal
- Choice of cardiac ultrasonography imaging window
  - Performed contemporaneously with needle insertion
  - Apical
  - Parasternal
  - Subcostal
- Using the subcostal approach for the pericardiocentesis procedure:
  - Needle traverses liver
  - Risk mainly of RV wall puncture
  - Use cardiac subcostal or apical window
  - Using subcostal imaging
    - Apply sterile probe cover
    - Can be performed by 1 person

- Using apical window
  - Second person needed
  - No sterile probe needed
  - Better view of needle entry
- Using the parasternal approach for the pericardiocentesis needle insertion
  - May use phased array, and even linear probe
  - Shorter distance of needle path
  - Risk mainly of left anterior descending, internal mammary artery, and cardiac puncture
  - Use modified parasternal imaging approach between PSLA and apical window
- Confirmation of central vascular catheter (CVC) placement[51–54]:
  - Used to detect optimal distal CVC tip position and suggest malposition
  - Can be used for internal jugular, subclavian, and femoral CVC
  - Real-time visualization of guidewire near to or within right heart chamber (before passage of catheter over guidewire) associated with proper CVC placement[55,56]
  - Direct visualization of distal CVC tip in superior vena cava (or IVC for femoral CVCs) is possible, but challenging, in a modified subcostal window
  - Agitated saline injection: turbulence detected entering RA then into RV
  - Saline flush: rapid flush of saline via distal CVC port with rapid appearance of turbulence entering RA and then RV (within 2 seconds of flush) using subcostal or apical 4-chamber windows (Video 27).

Transvenous Pacer placement

In 1 series, focused cardiac ultrasonography assisted in transvenous pacer placement.[57]

- Guided catheter advancement into the RV
- Identified catheter misplacement
- Confirmed successful repositioning.

Case

A well-dressed middle-aged man was rushed into the ED by ambulance with cardiopulmonary resuscitation (CPR) in progress. He had collapsed at church 5 minutes previously. He received prompt bystander CPR. His medical history was unknown. He was intubated and chest compressions continued. His cardiac monitor showed nonspecific electrical activity and no pulse was detected. He received epinephrine and intravenous fluids via the intraosseous line. He did not have shockable rhythm. Why did he have pulseless electrical activity? Would cardiac ultrasonography help or interfere with this resuscitation?

PERIARREST

Cardiac arrest is the extreme version of hypotension and shock. Periarrest requires the treating team to identify life-threatening causes of severe hemodynamic instability. Often, these causes are readily identified on the cardiac monitor as specific cardiac dysrhythmias that have specific interventions and guidelines for treatment within the Advanced Cardiac Life Support (ACLS) protocol. Nonspecific electrical activity with pulselessness (PEA) may be from other critical cardiorespiratory diagnoses. The ones that are reversible, time sensitive, and require specific medication or surgical therapeutic interventions include pericardial effusion, massive PE, severe hypovolemia, asystole or severely depressed LVF; sepsis; tension pneumothorax; severe hypokalemia, and so forth. Focused cardiac ultrasonography can rapidly identify, or strongly suggest, several of these serious conditions (**Table 11**).

This special application of focused cardiac ultrasonography is also referred to as periresuscitation echo.

- Periresuscitation echo is most effectively performed when assigned to a dedicated provider who is not performing chest compressions, airway management, or critical procedures such as central line, intraosseous line, or chest tube placements
- The subcostal window is the first option; parasternal is the second option
- Four-chamber views must be obtained quickly
- Performed during pulse checks (hold compressions)
- Acquire brief video clip (3 seconds) for review
- Incorporated and well integrated into ACLS without interruption to CPR cycles[58–61]
  - Clear commands to prepare, test, calibrate, and perform focused cardiac ultrasonography within 3 to 5 seconds, then resume CPR
  - Does not interrupt the advanced life support (ALS) management
  - Real-time evaluation of echo findings or after immediate review
  - Communication clear and concise communication of findings to CPR team
  - Augments quick identification of reversible causes

Table 11
Potential echo findings and clinical considerations during cardiac arrest resuscitation

Focused Cardiac Ultrasonography Finding	Pulse Check; Cardiac Monitor	Qualitative Interpretation	Management or Therapeutic Intervention Decision
No ventricular wall movement	Pulseless, asystole, other rhythm	Cardiac standstill	Resume CPR; continue ALS guidelines for asystole
Active organized ventricular wall movement	Weak or absent pulse	Circulation present	Hold chest compressions: evaluate for other causes of severe hypotension or shock
Isolated intermittent atrial contraction; valve movement; and no ventricular wall movement; blood stasis signs		Cardiac standstill	Continue CPR cycles and ALS and serial echo during pulse check; if persistent cardiac standstill, consider unsuccessful resuscitation
Occasional myocardial twitches to severe bradycardia and/or severely depressed systolic function	Pulseless; asystole; severe bradycardia	Myocardial shock	Adrenergic support; consider transcutaneous or transvenous pacing Serial echo to monitor response to medication or pacing
Pericardial effusion; note size; tamponade echo signs		Pericardial effusion: small or moderate/large; tamponade echo signs: consider if preexisting, new, or rapidly expanding effusion	Moderate/large: consider emergency pericardiocentesis if penetrating trauma and aortic dissection unlikely; small to large: urgent cardiothoracic surgery/trauma consultation if aortic dissection/ penetrating injury suspected
Small left ventricle; hyperdynamic; empty RA and ventricle	Pulseless or weak pulse, asystole or tachycardia on rhythm	Severe hypovolemia	Increased intravenous fluid administration; blood products; reversal of coagulopathy Evaluate for fluid loss on thorax and peritoneal spaces, hemorrhage, aorta disaster
Enlarged right ventricle cavity; septal flat or deviated toward left ventricle	Pulseless; asystole	Right heart strain	Consider massive PE or other causes of right heart strain. Consider thrombolytic therapy if no known contraindication
Poor images; impossible to get any image	Do not delay resuscitation	Indeterminate; retry with different window at next pulse check	Continue ALS without TTE assistance, consider use of TEE

- Improve patient safety with echo-guided procedural intervention; not long ago, PEA management could include blind pericardiocentesis with no knowledge of the presence or absence of a pericardial effusion
- Serial echo evaluations become important; serial focused cardiac ultrasound (FOCUS) performed throughout cardiac arrest resuscitation can reveal the following:
- Onset of organized cardiac activity before pulses can be palpated, electrical activity appears on the monitor, and return of measurable vital signs (ie, subclinical return of spontaneous circulation [ROSC]).
- Serial findings of cardiac standstill between CPR cycles, and ALS guidelines provide better information to rule out myocardial stunning and confirms an unsuccessful resuscitation
- Detect and monitor intermittent ROSC, responses to adrenergic agents, expansion of pericardial effusions, and progression to tamponade; monitor the responses to therapeutic interventions.

Primary Goals of Periresuscitation Echo

Patients with cardiac standstill identified by bedside cardiac ultrasonography at some point during ED resuscitation are unlikely to survive to hospital admission (Videos 28 and 29).

A single instance of LV standstill was 100% predictive of death in a study of 173 patients irrespective of the electrical rhythm on the cardiac monitor.[62] Minimal valvular activity with ventricular standstill was not considered to be a sign of viability or refute cardiac standstill. Slight valve twitches were considered a preterminal condition.

Survival was not zero with cardiac standstill on other studies.[62]

Focused cardiac ultrasonography during cardiac arrest works in concert with the cardiac monitor and ALS guidelines. The primary focus of the ultrasonography is the heart. It does not include IVC, aorta, thorax, or peritoneal assessments.

- Identification of a single view of cardiac standstill does not serve as a rule to declare the end of resuscitation attempts or declare death. Physician discretion is required.
- Myocardial stunning can occur
  - Ranges from temporary cardiac standstill to poor myocardial function
  - Causes of severe myocardial stunning include sepsis, massive myocardial infarction, acute drug toxicity, and noncardiogenic causes, such as intracranial bleed or seizures[63–65]

- Limitations of TTE during cardiac arrest include:
  - Not reliable or possible while chest compressions in progress
  - Heart evaluations are intermittent
  - Because of high acuity condition, optimal patient positioning is not possible
  - Sometimes any view of the heart is not possible
  - Suboptimal images, physician cannot obtain important anatomic details of the heart.
    - Do not delay CPR to struggle with a challenging view
    - When a good image is not possible or deemed indeterminate, move to a different window during the next pulse check and resume CPR resuscitation
- Other primary resuscitation goals of periarrest cardiac ultrasonography include detection of pericardial effusion, significant RV enlargement, and signs of severe hypovolemia

Case

Another patient arrived in cardiac arrest. The cardiac ultrasound views were poor. You could vaguely see cardiac activity. At the next few pulse checks, cardiac activity was briefly seen on a limited view but pulses were not felt. A transesophageal transducer was inserted and produced clear images of poor cardiac contractions but ineffective ongoing chest compressions. The provider gave instructions to improve chest compressions, resulting in more effective chest compressions as observed by TEE. Dobutamine and norepinephrine were infused with improved myocardial contractions. Chest compressions were discontinued. The patient survived to hospital admission but had an unsuccessful resuscitation several hours later.

TTE can be helpful during cardiac arrest resuscitations.[66] It is considered a more advanced application of focused cardiac ultrasonography, mainly because it is not commonly available to point-of-care physicians, the cardiac image orientation is different, and the cost of the transducer is high. It offers the following advantages over TTE.

- Improved anatomic detail and better assessment and interpretation of myocardial activity (eg, fine ventricular fibrillation on TEE vs cardiac standstill on TTE)
- Can be performed while chest compressions in progress

- Can be performed while defibrillation occurs
- Can better assess adequacy of chest compression
- Continuous viewing possible
  ○ May detect changes in rhythm and strength of contractions
  ○ Significant brief events (eg, clot in transit)
- Better at viewing pulmonary arteries and thoracic aorta

Hypotension

Although not as extreme as the periarrest resuscitation, hypotension, especially with signs and symptoms or shock, is a red flag that commands the physician's attention. The role of focused cardiac ultrasonography is well established. It is especially helpful when it can rule out specific cardiac causes of shock and quickly and accurate narrow the differential diagnosis.[67] The classic findings for severe hypovolemia, cardiogenic shock, and tamponade can be discovered.[2,58,68–71] It must be explicitly emphasized that patients arrive with preexisting medical conditions. In addition, cardiac profiles can evolve because of the current condition (like sepsis syndrome) or in response to therapeutic interventions such as volume loading or adrenergic medications. An example of this situation is that a patient with dilated cardiomyopathy does not have any classic severe hypovolemia echocardiographic features of a small hyperdynamic left ventricle with flat and collapsible IVC (Videos 30–35). Attributing positive ultrasonography findings as

the cause of dyspnea or hypotension can be a challenge, and such judgments require physician discretion (**Box 3**).

SUMMARY

The management of critically ill patients remains challenging, and the potential for harm abounds. Emergent life-threatening conditions must be quickly and carefully considered to allow for more informed resuscitation decisions. Focused cardiac ultrasonography provides emergency and critical care providers with a bedside modality to assess for immediate life threats and to gather essential, time-sensitive information. The clinical usefulness of focused cardiac ultrasonography is greatest in patients with dyspnea/hypoxia, hypotension/shock, tachycardia, and periarrest states. The core applications of focused cardiac ultrasonography confront these difficult states and include assessing left and right ventricular function, detecting the presence or absence of pericardial fluid, and assessing volume status/volume responsiveness. Although more advanced echocardiographic techniques exist, routine practice and clinical integration of these detailed applications are critical. Understanding the various limitations of focused cardiac ultrasonography is of equal importance and a key step toward realizing its many benefits.

SUPPLEMENTARY DATA

Videos related to this article can be found online at http://dx.doi.org/17.1016/j.cult.2014.01.010.

Box 3
Basic and advanced goals and findings of focused cardiac ultrasonography in emergent patient

Clinically Unstable or Emergent Patient:

- Periarrest condition
- Altered mental status
- Respiratory distress
- Hypotension (transient or persistent)
- Tachycardia
- Suspected CVP increase
- Suspected pericardial effusion

Pericardial Effusion?

If "yes":

Estimate effusion size:

Tamponade physiology?

Is IVC enlarged?

REFERENCES

1. American College of Emergency Physicians. Emergency ultrasound guidelines. 2008. Available at: http://www.acep.org. Accessed March 28, 2011.
2. Labovitz AJ, Noble VE, Bierig M, et al. Focused cardiac ultrasound in the emergent setting: a consensus statement of the American Society of Echocardiography and American College of Emergency Physicians. J Am Soc Echocardiogr 2010; 23:1225–30.
3. Lee T. Use of echocardiography: AHA/ACC guidelines summary. Heart disease: a textbook of cardiovascular medicine. p. 228–36.
4. Price S, Via G, Sloth E, et al. Echocardiography practice, training and accreditation in the intensive care: document for the World Interactive Network Focused on Critical Ultrasound (WINFOCUS). Cardiovasc Ultrasound 2008;6:49.
5. Adhikari S, Fiorello A, Stolz L, et al. Ability of EPs with advanced echocardiographic experience at a single center to identify complex

echocardiographic abnormalities. Am J Emerg Med 2013. http://dx.doi.org/10.1016/j.ajem.2013.12.010.

6. Lang RM, Bierig M, Devereux RB, et al. Recommendations for chamber quantification: a report from the American Society of Echocardiography's Guidelines and Standards Committee and the Chamber Quantification Writing Group, developed in conjunction with the European Association of Echocardiography, a branch of the European Society of Cardiology. J Am Soc Echocardiogr 2005;18:1440–63.

7. Anderson B. The normal examination and echocardiographic measurements. Wiley; 2006.

8. Qasim A, Raina A. Reference values. Available at: http://echocardiographer.org/Reference%20Values.html. Accessed January 13, 2014.

9. Weyman AE. Principles and practice of echocardiography. Philadelphia: Lea & Febiger; 1994.

10. 123sonography.com. Heart chambers and walls fact sheet. Available at: http://123sonography.com/sites/default/files/shortcourse_factsheets/Chapter%2003%20-%20Heart%20Chambers%20and%20Walls%20.pdf. Accessed January 13, 2014.

11. University of Nebraska Medical Center, College of Medicine Department of Anesthesiology. Available at: https://e-echocardiography.com/page/page.php?UID=1867001. Accessed January 13, 2014.

12. Kimura BJ, Parise CM, Monet Strachan G, et al. Diminished aortic excursion in chronic thromboembolic pulmonary hypertension. Echocardiography 2013. http://dx.doi.org/10.1111/echo.12252.

13. Unluer EE, Karagoz A, Bayata S, et al. An alternative approach to the bedside assessment of left ventricular systolic function in the emergency department: displacement of the aortic root. Acad Emerg Med 2013;20:367–73.

14. Nazerian P, Vanni S, Zanobetti M, et al. Diagnostic accuracy of emergency Doppler echocardiography for identification of acute left ventricular heart failure in patients with acute dyspnea: comparison with Boston criteria and N-terminal prohormone brain natriuretic peptide. Acad Emerg Med 2010;17:18–26.

15. Mandavia DP, Hoffner RJ, Mahaney K, et al. Bedside echocardiography by emergency physicians. Ann Emerg Med 2001;38:377–82.

16. Rozycki GS, Feliciano DV, Ochsner MG, et al. The role of ultrasound in patients with possible penetrating cardiac wounds: a prospective multicenter study. J Trauma 1999;46:543–51 [discussion: 51–2].

17. Tayal VS, Beatty MA, Marx JA, et al. FAST (focused assessment with sonography in trauma) accurate for cardiac and intraperitoneal injury in penetrating anterior chest trauma. J Ultrasound Med 2004;23:467–72.

18. Ball CG, Williams BH, Wyrzykowski AD, et al. A caveat to the performance of pericardial ultrasound in patients with penetrating cardiac wounds. J Trauma 2009;67:1123–4.

19. Goodman A, Perera P, Mailhot T, et al. The role of bedside ultrasound in the diagnosis of pericardial effusion and cardiac tamponade. J Emerg Trauma Shock 2012;5:72–5.

20. Nagdev A, Stone MB. Point-of-care ultrasound evaluation of pericardial effusions: does this patient have cardiac tamponade? Resuscitation 2011;82(6):671–3.

21. Kline JA, Steuerwald MT, Marchick MR, et al. Prospective evaluation of right ventricular function and functional status 6 months after acute submassive PE: frequency of persistent or subsequent elevation in estimated pulmonary artery pressure. Chest 2009;136:1202–10.

22. Jackson RE, Rudoni RR, Hauser AM, et al. Prospective evaluation of two-dimensional transthoracic echocardiography in emergency department patients with suspected PE. Acad Emerg Med 2000;7:994–8.

23. Dresden S, Mitchell P, Rahimi L, et al. Right ventricular dilatation on bedside echocardiography performed by emergency physicians aids in the diagnosis of PE. Ann Emerg Med 2014;63:16–24.

24. Toosi MS, Merlino JD, Leeper KV. Prognostic value of the shock index along with transthoracic echocardiography in risk stratification of patients with acute PE. Am J Cardiol 2008;101:700–5.

25. Jaff MR, McMurtry MS, Archer SL, et al. Management of massive and submassive PE, iliofemoral deep vein thrombosis, and chronic thromboembolic pulmonary hypertension: a scientific statement from the American Heart Association. Circulation 2011;123:1788–830.

26. Rudski LG, Lai WW, Afilalo J, et al. Guidelines for the echocardiographic assessment of the right heart in adults: a report from the American Society of Echocardiography endorsed by the European Association of Echocardiography, a registered branch of the European Society of Cardiology, and the Canadian Society of Echocardiography. J Am Soc Echocardiogr 2010;23:685–713 [quiz: 86–8].

27. Meredith EL, Masani ND. Echocardiography in the emergency assessment of acute aortic syndromes. Eur J Echocardiogr 2009;10:i31–9.

28. Erbel R, Engberding R, Daniel W, et al. Echocardiography in diagnosis of aortic dissection. Lancet 1989;1:457–61.

29. Rogers RL, McCormack R. Aortic disasters. Emerg Med Clin North Am 2004;22:887–908.

30. Evangelista A, Flachskampf FA, Erbel R, et al. Echocardiography in aortic diseases: EAE

recommendations for clinical practice. Eur J Echocardiogr 2010;11:645–58.

31. Erbel R, Alfonso F, Boileau C, et al. Diagnosis and management of aortic dissection. Eur Heart J 2001; 22:1642–81.

32. Dellinger RP, Levy MM, Carlet JM, et al. Surviving Sepsis Campaign: international guidelines for management of severe sepsis and septic shock: 2008. Crit Care Med 2008;36:296–327.

33. Michard F, Teboul JL. Predicting fluid responsiveness in ICU patients: a critical analysis of the evidence. Chest 2002;121:2000–8.

34. Kircher BJ, Himelman RB, Schiller NB. Noninvasive estimation of right atrial pressure from the inspiratory collapse of the inferior vena cava. Am J Cardiol 1990;66:493–6.

35. Weekes AJ, Lewis MR, Kahler ZP, et al. Comparison of baseline aortic velocity profiles and response to weight-based volume loading in fasting subjects. Acad Emerg Med 2012;19:S52.

36. Lanspa MJ, Grissom CK, Hirshberg EL, et al. Applying dynamic parameters to predict hemodynamic response to volume expansion in spontaneously breathing patients with septic shock: reply. Shock 2013;39:462.

37. Barbier C, Loubieres Y, Schmit C, et al. Respiratory changes in inferior vena cava diameter are helpful in predicting fluid responsiveness in ventilated septic patients. Intensive Care Med 2004;30: 1740–6.

38. Moretti R, Pizzi B. Inferior vena cava distensibility as a predictor of fluid responsiveness in patients with subarachnoid hemorrhage. Neurocrit Care 2010;13:3–9.

39. Nagdev AD, Merchant RC, Tirado-Gonzalez A, et al. Emergency department bedside ultrasonographic measurement of the caval index for noninvasive determination of low central venous pressure. Ann Emerg Med 2010;55:290–5.

40. Brennan JM, Blair JE, Goonewardena S, et al. Reappraisal of the use of inferior vena cava for estimating right atrial pressure. J Am Soc Echocardiogr 2007;20:857–61.

41. Weekes AJ, Lewis MR, Kahler ZP, et al. The effect of weight-based volume loading on the inferior vena cava in fasting subjects: a prospective randomized double-blinded trial. Acad Emerg Med 2012;19:901–7.

42. Muller L, Bobbia X, Toumi M, et al. Respiratory variations of inferior vena cava diameter to predict fluid responsiveness in spontaneously breathing patients with acute circulatory failure: need for a cautious use. Crit Care 2012;16:R188.

43. Feissel M, Michard F, Faller JP, et al. The respiratory variation in inferior vena cava diameter as a guide to fluid therapy. Intensive Care Med 2004; 30:1834–7.

44. Pinsky MR, Teboul JL. Assessment of indices of preload and volume responsiveness. Curr Opin Crit Care 2005;11:235–9.

45. Pinsky MR, Payen D. Functional hemodynamic monitoring. Crit Care 2005;9:566–72.

46. Muller L, Toumi M, Bousquet PJ, et al. An increase in aortic blood flow after an infusion of 100 ml colloid over 1 minute can predict fluid responsiveness: the mini-fluid challenge study. Anesthesiology 2011;115:541–7.

47. Feissel M, Michard F, Mangin I, et al. Respiratory changes in aortic blood velocity as an indicator of fluid responsiveness in ventilated patients with septic shock. Chest 2001;119: 867–73.

48. Thiel SW, Kollef MH, Isakow W. Non-invasive stroke volume measurement and passive leg raising predict volume responsiveness in medical ICU patients: an observational cohort study. Crit Care 2009;13:R111.

49. Lafanechere A, Pene F, Goulenok C, et al. Changes in aortic blood flow induced by passive leg raising predict fluid responsiveness in critically ill patients. Crit Care 2006;10:R132.

50. Kimura BJ, Kedar E, Weiss DE, et al. A bedside ultrasound sign of cardiac disease: the left atrium-to-aorta diastolic diameter ratio. Am J Emerg Med 2010;28:203–7.

51. Maury E, Guglielminotti J, Alzieu M, et al. Ultrasonic examination: an alternative to chest radiography after central venous catheter insertion? Am J Respir Crit Care Med 2001;164:403–5.

52. Vezzani A, Brusasco C, Palermo S, et al. Ultrasound localization of central vein catheter and detection of postprocedural pneumothorax: an alternative to chest radiography. Crit Care Med 2010;38:533–8.

53. Weekes AJ, Johnson D, Keller SM, et al. Central vascular catheter placement evaluation using saline flush and bedside echocardiography. Acad Emerg Med;21(1):65–72.

54. Zanobetti M, Coppa A, Bulletti F, et al. Verification of correct central venous catheter placement in the emergency department: comparison between ultrasonography and chest radiography. Intern Emerg Med 2013;8:173–80.

55. Bedel J, Vallee F, Mari A, et al. Guidewire localization by transthoracic echocardiography during central venous catheter insertion: a periprocedural method to evaluate catheter placement. Intensive Care Med 2013;39:1932–7.

56. Kim SC, Heinze I, Schmiedel A, et al. Ultrasound confirmation of central venous catheter position via a right supraclavicular fossa view using a microconvex probe: a observational pilot study. Eur J Anaesthesiol 2013. [Epub ahead of print].

57. Aguilera PA, Durham BA, Riley DA. Emergency transvenous cardiac pacing placement using ultrasound guidance. Ann Emerg Med 2000;36:224–7.

58. Breitkreutz R, Walcher F, Seeger FH. Focused echocardiographic evaluation in resuscitation management: concept of an advanced life support-conformed algorithm. Crit Care Med 2007;35: S150–61.

59. Hernandez C, Shuler K, Hannan H, et al. C.A.U.S.E.: cardiac arrest ultra-sound exam–a better approach to managing patients in primary non-arrhythmogenic cardiac arrest. Resuscitation 2008; 76:198–206.

60. Price S, Uddin S, Quinn T. Echocardiography in cardiac arrest. Curr Opin Crit Care 2010;16:211–5.

61. Shah BN, Ahmadvazir S, Pabla JS, et al. The role of urgent transthoracic echocardiography in the evaluation of patients presenting with acute chest pain. Eur J Emerg Med 2012;19:277–83.

62. Salen P, Melniker L, Chooljian C, et al. Does the presence or absence of sonographically identified cardiac activity predict resuscitation outcomes of cardiac arrest patients? Am J Emerg Med 2005; 23:459–62.

63. Kan H, Failinger CF, Fang Q, et al. Reversible myocardial dysfunction in sepsis and ischemia. Crit Care Med 2005;33:2845–7.

64. Laurent I, Monchi M, Chiche JD, et al. Reversible myocardial dysfunction in survivors of out-of-hospital cardiac arrest. J Am Coll Cardiol 2002; 40:2110–6.

65. Ruiz Bailen M. Reversible myocardial dysfunction in critically ill, noncardiac patients: a review. Crit Care Med 2002;30:1280–90.

66. Blaivas M. Transesophageal echocardiography during cardiopulmonary arrest in the emergency department. Resuscitation 2008;78:135–40.

67. Jones AE, Tayal VS, Sullivan DM, et al. Randomized, controlled trial of immediate versus delayed goal-directed ultrasound to identify the cause of nontraumatic hypotension in emergency department patients. Crit Care Med 2004;32:1703–8.

68. Marcelino P, Marum S, Fernandes AP, et al. Transthoracic echocardiography for evaluation of hypotensive critically ill patient. Acta Med Port 2006; 19:363–71 [in Portuguese].

69. Perera P, Mailhot T, Riley D, et al. The RUSH exam: Rapid Ultrasound in SHock in the evaluation of the critically ill. Emerg Med Clin North Am 2010;28:29–56, vii.

70. Pershad J, Myers S, Plouman C, et al. Bedside limited echocardiography by the emergency physician is accurate during evaluation of the critically ill patient. Pediatrics 2004;114:e667–71.

71. Rose JS, Bair AE, Mandavia D, et al. The UHP ultrasound protocol: a novel ultrasound approach to the empiric evaluation of the undifferentiated hypotensive patient. Am J Emerg Med 2001;19:299–302.

Point-of-Care Pelvic Ultrasonography in Emergency Medicine

Lori A. Stolz, MD[a],*, Refky Nicola, MS, DO[b]

KEYWORDS

- Point-of-care ultrasonography • Obstetrics • Acute pelvic pain • Pelvic imaging • Vaginal bleeding

KEY POINTS

- Visualization of the yolk sac on transvaginal ultrasonography should be used as a criterion for diagnosing intrauterine pregnancy by emergency physicians.
- Values of β–human chorionic gonadotropin should not be used to exclude the diagnosis of ectopic pregnancy in patients with a nondiagnostic ultrasonogram.
- The presence of arterial waveforms on Doppler imaging of the ovaries does not rule out adnexal torsion.
- The use of clinical algorithms that include ultrasonography in the diagnosis of appendicitis can decrease ionizing radiation without decreasing diagnostic accuracy.

INTRODUCTION

Point-of-care (POC) pelvic ultrasound by emergency physicians allows for a rapid and safe diagnosis of a multitude of pathologies during the acute phase of disease in both the obstetric and nonobstetric patient. Ultrasonography has become the gold standard for evaluation of acute pelvic pathology. History and physical examination are notoriously unreliable, with poor interexaminer reliability.[1,2] Emergency medicine physicians' expertise in performing POC ultrsonography has been well-documented in the literature on a wide variety of applications. Its integration into clinical practice is supported by the American College of Emergency Physicians (ACEP).[3]

INDICATIONS

Patients presenting with complaints of pelvic pain, abdominal pain, abdominal distention, palpable abdominal mass, vaginal bleeding, or decreased fetal movement are amenable to evaluation with POC ultrasonography. Additionally, undifferentiated patients with a history of traumatic injury, hemodynamic instability, vague symptoms of syncope, fatigue, dizziness, back pain, or flank pain may benefit from the use of POC pelvic ultrasonography.

SONOGRAPHIC TECHNIQUE

Transabdominal sonography (TAS) and transvaginal sonography (TVS) are the gold standard for the evaluation of the pelvic organs. However, both have inherent limitations and advantages that need to be weighed by the clinician. TAS provides a greater field of view, allowing the clinician to evaluate the surrounding structures such as the splenorenal and hepatorenal spaces for free peritoneal fluid. It allows for assessment of the spatial relationship of the pelvic organs to other abdominal structures, which is ideal for imaging

Funding Sources: None.
Conflict of Interest: None.
[a] Department of Emergency Medicine, University of Arizona, 1501 North Campbell Avenue, Tucson, AZ 85724-5057, USA; [b] Department of Imaging Sciences and Emergency Medicine, University of Rochester Medical Center, University of Rochester, 601 Elmwood Avenue, PO Box 648, Rochester, NY 14642, USA
* Corresponding author.
E-mail address: lstolz@aemrc.arizona.edu

ultrasound.theclinics.com

large masses. In addition, it is more rapidly performed at the bedside and can be used as a preliminary assessment when TVS is planned. Alternatively, TVS provides better visualization of the pelvic organs, owing to the proximity of the probe to the pelvic organs, as well as improved spatial resolution, as it is a higher-frequency probe; this is particularly true in obese patients whose pelvic organs may not be visualized on TAS. Also, the endocavitary probe can be used to separate pelvic organs, revealing additional abnormalities such as an ectopic pregnancy. The endocavitary probe may also directly probe organs of interest to see if they are the cause of a patient's pain, in effect performing a hyperaccurate physical or bimanual examination. However, TVS is limited in its field of view, requires patient positioning and cooperation, and is a more invasive examination. These two modalities are complementary. In most robust emergency medicine practices the endovaginal examination is done immediately at the time of the pelvic evaluation and TAS is performed only if additional views are needed.[4,5]

For TAS, the bladder should be full, as it provides an optimal acoustic window to visualize the uterus and adnexa. The bladder should not be overly distended because this results in the pelvic organs being displaced posteriorly, thus negatively affecting imaging quality. By contrast, TVS is best performed with a completely empty bladder. A distended bladder pushes the uterus posteriorly and distorts the anatomy, pushing it further from the probe.

Special considerations are necessary for the patient's comfort when performing TVS. Consent should be obtained. The procedure should be explained in detail to the patient, as well as the possible need for additional imaging by other specialties (Radiology or Obstetrics/Gynecology [OB/-GYN]). Analgesia may be required by some patients with pelvic pain. For the patient's comfort,

the examination can be performed along with the speculum and bimanual examination. In addition, the patient needs to be positioned appropriately to allow unobstructed motion of the endocavitary probe, which involves the use of a bed with stirrups. If one is not available it is possible, though not ideal, to elevate the patient's pelvis by using several folded blankets or a blanket-wrapped, face-down bedpan. The motor skills required for successful TVS are unlike those for most emergency sonography. The endocavitary probe is directed to different areas of the pelvis using the midpoint of the probe as a fulcrum in such a way that to visualize anteriorly, the probe handle should be moved posteriorly, and to visualize to the left the probe handle is directed to the right.

The operator should obtain two orthogonal views of each organ and structure, sweeping the ultrasound probe to fully evaluate the entire organ. Images of the uterus should be obtained in the sagittal and transverse planes, identifying the cervix, the fundus, and the endometrial stripe. The characteristics of the endometrial stripe change throughout the ovulatory cycle. Before ovulation, it is thin and has a multilayered appearance. During the secretory phase, it becomes thicker and more echogenic.[6] For the evaluation of the adnexa, the iliac vessels are used as a landmark. The ovaries normally lie adjacent or anterior to the iliac vessels. Ovaries are identified by their characteristic oval appearance with multiple hypoechoic follicles within the isoechoic ovarian tissue (**Fig. 1**). The ovaries should be assessed in two planes. Adjacent structures, free fluid, complex fluid collections, and masses should be sought and documented.

THE OBSTETRIC PATIENT

Vaginal bleeding or pelvic pain in a first-trimester pregnancy is a common presenting complaint in

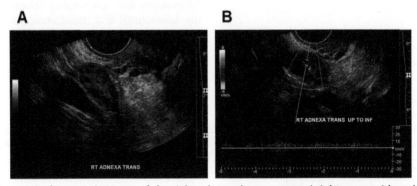

Fig. 1. (*A*) Transvaginal gray-scale image of the right adnexa shows a normal right ovary with multiple follicles. (*B*) Spectral Doppler flow image of the right ovary shows a normal venous waveform.

the emergency department (ED). Evaluation for ectopic pregnancy is the first priority for these patients, followed by evaluation for spontaneous abortion. The sensitivity of ED POC ultrasonography in the diagnosis of intrauterine pregnancy (IUP) ranges from 67% to 91% and the specificity ranges from 92% to 100%.[7–11] The sonographic signs of normal pregnancy progression are predictable, with visualization of the gestational sac occurring at 4 to 5 weeks, the yolk sac at 5 to 6 weeks, and the fetal pole at 6 to 7 weeks (**Figs. 2** and **3A**). Cardiac activity can be seen as early as 5 weeks (see **Fig. 3B**). The first definitive sign of an intrauterine gestation is the yolk sac. Although the earliest sonographic sign of a pregnancy is an intrauterine gestational sac, this is not definitive evidence of an IUP. The double decidual sign, two hyperechoic rings surrounding the gestational sac separated by one hypoechoic ring, can be used to suggest an early IUP. However, it should not be the only sign used by emergency physicians as diagnosis of an IUP, as it lacks sufficient sensitivity and specificity, especially with less advanced ultrasound equipment (**Fig. 4**).

Ectopic Pregnancy

Ectopic pregnancy is a true emergency and is a diagnostic consideration in any symptomatic first-trimester patient. In patients presenting to the ED the incidence of ectopic pregnancy is between 3% and 13%, which is higher than the overall frequency among all recognized pregnancies at approximately 2%.[10,12,13] History and physical examination are not accurate in determining the presence of an ectopic pregnancy, so ultrasonography is a necessary tool for evaluating women with abdominal pain or bleeding in early pregnancy. In one large systematic review, no elements of the history had a likelihood ratio greater than 1.5.[14] Traditionally the historical features of prior ectopic pregnancy, history of pelvic inflammatory disease (PID), history of intrauterine device

use, and history of tubal surgery should raise the suspicion of ectopic pregnancy, although half of all patients with ectopic pregnancy have none of these features.[15,16]

Previously many physicians practiced by the axiom that an IUP producing serum β–human chorionic gonadotropin (β-hCG) above a certain level, termed the discriminatory zone, would be visualized sonographically, whereas below this level the absence of a visualized IUP was of less concern. The use of the discriminatory zone has been dismissed and is no longer considered valid, because no β-hCG level can reliably distinguish between ectopic, viable, and nonviable pregnancy. The ACEP clinical policy on the management of patients with early pregnancy recommends that β-hCG values should not be used to exclude the diagnosis of ectopic pregnancy in patients with an indeterminate sonogram. In addition, the policy recommends obtaining or performing pelvic ultrasonography for symptomatic patients with a β-hCG level below any discriminatory threshold.[17] Even when a patient's β-hCG is very low, TVS is indicated. Ectopic pregnancies have been documented at β-hCG levels as low as 100 mIU/mL. A β-hCG discriminatory zone of 3000 mIU/mL has been shown to have poor test characteristics for identification of patients with ectopic pregnancy who present to the ED, with a sensitivity of 35% and specificity of 58%.[10]

In patients with ectopic pregnancy, the sensitivity of POC ultrasonography in identifying the absence of IUP is 99.3%, with a negative predictive value (NPV) of 99.6%.[18] Sonographic features of ectopic pregnancy include the following: extrauterine gestational sac with yolk sac or embryo, extrauterine fetal cardiac activity, tubal ring, complex pelvic mass, and free peritoneal fluid.[4] Discovery of a live extrauterine pregnancy is the most specific finding, although it is rare (**Fig. 5**). An adnexal mass is the most common finding.[12] The presence of an adnexal mass in the absence of an IUP on TVS has a likelihood ratio of 111 for

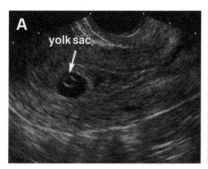 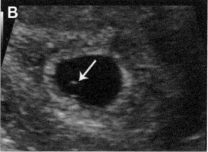

Fig. 2. (*A*) Transvaginal sonogram of a young woman who complained of pelvic pain shows a normal yolk sac. (*B*) Transvaginal sonogram shows a dedicated cone-down view of the gestational sac (*arrow*).

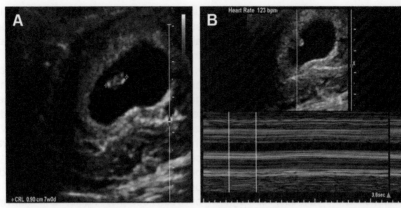

Fig. 3. (*A*) A Gray-scale image of the uterus 7-week fetal pole with cardiac activity. (*B*) Fetal heart rate in M-mode shows a heart rate of 123 beats/min.

ectopic pregnancy.[14] A tubal ring is a hypoechoic circular structure with a hyperechoic border that is outside the ovary and within the adnexa. It can appear directly adjacent to the ovary, and may mimic a corpus luteum cyst. The two structures are very difficult to distinguish based on purely visual sonographic features; however, a tubal ring may be separated from the ovary using pressure with the endocavitary probe.[12,19] The NPV for ectopic pregnancy when the mass and ovary cannot be separated is 96.1% and the PPV for ectopic pregnancy is 77.8% with mass separation.[20] Presence of fluid within the uterus does not exclude the possibility of an ectopic pregnancy. As mentioned previously, a yolk sac visualized within a gestational sac is the first definitive

sign of IUP. Intrauterine fluid can be seen in 16% of patients with an ectopic pregnancy.[21] A few rare forms of ectopic pregnancy may closely mimic IUP, and are difficult to recognize and diagnose. These forms include interstitial ectopic (pregnancy imbedded within the uterine tissue), cornual ectopic (pregnancy in either of the cornua or uterine horns), and cervical ectopic. Any suggestion of these entities should prompt a comprehensive radiologic study or prompt obstetric consultation.

When ectopic pregnancy is a diagnostic consideration, the abdomen should be evaluated for free fluid in both the posterior cul-de-sac and the hepatorenal space, also known as Morrison's pouch. Any abdominal free fluid in any location in a symptomatic pregnant patient is suggestive of an ectopic pregnancy.[22] The presence of free fluid in Morrison's pouch strongly predicts the need for operative intervention in patients with ectopic

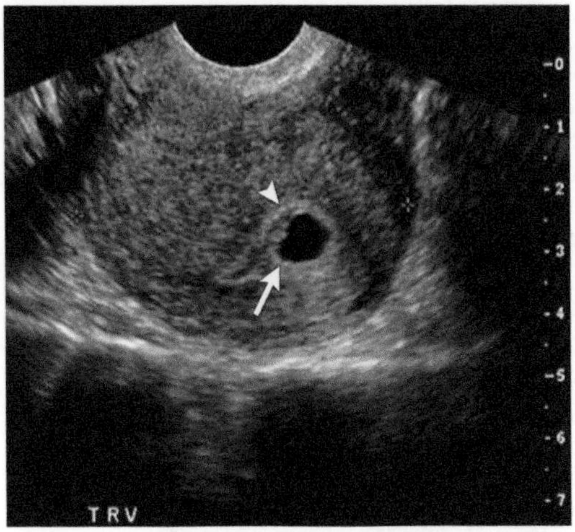

Fig. 4. Gray-scale ultrasonography image shows 2 hyperechoic concentric rings surrounding an anechoic gestational sac. The decidua parietalis, which lines the uterine cavity (*arrowhead*) and the decidua capsularis which lines the gestational sac (*arrow*) together are known as the double decidual sign.

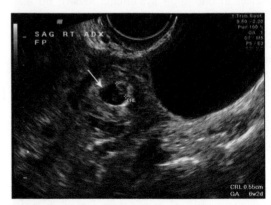

Fig. 5. Transabdominal ultrasonogram of a young woman who complained of pain and bleeding in the right lower quadrant. Gray-scale image shows a complex heterogeneous adnexal mass with evidence of a fetal pole (*arrow*); this is an ectopic pregnancy.

pregnancy.[23] Patients with ectopic pregnancy who have had right upper quadrant POC ultrasonography performed to assess for free fluid have a significantly shorter time to operative management than patients who have not, making this a critical step in evaluating patients with suspected ectopic pregnancy.[24]

Pregnancy of Unknown Location

Pelvic ultrasonography of a first-trimester patient may reveal a normal IUP, ectopic pregnancy, molar pregnancy, or none of these. An indeterminate ultrasonography examination occurs frequently. These patients could have an ectopic pregnancy, a normal early IUP, or a completed abortion. This indeterminate result occurs in 20% of ED patients undergoing POC ultrasonography. The final outcomes of these pregnancies in one prospective study was found to be embryonic demise in 53% of patients, ectopic pregnancy in 15%, and IUP in 29%.[25] Another retrospective review found spontaneous abortion in 65% of patients and ectopic pregnancy in 10%; 23% of patients carried the pregnancy to 20 weeks and beyond.[26] These numbers are important when discussing prognosis and likely outcome with patients and ensuring follow-up. Only roughly one-fourth of these patients will ultimately have a normal pregnancy. Given the high rates of ectopic pregnancy among these patients, this population needs close follow-up. In addition, there is a subset of patients with pregnancy of unknown location who are mistakenly presumed to have ectopic pregnancy when there is a viable pregnancy. The erroneous administration of methotrexate in these patients poses a great risk for fetal anomalies and fetal demise. All patients with a pregnancy of unknown location require close follow-up and management by OB/GYN.[27]

Heterotopic Pregnancy

Heterotopic pregnancy, the simultaneous occurrence of an intrauterine gestation and an extrauterine gestation, poses a serious diagnostic challenge for physicians evaluating patients in early pregnancy. It is a rare event in the general population, with a frequency ranging from 1 in 3000 to 1 in 8000 pregnant patients. However, in patients who have undergone in vitro fertilization the risk is 100-fold higher, at 1% to 3%.[28] Other risk factors include PID, prior ectopic pregnancy, prior adnexal surgery, and ovarian stimulation. Twenty-nine percent of heterotopic pregnancies have no preexisting risk factors.[28] Even when an IUP is diagnosed in a symptomatic first-trimester patient, heterotopic pregnancy

cannot be fully excluded. Therefore, the sonographic signs of ectopic pregnancy should be sought during every ultrasonography evaluation even when an IUP is identified. The clinician should consider the risk factors for heterotopic pregnancy and the clinical presentation in every pregnant patient.

Nonviable Pregnancy

The diagnostic criteria for identifying a nonviable pregnancy have recently been revised.[29] Because of the growing concern and increasing liability over treatment of viable IUPs with methotrexate or dilatation and curettage, the criteria have been expanded to produce a PPV and specificity of nearly 100%. These criteria are defined with TVS and are listed in **Box 1** as well as criteria that are suspicious, though not diagnostic, for nonviable pregnancy. Patients that meet any of these criteria require consultation with OB/GYN regarding further management. There are additional criteria that define a nonviable pregnancy on serial ultrasonography examinations, although these rarely apply to patients seen in the emergency setting.

Spontaneous Abortion

Vaginal bleeding will occur in one-fourth of all early pregnancies, and one-half of these pregnancies

---

Box 1
Ultrasonographic findings of pregnancy failure

Findings Diagnostic of Pregnancy Failure

Crown-rump length greater than or equal to 7 mm with no cardiac activity

Mean gestational sac diameter[a] of greater than 25 mm with no visible embryo

Findings Suspicious for Pregnancy Failure

Crown-rump length of less than 7 mm and no heartbeat

Mean gestational sac diameter of 16 to 24 mm and no embryo

Enlarged yolk sac (>7 mm)

Small gestational sac in relation to the size of the embryo (<5 mm difference between mean sac diameter and crown-rump length)

---

[a] Mean sac diameter is calculated by measuring the diameter of the gestational sac in three planes and obtaining the average.

Adapted from Doubilet PM, Benson CB, Bourne T, et al. Diagnostic criteria for nonviable pregnancy early in the first trimester. N Engl J Med 2013;369(15):1446; with permission.

will end in spontaneous abortion.[30] Many of the patients are evaluated in the ED for their symptoms. Seventy percent of patients presenting with vaginal bleeding or pelvic pain who have a visualized yolk sac will carry their pregnancy beyond 20 weeks.[31] In this cohort, women with vaginal bleeding have a higher rate of miscarriage than patients with pain alone. In symptomatic patients with a documented live IUP, spontaneous abortion occurred in 9.2% of patients overall, 13.8% of patients with vaginal bleeding, and 2.5% of patients without vaginal bleeding (**Table 1**).[32]

Subchorionic Hemorrhage

Subchorionic hemorrhage may be seen on ultrasonography in symptomatic or asymptomatic pregnant patients presenting to the ED. On ultrasonography, subchorionic hemorrhage is a collection of blood between the placenta and the uterus, which can appear hyperechoic or isoechoic acutely and becomes hypoechoic to anechoic over time (**Fig. 6**). It can be found at any stage of pregnancy, and the reported frequency varies widely. Several studies have examined the pregnancy outcomes for patients with subchorionic hemorrhage noted on ultrasonography. One meta-analysis found an increased risk of spontaneous abortion (odds ratio [OR] 2.18), stillbirth (OR 2.09), abruption (OR 5.71), preterm delivery (OR 1.40), and preterm premature rupture of membranes (OR 1.64).[33] In the first trimester, the rate of spontaneous abortion in patients with identified subchorionic hemorrhage is 9.3% and is further increased with advanced maternal age, large hemorrhage, and a gestational age less than 8 weeks.[34] These patients are managed with supportive care and close follow-up with OB/GYN.

Evaluating Fetal Heart Rate

There are several clinical scenarios in which the fetal heart rate should be assessed, such as abdominal or pelvic trauma, early-pregnancy bleeding, decreased fetal movement, or maternal illness. M-mode is the preferred method for evaluation of fetal heart rate. Doppler evaluation is not recommended in the emergency setting because it poses a theoretical risk of thermal injury to sensitive developing tissue, without benefit.[35] Fetal heart rates below 120 bpm are associated with poor prognosis, with a PPV for fetal demise of 72%.[36] Fetuses with heart rates lower than 85 bpm rarely, if ever, survive.[37]

THE NONOBSTETRIC PATIENT

The sonographic evaluation of the pelvic organs for uterine and adnexal abnormality is an advanced and emerging POC ultrasonography application. Diagnostic considerations include rupture of ovarian cyst, ovarian torsion, adnexal masses, uterine masses, tubo-ovarian abscess, and PID. Routine evaluation for these entities does not often fall within the scope of emergency medicine. However, there are clinical scenarios in which there is a need for timely diagnosis and no other immediately available imaging options. Occasionally, POC ultrasonography can aid in the decision to refer to on-call sonography technologists for evaluation by a radiologist.

Hemorrhage or Rupture of Ovarian Cyst

Ovarian cysts may be detected incidentally on bedside ultrasonography or may be sought as a cause of a patient's presenting symptoms. The characteristics of an ovarian cyst should be specifically noted, including size, echogenicity, homogeneity (cystic, solid, or mixed), and evidence of septations. Functional simple cysts are the most common ovarian cysts. These cysts are considered physiologic until they reach a diameter greater than 2.5 cms (**Fig. 7**).[4] Typical presentation of a patient with a hemorrhagic ovarian cyst is sudden onset of pelvic pain, although this can mimic several other pathologic conditions. The characteristic sonographic features are a heterogeneous mass within the ovary with a thick rim, septations,

Table 1
Pregnancy outcome of symptomatic first-trimester patients presenting to the emergency department

	Normal Gestation (%)[a]	Fetal Loss (%)	Ectopic Pregnancy (%)
No documented IUP	23–29	53–65	10–15
Yolk-sac IUP	70	30	NA
Live IUP	90.8	9.2–14.8	NA

Abbreviations: IUP, intrauterine pregnancy; NA, not applicable.
[a] Defined as IUP in Ref.[25] and pregnancy carried to >20 weeks' gestation in remaining studies.
Data from Refs.[25,26,31,32,71]

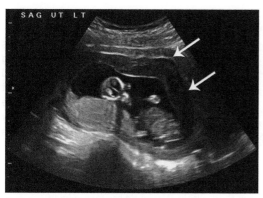

Fig. 6. Gray-scale ultrasonography image shows heterogeneous fluid collection between the uterine wall and chorionic membrane (*arrows*), consistent with a subchorionic hematoma.

internal echoes, and moderate amount of free fluid in the posterior cul-de-sac (**Fig. 8**).[38] Rarely these hemorrhagic cysts can rupture into the peritoneum, causing massive hemoperitoneum. If there is continued hemorrhage, this can be life-threatening because of hemorrhagic shock and hemodynamic instability. Diagnosis of cyst rupture can be complicated by the possibility that the ruptured cyst will no longer be visible.

Ovarian Torsion

Ovarian torsion is the twisting of the adnexa and ovary on its ligamentous support, consisting of lymphatics, veins, and arteries. This twisting results in an initial obstruction of lymphatic supply, which causes an increase in capillary pressure and massive edema of the ovaries. If left untreated torsion will progress to venous obstruction and, ultimately, hemorrhagic infarction of the ovary.[39]

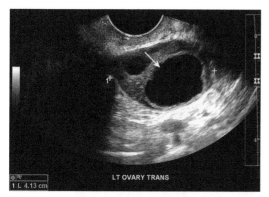

Fig. 7. Gray-scale ultrasonography image of a young woman who complained of mild pain in the left lower quadrant for 2 days, showing a large anechoic cyst in the left ovary (*arrow*); this is most likely a functional cyst.

Complete infarction of the ovary can lead to a systemic infection and inflammatory response.[40,41] Ovarian torsion is most prevalent in women during their reproductive years, with 17% to 20% of cases occurring during pregnancy. Additional risk factors include ovarian teratoma, hemorrhagic cyst, ovarian malignancy, and ovarian hyperstimulation syndrome. Some studies have suggested that the right ovary is more susceptible to torsion because the space occupied by the sigmoid colon on the left side offers a protective effect to the left ovary.[42,43] The symptoms of ovarian torsion are nonspecific and include nausea, vomiting, sharp localized right or left lower abdominal pain, and tenderness. Patients may complain of constant or intermittent pain according to whether there is complete torsion or torsion-detorsion of the ovary.

The gold standard for the evaluation of patients with adnexal torsion is TAS and TVS. The most common initial sonographic finding is markedly enlarged ovaries (>4 cm) with a volume measuring up to 12 to 20 times the normal size.[44] Gray-scale ultrasonography will also show multiple follicles along the periphery of the engorged ovary, attributable to the marked edema and venous congestion.[39,45,46] There is free fluid within the cul-de-sac in 87% of cases.[45–47] On color Doppler imaging, the classic appearance is of complete absence of arterial flow. However, this is only present in a minority of cases, with 60% having normal color Doppler flow findings.[43,47] The most common findings are either a decrease or absence of venous flow.[47] Arterial waveforms may be present because of dual vascular supply to the ovary, but it is the venous congestion that causes edema and eventual infarction. The presence of arterial flow does not rule out the diagnosis of ovarian torsion (**Fig. 9**).

Another finding associated with ovarian torsion is the twisted pedicle or the whirlpool sign. Initially described by Lee and colleagues,[48] the whirlpool sign features a twisted pedicle with feeding vessels wrapping around a central axis on color Doppler ultrasonography. This feature is detected in 88% of cases of ovarian torsion. Absence of flow within the twisted pedicle predicts ovarian infarction, and is a strong preoperative predictor of loss of ovarian viability.[49,50]

The diagnosis of ovarian torsion is complex, and involves interrogation and comparison of the venous and arterial waveforms of the bilateral ovaries with color Doppler imaging. Because of the complex nature of the examination, it is not a diagnosis that typically falls within the realm of POC ultrasonography. Understanding these findings may aid a clinician in the use of appropriate resources and interpreting radiologic studies.

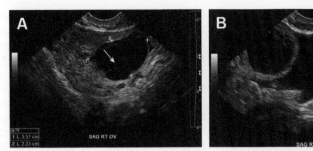

Fig. 8. Gray-scale ultrasonography images of a young woman who complained of pain in the right lower quadrant pain for 2 days. (*A*) There is a complex cystic mass in the right ovary with low-level echoes (*arrow*). There are fine interdigitating septations, which give the appearance of fishnet weave or a fine reticular appearance. (*B*) Adacent to the right ovary, there is a moderate amount of free fluid within the cul-de-sac (*arrowhead*).

When the diagnosis is considered or any findings are noted on sonographic examination, emergent OB/GYN consultation is necessary.

Pelvic Inflammatory Disease

PID is one of the most common causes of acute pelvic pain in women of reproductive age, and affects approximately 1 million women per year.[51] PID is an ascending infection that can involve the endometrium, fallopian tubes, and ovaries. PID includes a wide spectrum of disease entities from salpingitis, pylosalpinx, tubo-ovarian complex, tubo-ovarian abscess, and hydrosalpinx. The infection is commonly caused by *Chlamydia trachomatis* and *Neisseria gonorrhoeae*, which spreads along the uterine cervix and the endometrium to fallopian tube, ovaries, and peritoneal cavity.

Women who have a history of sexually transmitted diseases and multiple sexual partners, and sexually active adolescent girls are all at risk for PID.[52] Recent placement of an intrauterine contraceptive device is a significant additional risk factor. PID affects 10% to 15% of women in the United States and is a serious threat because

of complications such as infertility, chronic pelvic pain, ectopic pregnancy, Fitz-Hugh-Curtis syndrome, and perihepatitis.[53] Women with PID present with pelvic pain, fever, leukocytosis, foul-smelling discharge, and cervical motion tenderness.

The gold standard for diagnosis is laparoscopy (sensitivity 100%); however, the diagnosis is often made clinically (sensitivity 87%).[54] The utility of TVS in the diagnosis of PID is limited (30% sensitivity and 67% specificity), although it is often used to identify complications requiring surgical or percutaneous management. TVS has an overall accuracy of 93% for the detection of tubal or ovarian complications.[55]

Salpingitis usually sonographically manifests as a thickening of 5 mm or more of the imperceptible wall of the tubes without intraluminal pus. On ultrasonography it can appear as an indistinct elongated adnexal mass adjacent to the ovary, but separate from it. As the infection progresses, distal occlusion leads to the formation of pyosalpinx, which is the presence of low-level echoes or layering with a fluid debris level in a dilated fluid-filled tube. When the infection involves the fallopian

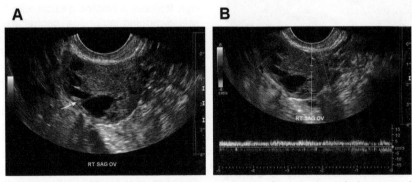

Fig. 9. (*A*) Gray-scale sonogram of a young woman who complained of pain in the right lower quadrant, showing an enlarged ovary with multiple follicles along the periphery (*arrow*); this is known as the string of pearls sign. (*B*) Spectral Doppler waveforms show dampening of venous waveforms in the right ovary, suggestive of ovarian torsion/detorsion of the right ovary.

tubes and ovaries, a tubo-ovarian complex develops. Tubo-ovarian complexes may respond better than tubo-ovarian abscesses to antibiotic therapy alone, which generally require surgical management. A tubo-ovarian abscess is a large complex adnexal mass that engulfs the tube and ovary with destruction of the normal architecture. Color and power Doppler show an increase in vascularity with low-resistance arterial waveforms around the adnexal mass, reflecting hyperemia of acute inflammation. Without treatment, a tubo-ovarian abscess can result in peritonitis and multiple intra-abdominal abscesses (**Fig. 10**).

Untreated PID can result in a hydrosalpinx (the dilatation of the fallopian tubes with fluid), which can develop secondary to obstruction from pelvic adhesions and appears as a tubular anechoic adnexal structure in a C-shape or S-shape. The dilated tube can have a cogwheel appearance on transverse images, with multiple tiny mural protrusions representing the inflamed folded/redundant tubal mucosa.[56]

Acute Appendicitis

Acute appendicitis is the most common cause of nongynecologic acute pain in the pelvis and right lower quadrant, and is often considered concurrently with many of the disorders already mentioned. The lifetime risk of appendicitis is approximately 7%, with a current incidence of 86 cases per 100,000 patients per year.[57] The overall mortality rate for appendicitis is less than 1%, but this increases to 3% if the appendix is ruptured, and approaches 15% in the elderly.[58] Early diagnosis of appendicitis is paramount because patient morbidity rapidly increases once appendicitis becomes complicated by abscess and perforation. Appendicitis occurs when the

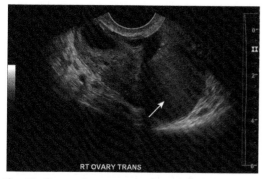

Fig. 10. Gray-scale sonogram of a young woman with pain in the right lower quadrant and cervical motion tenderness, showing an enlarged right ovary with a complex mass in the right adnexa with low-level internal echoes and debris (*arrow*), consistent with a pyosalpinx.

appendix becomes obstructed or inflamed. It becomes distended as mucosal secretion and bacterial proliferation continue in the face of the obstructed lumen, causing inflammatory changes in the surrounding tissues such as the pericecal fat and peritoneum.

Appendicitis classically presents as a vague abdominal pain in the periumbilical area secondary to visceral afferent nerves, which then localizes to the right lower quadrant. Associated symptoms include nausea, vomiting, anorexia, and fever. Because there is variability in the position of the appendix, the classic presentation is not always present. The appendix may lie in a retrocecal, retroiliac, or pelvic location, leading to pain in the right flank, pelvis, suprapubic region, or even left lower quadrant if the appendix crosses the midline. These variable positions and symptoms can result in a delay in the diagnosis, thus increasing the risk of gangrene or perforation.[59]

Over the years, ultrasonography has gained acceptance as a modality for the evaluation of appendicitis, especially in children, women of reproductive age, and pregnant women, owing to the avoidance of nonionizing radiation. Puylaert[60] first described the technique of graded compression ultrasonography to diagnose acute appendicitis in 1986, which has since been validated by multiple other studies. Using a linear or curvilinear transducer, the operator examines the right lower quadrant by applying gradually increasing pressure over the cecum with the patient in the supine position. The diagnosis of appendicitis is confirmed by showing a noncompressible, blind-ending loop measuring greater than 6 mm without peristalsis.[61] The presence of an appendicolith (a hyperechoic, shadowing focus within the appendix), focal tenderness, trace amounts of surrounding free fluid, and guarding under the transducer are additional important signs. Color or power Doppler typically shows hyperemia in the appendiceal wall, with a sensitivity of 87% for appendicitis. However, the Doppler signal diminishes when the appendix is gangrenous or necrotic (**Fig. 11**).[62]

There are several additional maneuvers that have been shown to facilitate the visualization of the appendix. Applying pressure posteriorly with the left hand directed toward the transducer helps improve the degree of compression, and is reported to increase the rate of visualization of the appendix to 95%.[63] Lee and colleagues[64] have suggested another maneuver called upward graded compression. This technique consists of forceful upward sweeps with the transducer to displace the cecum and appendix upward. This method is particularly helpful when the appendix is low-lying or in the pelvis. Another maneuver is

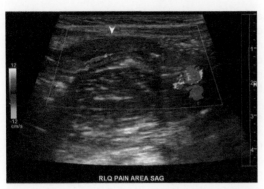

Fig. 11. Gray-scale ultrasonography image of the right lower quadrant shows an enlarged and thickened appendix (*arrowhead*) with increased Doppler flow, consistent with acute appendicitis.

placing the patient in the left lateral decubitus position to visualize a retrocecal appendix.[65]

Because TVS is frequently performed to evaluate acute pelvic pain, an evaluation of the appendix can be done at the same time.[66,67] Unfortunately there are limitations when performing ultrasonography of the appendix, such as a large body habitus, operator experience, and atypical location of the appendix in a retrocecal position or deep in the pelvis. Secondary to these limitations, graded compression ultrasonography has a lower sensitivity and specificity than contrast-enhanced computed tomography or magnetic resonance imaging.[68] Clinical algorithms that incorporate ultrasonography first with progression to advanced imaging have been shown to successfully reduce the overall use of ionizing radiation without decreasing diagnostic accuracy.[69,70]

SUMMARY

POC ultrasonography is an especially useful tool for emergency physicians. It allows prompt, accurate diagnosis of several acute pelvic abnormalities. Knowledge of the sonographic features of these disease processes is necessary if one is to incorporate bedside sonography into practice. The literature has demonstrated that POC ultrasonography performed by the emergency physician is accurate and beneficial for patient care. Every emergency physician should understand the benefits, scope, and limitations of POC pelvic ultrasonography, and the need for further evaluation if necessary.

ACKNOWLEDGMENTS

Special thanks to Erin Lemcke-Berno RDMS, MPH, Division of Maternal-Fetal Medicine, and Sarah Peangatelli, Radiology Graphics Imaging Specialist, Department of Imaging Sciences, from the University of Rochester Medical Center for their assistance in the preparation of this article.

REFERENCES

1. Lundberg WI, Wall JE, Mathers JE. Laparoscopy in evaluation of pelvic pain. Obstet Gynecol 1973; 42(6):872–6.
2. Close RJ, Sachs CJ, Dyne PL. Reliability of bimanual pelvic examinations performed in emergency departments. West J Med 2001;175(4): 240–4 [discussion: 244–5].
3. American College of Emergency Physicians. Emergency ultrasound guidelines. Ann Emerg Med 2009;53(4):550–70.
4. Ma OJ, Mateer JR, Blaivas M, editors. Emergency ultrasound. 2nd edition. New York: McGraw-Hill; 2008.
5. Sabbagha RE, editor. Diagnostic ultrasound applied to obstetrics and gynecology. 3rd edition. Philadelphia: J. B. Lippincott Company; 1994.
6. Goldstein SR, Timor-Tritsch IE. Ultrasound in gynecology. New York: Churchill Livingstone; 1995.
7. Durham B, Lane B, Burbridge L, et al. Pelvic ultrasound performed by emergency physicians for the detection of ectopic pregnancy in complicated first-trimester pregnancies. Ann Emerg Med 1997; 29(3):338–47.
8. Mateer JR, Valley VT, Aiman EJ, et al. Outcome analysis of a protocol including bedside endovaginal sonography in patients at risk for ectopic pregnancy. Ann Emerg Med 1996;27(3):283–9.
9. Wong TW, Lau CC, Yeung A, et al. Efficacy of transabdominal ultrasound examination in the diagnosis of early pregnancy complications in an emergency department. J Accid Emerg Med 1998;15(3):155–8.
10. Wang R, Reynolds TA, West HH, et al. Use of a beta-hCG discriminatory zone with bedside pelvic ultrasonography. Ann Emerg Med 2011; 58(1):12–20.
11. McRae A, Murray H, Edmonds M. Diagnostic accuracy and clinical utility of emergency department targeted ultrasonography in the evaluation of first-trimester pelvic pain and bleeding: a systematic review. CJEM 2009;11(4):355–64.
12. Adhikari S, Blaivas M, Lyon M. Diagnosis and management of ectopic pregnancy using bedside transvaginal ultrasonography in the ED: a 2-year experience. Am J Emerg Med 2007;25(6):591–6.
13. Marion LL, Meeks GR. Ectopic pregnancy: history, incidence, epidemiology, and risk factors. Clin Obstet Gynecol 2012;55(2):376–86.
14. Crochet JR, Bastian LA, Chireau MV. Does this woman have an ectopic pregnancy?: the rational

clinical examination systematic review. JAMA 2013;309(16):1722–9.

15. Della-Giustina D, Denny M. Ectopic pregnancy. Emerg Med Clin North Am 2003;21(3):565–84.

16. Spandorfer SD, Barnhart KT. Role of previous ectopic pregnancy in altering the presentation of suspected ectopic pregnancy. J Reprod Med 2003;48(3):133–6.

17. Hahn SA, Lavonas EJ, Mace SE, et al. Clinical policy: critical issues in the initial evaluation and management of patients presenting to the emergency department in early pregnancy. Ann Emerg Med 2012;60(3):381–90.e28.

18. Stein JC, Wang R, Adler N, et al. Emergency physician ultrasonography for evaluating patients at risk for ectopic pregnancy: a meta-analysis. Ann Emerg Med 2010;56(6):674–83.

19. Stein MW, Ricci ZJ, Novak L, et al. Sonographic comparison of the tubal ring of ectopic pregnancy with the corpus luteum. J Ultrasound Med 2004;23(1):57–62.

20. Blaivas M, Lyon M. Reliability of adnexal mass mobility in distinguishing possible ectopic pregnancy from corpus luteum cysts. J Ultrasound Med 2005;24(5):599–603.

21. Benson CB, Doubilet PM, Peters HE, et al. Intrauterine fluid with ectopic pregnancy: a reappraisal. J Ultrasound Med 2013;32(3):389–93.

22. Nyberg DA, Hughes MP, Mack LA, et al. Extrauterine findings of ectopic pregnancy of transvaginal US: importance of echogenic fluid. Radiology 1991;178(3):823–6.

23. Moore C, Todd WM, O'Brien E, et al. Free fluid in Morison's pouch on bedside ultrasound predicts need for operative intervention in suspected ectopic pregnancy. Acad Emerg Med 2007;14(8):755–8.

24. Rodgerson JD, Heegaard WG, Plummer D, et al. Emergency department right upper quadrant ultrasound is associated with a reduced time to diagnosis and treatment of ruptured ectopic pregnancies. Acad Emerg Med 2001;8(4):331–6.

25. Tayal VS, Cohen H, Norton HJ. Outcome of patients with an indeterminate emergency department first-trimester pelvic ultrasound to rule out ectopic pregnancy. Acad Emerg Med 2004;11(9):912–7.

26. Juliano ML, Sauter BM. Fetal outcomes in first trimester pregnancies with an indeterminate ultrasound. J Emerg Med 2012;43(3):417–22.

27. Barnhart KT. Early pregnancy failure: beware of the pitfalls of modern management. Fertil Steril 2012;98(5):1061–5.

28. Talbot K, Simpson R, Price N, et al. Heterotopic pregnancy. J Obstet Gynaecol 2011;31(1):7–12.

29. Doubilet PM, Benson CB, Bourne T, et al. Diagnostic criteria for nonviable pregnancy early in the first trimester. N Engl J Med 2013;369(15):1443–51.

30. Eyvazzadeh AD, Levine D. Imaging of pelvic pain in the first trimester of pregnancy. Radiol Clin North Am 2006;44(6):863–77.

31. Hessert MJ, Juliano M. Fetal loss in symptomatic first-trimester pregnancy with documented yolk sac intrauterine pregnancy. Am J Emerg Med 2012;30(3):399–404.

32. Juliano M, Dabulis S, Heffner A. Characteristics of women with fetal loss in symptomatic first trimester pregnancies with documented fetal cardiac activity. Ann Emerg Med 2008;52(2):143–7.

33. Tuuli MG, Norman SM, Odibo AO, et al. Perinatal outcomes in women with subchorionic hematoma: a systematic review and meta-analysis. Obstet Gynecol 2011;117(5):1205–12.

34. Bennett GL, Bromley B, Lieberman E, et al. Subchorionic hemorrhage in first-trimester pregnancies: prediction of pregnancy outcome with sonography. Radiology 1996;200(3):803–6.

35. Salvesen K, Lees C, Abramowicz J, et al. ISUOG statement on the safe use of Doppler in the 11 to 13 +6-week fetal ultrasound examination. Ultrasound Obstet Gynecol 2011;37(6):628.

36. Chittacharoen A, Herabutya Y. Slow fetal heart rate may predict pregnancy outcome in first-trimester threatened abortion. Fertil Steril 2004;82(1):227–9.

37. Stefos TI, Lolis DE, Sotiriadis AJ, et al. Embryonic heart rate in early pregnancy. J Clin Ultrasound 1998;26(1):33–6.

38. Baltarowich OH, Kurtz AB, Pasto ME, et al. The spectrum of sonographic findings in hemorrhagic ovarian cysts. AJR Am J Roentgenol 1987;148(5):901–5.

39. Graif M, Itzchak Y. Sonographic evaluation of ovarian torsion in childhood and adolescence. AJR Am J Roentgenol 1988;150(3):647–9.

40. Oelsner G, Shashar D. Adnexal torsion. Clin Obstet Gynecol 2006;49(3):459–63.

41. Rosado WM Jr, Trambert MA, Gosink BB, et al. Adnexal torsion: diagnosis by using Doppler sonography. AJR Am J Roentgenol 1992;159(6):1251–3.

42. Nichols DH, Julian PJ. Torsion of the adnexa. Clin Obstet Gynecol 1985;28(2):375–80.

43. Pena JE, Ufberg D, Cooney N, et al. Usefulness of Doppler sonography in the diagnosis of ovarian torsion. Fertil Steril 2000;73(5):1047–50.

44. Servaes S, Zurakowski D, Laufer MR, et al. Sonographic findings of ovarian torsion in children. Pediatr Radiol 2007;37(5):446–51.

45. Stark JE, Siegel MJ. Ovarian torsion in prepubertal and pubertal girls: sonographic findings. AJR Am J Roentgenol 1994;163(6):1479–82.

46. Graif M, Shalev J, Strauss S, et al. Torsion of the ovary: sonographic features. AJR Am J Roentgenol 1984;143(6):1331–4.

47. Albayram F, Hamper UM. Ovarian and adnexal torsion: spectrum of sonographic findings with

pathologic correlation. J Ultrasound Med 2001;
20(10):1083–9.

48. Lee EJ, Kwon HC, Joo HJ, et al. Diagnosis of ovarian torsion with color Doppler sonography: depiction of twisted vascular pedicle. J Ultrasound Med 1998; 17(2):83–9.

49. Vijayaraghavan SB. Sonographic whirlpool sign in ovarian torsion. J Ultrasound Med 2004;23(12): 1643–9 [quiz: 1650–1].

50. Chang HC, Bhatt S, Dogra VS. Pearls and pitfalls in diagnosis of ovarian torsion. Radiographics 2008; 28(5):1355–68.

51. Ghiatas AA. The spectrum of pelvic inflammatory disease. Eur Radiol 2004;14(Suppl 3):E184–92.

52. Sam JW, Jacobs JE, Birnbaum BA. Spectrum of CT findings in acute pyogenic pelvic inflammatory disease. Radiographics 2002;22(6):1327–34.

53. Timor-Tritsch IE, Lerner JP, Monteagudo A, et al. Transvaginal sonographic markers of tubal inflammatory disease. Ultrasound Obstet Gynecol 1998; 12(1):56–66.

54. Gaitan H, Angel E, Diaz R, et al. Accuracy of five different diagnostic techniques in mild-to-moderate pelvic inflammatory disease. Infect Dis Obstet Gynecol 2002;10(4):171–80.

55. Patten RM, Vincent LM, Wolner-Hanssen P, et al. Pelvic inflammatory disease. Endovaginal sonography with laparoscopic correlation. J Ultrasound Med 1990;9(12):681–9.

56. Cicchiello LA, Hamper UM, Scoutt LM. Ultrasound evaluation of gynecologic causes of pelvic pain. Obstet Gynecol Clin North Am 2011;38(1): 85–114, viii.

57. Korner H, Sondenaa K, Soreide JA, et al. Incidence of acute nonperforated and perforated appendicitis: age-specific and sex-specific analysis. World J Surg 1997;21(3):313–7.

58. Yeh B. Evidence-based emergency medicine/rational clinical examination abstract. Does this adult patient have appendicitis? Ann Emerg Med 2008;52(3):301–3.

59. Guidry SP, Poole GV. The anatomy of appendicitis. Am Surg 1994;60(1):68–71.

60. Puylaert JB. Acute appendicitis: US evaluation using graded compression. Radiology 1986;158(2): 355–60.

61. Jeffrey RB Jr, Laing FC, Townsend RR. Acute appendicitis: sonographic criteria based on 250 cases. Radiology 1988;167(2):327–9.

62. Rybkin AV, Thoeni RF. Current concepts in imaging of appendicitis. Radiol Clin North Am 2007;45(3): 411–22, vii.

63. Lee JH, Jeong YK, Hwang JC, et al. Graded compression sonography with adjuvant use of a posterior manual compression technique in the sonographic diagnosis of acute appendicitis. AJR Am J Roentgenol 2002;178(4):863–8.

64. Lee JH, Jeong YK, Park KB, et al. Operator-dependent techniques for graded compression sonography to detect the appendix and diagnose acute appendicitis. AJR Am J Roentgenol 2005;184(1): 91–7.

65. Rioux M. Sonographic detection of the normal and abnormal appendix. AJR Am J Roentgenol 1992; 158(4):773–8.

66. Bramante R, Radomski M, Nelson M, et al. Appendicitis diagnosed by emergency physician performed point-of-care transvaginal ultrasound: case series. West J Emerg Med 2013;14(5): 415–8.

67. Tayal VS, Bullard M, Swanson DR, et al. ED endovaginal pelvic ultrasound in nonpregnant women with right lower quadrant pain. Am J Emerg Med 2008;26(1):81–5.

68. van Randen A, Bipat S, Zwinderman AH, et al. Acute appendicitis: meta-analysis of diagnostic performance of CT and graded compression US related to prevalence of disease. Radiology 2008; 249(1):97–106.

69. Russell WS, Schuh AM, Hill JG, et al. Clinical practice guidelines for pediatric appendicitis evaluation can decrease computed tomography utilization while maintaining diagnostic accuracy. Pediatr Emerg Care 2013;29(5):568–73.

70. Santillanes G, Simms S, Gausche-Hill M, et al. Prospective evaluation of a clinical practice guideline for diagnosis of appendicitis in children. Acad Emerg Med 2012;19(8):886–93.

71. Mallin M, Dawson M, Schroeder E, et al. Prospective outcomes of pregnant ED patients with documented fetal cardiac activity on ultrasound. Am J Emerg Med 2012;30(3):472–5.

Emergency Ultrasonography
Vascular Applications

Christopher Vaughn, MD[a], James Moak, MD, RDMS[b],*

KEYWORDS

- Doppler • Deep venous thrombosis • Compression • Abdominal aortic aneurysm
- Inferior vena cava • Septic thrombophlebitis • Intima-media thickness

KEY POINTS

- Evaluation for deep venous thrombosis is indicated in symptomatic patients.
- Diagnosis of deep venous thrombosis relies on compression.
- Two-point compression is adequate for evaluation of deep venous thrombosis.
- Thromboses distal to the popliteal vein are generally not treated with anticoagulation.
- Abdominal aortic aneurysms may present with nonspecific symptoms.
- Most aneurysms occur distal to the renal arteries.
- Abdominal aortic aneurysm rupture has high mortality.
- Evaluation of the inferior vena cava may help determine intravascular volume status.
- Inferior vena cava diameter varies with respiration.

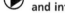 Videos identifying the deep venous system of the lower extremities as well as the abdominal aorta and inferior vena cava accompany this article at http://www.ultrasound.theclinics.com/

INTRODUCTION

Point-of-care ultrasonography of vascular structures such as the aorta and lower extremity deep venous system to evaluate for aneurysm and deep venous thrombosis (DVT), respectively, are core applications of emergency ultrasonography, as outlined by the American College of Emergency Physician's *Emergency Ultrasound Guidelines*.[1]

In this article, these applications as well as imaging of the inferior vena cava (IVC) and potential future applications of emergency ultrasonography are discussed. Standard water-based ultrasound gel should be used as an ultrasound medium with all of the following studies.

DVT
Clinical Problem/Statistics

The incidence of symptomatic DVT in the United States is estimated to be approximately 250,000 adults per year.[2] Ultrasonography use for diagnosis of DVT was just more than 25% in the emergency department (ED) in 2006, and ED patients were nearly 2 times more likely to receive ultrasonography for diagnosis.[3] Approximately 60,000 to 100,000 Americans are estimated to die each year from DVT or pulmonary embolism (PE), 10% to 30% of whom die within 1 month of diagnosis.[4] One-third of patients with a PE present with symptoms of DVT.[5] With the comorbidity

The authors have nothing to disclose.
[a] Department of Emergency Medicine, University of Wisconsin School of Medicine and Public Health, Madison, WI 53792, USA; [b] Department of Emergency Medicine, School of Medicine, University of Virginia, PO Box 800699, Charlottesville, VA 22908, USA
* Corresponding author.
E-mail address: JHM7Q@hscmail.mcc.virginia.edu

and mortality associated with venous thromboembolism, recognizing warning signs and symptoms, as well as timely evaluation of potential DVT, is an important skill set in the practice of emergency medicine. Limited access to formal ultrasonography to evaluate for DVT can lead to delays in care or subject patients to the risk of anticoagulation, given the necessity to treat despite diagnostic uncertainty.

Although formal radiology Doppler studies have traditionally imaged the entire proximal deep venous system from the common femoral vein to the termination of the popliteal vein, studies have shown that compression at 2 points, the common femoral vein and the popliteal vein, is just as sensitive and specific as imaging the entire proximal deep venous system using duplex ultrasonography for diagnosis of DVT in symptomatic patients.[6,7] In patients with a high pretest probability of DVT, 1 study has shown that combining compression ultrasonography in the ED has a high likelihood ratio for DVT as well.[8,9] ED physicians have a significant agreement with radiology in the interpretation of ED ultrasonography for evaluation of DVT.[10] In addition, a correlation between vascular laboratory studies has been seen with the added benefit of increased speed with ED bedside ultrasonography.[11,12]

Anatomy

Proximally to distally

As the external iliac vein crosses the inguinal ligament, it becomes the common femoral vein and subsequently bifurcates into the superficial and deep femoral veins, both classified as parts of the deep venous system. The femoral vein is found just lateral to the common femoral artery immediately after the inguinal ligament and before the common femoral artery and vein take an anterior-posterior relationship, respectively. Similar to the vein, the common femoral artery then bifurcates into the superficial and deep femoral arteries.

The popliteal vein begins in the proximal popliteal fossa and terminates as it diverges in the anterior and posterior tibial veins.

Imaging Protocols

Transducer

A linear transducer ranging from 7.5 to 10 MHz.

Positioning

The patient may be placed in a supine position or sit on the edge of a gurney or examining table, with knees flexed at 90°. If the patient is supine,

leg should be mildly abducted and externally rotated at the hip to provide convenient access to the common femoral vein and its proximal branches. In this position, the knee may be passively flexed from 30° to 80°, allowing for comfort and evaluation of the popliteal fossa. Depending on the side being imaged, the sonologist may choose to stand to the patient's left or right side. An easy way to find the best starting position when evaluating the common femoral vein is by palpating the common femoral artery pulse a few centimeters distal to the inguinal crease. The transducer should be placed perpendicular to the skin, with the indicator toward the patient's right.

It is important to remember anatomic relationships when differentiating between the common femoral artery and vein, particularly their relationship to one another. The common femoral vein is medial to the artery. When comparing sides, the ultrasonographic images appear as mirror images of each other. Other factors allowing for differentiation include the relatively thick walls and pulsatile nature of the artery (which may be more apparent with the use of color flow Doppler). The vein should be more compressible than the artery, but in the presence of a DVT, this is not always a reliable characteristic. Pulse wave Doppler may be used for further differentiation of the artery and vein.

1. Identify the common femoral artery and common femoral vein (**Fig. 1**, Video 1).
2. Identify the greater saphenous vein joining the common femoral vein medially and compress at this level. The amount of pressure applied should not collapse the artery (Video 2).
3. Proceed distally to the branching of the common femoral vein into the superficial and deep femoral veins and evaluate compressibility at the bifurcation and proximal segments of each vein. Thromboses may be more prone to form around points of divergence (when assuming a proximal to distal viewpoint) in the vascular system (eg, as the common femoral vein bifurcates to form the superficial and deep femoral veins) (Video 3).

Proceed to the popliteal fossa:
1. Place the transducer in the proximal popliteal fossa. The popliteal vein and artery typically have an anterior-posterior relationship, respectively. In the ultrasonographic image, the vein appears more superficial (**Fig. 2**).
2. Follow the popliteal vein down, and intermittently compress every 1 cm until it divides into the fibular vein and the posterior and anterior tibial veins (Videos 4 and 5).

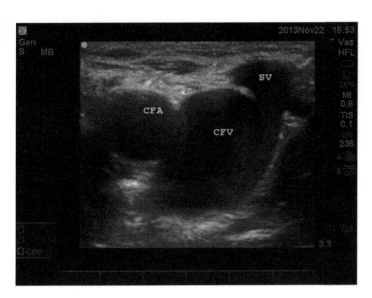

Fig. 1. Identify the common femoral artery and common femoral vein.

Diagnostic Criteria

The primary diagnostic criterion in the evaluation of DVT is compressibility. The criterion for a negative study is complete compressibility of the vein. Previous studies have shown that although color flow Doppler may be helpful in locating the vessels, neither it nor augmentation is more accurate in the diagnosis of DVT than compressibility.[13,14]

Pathology

Clinically significant DVTs are found in or proximal to the popliteal divergence in the deep venous system, extending from the common femoral vein to the popliteal vein. Thromboses in this area are at increased risk for embolization and are therefore generally treated with anticoagulation, thrombectomy, or filter placement.

Pearls, Pitfalls, and Variants

Pearls

- Color flow Doppler and pulse wave Doppler may assist in differentiating the artery and vein (**Figs. 3** and **4**, Video 6).
- An inability to compress the vein with augmentation of the artery is concerning for a DVT.
- Follow-up ultrasonography of the deep venous system in approximately 1 week is suggested to evaluate for propagation of thrombus distal to the popliteal vein.

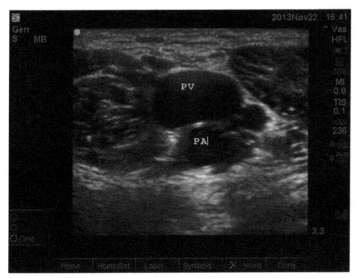

Fig. 2. Place the transducer in the proximal popliteal fossa. The popliteal vein and artery typically have an anterior-posterior relationship, respectively. In the ultrasonographic image, the vein appears more superficial.

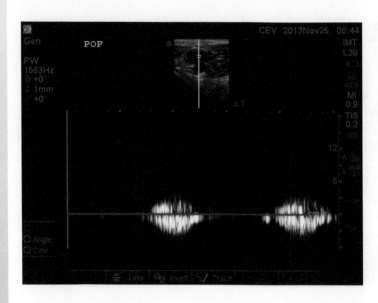

Fig. 3. Color flow Doppler and pulse wave Doppler may assist in differentiating the artery and vein. Pulse wave doppler of the popliteal vein is shown.

- A suggested algorithm for evaluation of DVT is shown in **Fig. 5**.[9]

Pitfalls
- Obesity may obscure deeper structures.
- Significant venous wall noncompliance may make compression difficult.

Variants
- Veins may converge at different locations in patients.
- Duplication of venous systems may occur and is a normal variant particularly with the superficial femoral vein and the popliteal vein.[15]

What the Treating Physician Needs to Know

1. Compressibility is key; although some clots may be visualized, they are not necessary for diagnosis.

2. Two-point compression has been shown to be sensitive and specific for the evaluation of DVT.
3. Point-of-care ultrasonography for DVT may save patients unneeded anticoagulation and decrease length of stay in the ED.

Ultrasonography for Upper Extremity DVT

The deep venous system of the upper extremity is amenable to ultrasonographic evaluation, and more research has been focused on the diagnosis, treatment, morbidity and mortality of upper extremity DVTs (UEDVTs) over the last 5 to 10 years. UEDVTs account for 18% of all DVTs and have a 9% incidence rate of PE.[16,17] Risk factors include central venous catheters, malignancy, and pacemaker wires.[17,18] Secondary DVTs are caused by these risk factors and are more common than

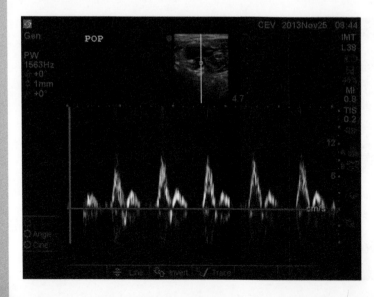

Fig. 4. Another example of how color flow Doppler and pulse wave Doppler may assist in differentiating the artery and vein. Pulse wave doppler of the popliteal artery is shown.

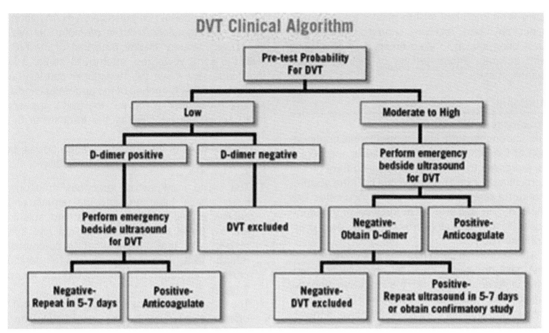

Fig. 5. A suggested algorithm for evaluation of DVT. (*From* Rios M, Lewiss R, Saul T. Focus on: emergency ultrasound for deep vein thrombosis. 2009. Available at: http://www.acep.org/content.aspx?id=44490. Access November 18, 2013; with permission.)

primary DVTs, which include causes such as Paget-Schroetter disease, anatomic abnormality, or idiopathic.[19–21]

The evaluation of upper extremity with ultrasonography relies on the same principles of compressibility as evaluation for lower extremity DVT with a sensitivity and specificity for compression-only ultrasonography of 97% and 100%, respectively.[22] From proximal to distal, the deep venous system of the upper extremity consists of the brachiocephalic veins, internal jugular vein, subclavian vein, axillary vein, brachial veins, ulnar vein, radial vein, and interosseous veins. Evaluation consists of graded compression proximally to distally at recommended intervals of 1 cm. Visualization may be aided by positioning the patient in such a manner that allows for distension of the upper extremity venous system (eg, Trendelenburg position when evaluating the internal jugular vein). Given the anatomy of the upper extremity, shoulder, and thorax, visualization may be impaired at times when attempting to view the subclavian vein and proximal portion of the axillary vein.[21]

Initial treatment involves removing the inciting factor, such as a central venous catheter, if possible. Given the risk for embolization and associated rates of morbidity and mortality, anticoagulation is recommended for the treatment UEDVTs. In cases of recurrence, surgical decompression,

superior vena cava filter placement or venous angioplasty may be beneficial.[23]

ABDOMINAL AORTA
Clinical Problem/Statistics

Abdominal aortic aneurysm (AAA) has an approximately 90% mortality. The risks of rupture of an AAA with diameters greater than 5 cm, 6 cm, and 7 cm are approximately 20%, 40%, and 50%, respectively. They are more prevalent in men than women and more commonly found in people older than 65 years.[24] The classic triad of symptoms related to AAA rupture consists of hypotension, pain, and a pulsatile abdominal mass, although patients may commonly have more insidious presentations and are frequently misdiagnosed.[25] Less than 50% of patients present with all 3 classic symptoms.[26,27] Most AAAs occur infrarenally.

Beside ultrasonography performed by emergency physicians has been shown to be sensitive and specific in the evaluation of AAA in symptomatic patients in the ED compared with formal ultrasonography performed by radiology or computed tomography.[28–31] Studies have also shown that simple screening ultrasonography of at-risk patients may be quick and beneficial in the ED setting, allowing for appropriate follow-up.[32,33] Although bedside ultrasonography of the abdominal aorta is an important skill to master for the emergency physician, relatively short training periods have been shown to yield emergency physicians with accurate interpretations of their ultrasonographic images.[34]

Anatomy

Proximally to distally

The abdominal aorta is a retroperitoneal continuation of the descending thoracic aorta and begins as it crosses the diaphragm traveling through the aortic hiatus. Lying just left of the IVC, the abdominal aorta terminates distally as it bifurcates into the common iliac arteries at the level of the umbilicus, fourth lumbar vertebra, and iliac crest approximately.

The abdominal aorta has multiple branches, the first being the celiac trunk, which projects anteriorly, before dividing into the common hepatic, left gastric, and splenic arteries. The superior mesenteric artery is the second branch and travels caudally to supply blood to much of the small and large intestine as well as the pancreas. The renal arteries project laterally, the right traveling between the IVC and spine, whereas the left originates slightly more distal than the right.

Imaging Protocols

Positioning

The patient should be placed in a supine position with the sonologist positioned to the patient's right. Holding the ultrasound transducer in the right hand allows freedom to operate the machine with the left. The patient may be draped to preserve modesty, as with the basic physical examination.

Transducer

A phased array or curvilinear transducer ranging from 3.5 to 5 MHz.

Technique

Place the transducer just below the xiphoid process in a transverse plane. The vertebral column is a key landmark when locating the abdominal aorta. The vertebrae appear hyperechoic superficially secondary to the periosteum before appearing hypoechoic deep to the periosteum. Minimize the depth on the image so the vertebral column is just in view at the bottom. The IVC and aorta are located just superficial to, or on top of, the vertebral column. In a transverse plane, the IVC is commonly noted to be shaped as a sideways teardrop located on the patient's right instead of a more rigid, uniform circle like the aorta. The shape of the IVC may change depending on the patient's volume status and at times may appear flattened or effaced. The aorta is located to the left of the IVC, should be pulsatile on examination, and is approximately 2 cm in diameter. Its wall should also appear thicker than that of the IVC. With the aorta visualized, attempt to center it in the image and move the transducer caudally to evaluate the first branches of the abdominal aorta. As the transducer is moved, the aorta appears more superficial because of the lordosis of the lumbar spine.

The branches of the abdominal aorta appear in order as follows, from proximally to distally:

1. The celiac trunk, which branches anteriorly, subsequently bifurcates into the hepatic and splenic arteries. As the hepatic and splenic arteries travel to the patient's right and left, respectively, they create what is commonly referred to as the seagull sign. The left gastric artery is not commonly visualized (**Figs. 6** and **7**, Video 7).
2. The superior mesenteric artery, which initially branches anteriorly before immediately traveling caudally parallel to the aorta, is seen in cross-section while imaging in a transverse plane (**Fig. 8**).
3. The right renal artery travels between the IVC and vertebral column perpendicular to the aorta.
4. The left renal artery travels perpendicular to the aorta (**Figs. 9** and **10**).
5. The common iliac arteries branch approximately at the level of the umbilicus. The upper limit of normal for the external iliac diameter is 1.5 cm. Just before a clear bifurcation, the aorta may look ovoid, with the long axis extending laterally (**Fig. 10**; **Fig. 11**, Video 8).

Measure the proximal and distal aorta in a transverse plane (indicator to the right) from anterior to posterior from outer wall to outer wall. It is important to measure from the outer walls, given the possibility of intramural clot creating a false lumen with a diameter appearing to be within normal limits. Measurements should be taken at the proximal, mid, and distal abdominal aorta.

Diagnostic Criteria

AAA is defined as a diameter greater than 3 cm when measuring from outer arterial wall to outer arterial wall. While viewing the aorta in a longitudinal plane, the ultrasound beam may have a tangential relationship with the aorta, and the anterior-posterior diameter may not be accurate. As mentioned earlier, most AAAs occur infrarenally.

Pathology

A fusiform aneurysm involves all 3 layers of the aortic wall resulting in a uniform aneurysm and is

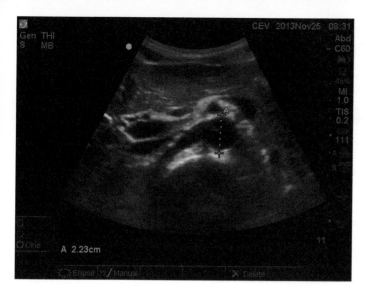

Fig. 6. The celiac trunk, which branches anteriorly, subsequently divides into the hepatic and splenic arteries. As the hepatic and splenic arteries travel to the patient's right and left, respectively, they create what is commonly referred to as the seagull sign (not shown here). The left gastric artery is not commonly visualized. The aorta is measured from outer wall to outer wall.

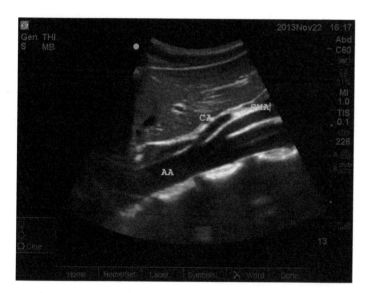

Fig. 7. An additional example of the celiac trunk, superior mesenteric artery and proximal aorta viewed longitudinally.

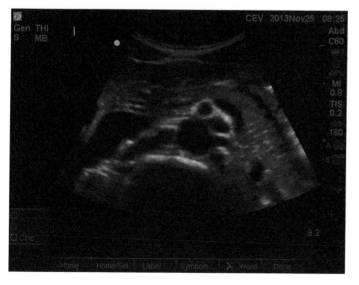

Fig. 8. The superior mesenteric artery, which initially branches anteriorly before immediately traveling caudally and parallel with the aorta, is seen in cross-section while imaging in a transverse plane.

192

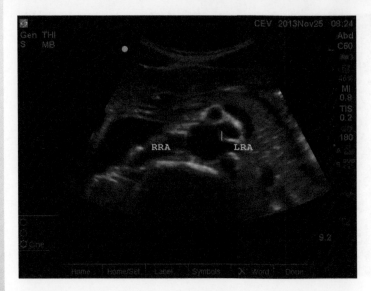

Fig. 9. The left renal artery travels perpendicular to the aorta.

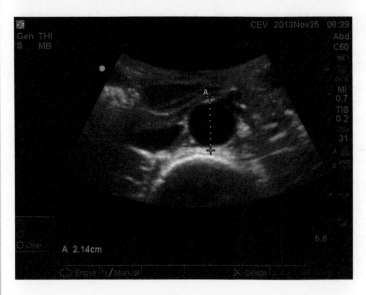

Fig. 10. Additional example of the left renal artery.

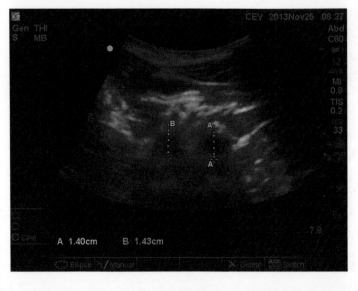

Fig. 11. The common iliac arteries branch approximately at the level of the umbilicus. The upper limit of normal for the external iliac diameter is 1.5 cm. Just before a clear bifurcation, the aorta may look ovoid, with the long axis extending laterally.

the commonest. Saccular aneurysms affect a portion of the aortic wall, resulting in a relative out-pouching, and are relatively uncommon compared with fusiform aneurysms.

Pearls, Pitfalls, and Variants

- Pearls
  - Perform a FAST (focused assessment with sonography for trauma) examination in concert with the finding of an AAA in a symptomatic patient.
  - Use color or pulse wave Doppler to help identify the aorta (**Fig. 12**, Video 9).
  - False-positive results are rare.[35]
- Pitfalls
  - Bowel gas may obscure underlying structures. Pressure and rocking the transducer back and forth may help displace some of the gas; one may also reposition the probe and use the liver as a window. Despite these measures, incomplete evaluation of the abdominal aorta may occur.[36]
  - Significant obesity may impede visualization of deeper structures.

What the Referring Physician Needs to Know

1. Consider performing a FAST scan on an unstable patient to look for free fluid in the presence of an aortic aneurysm.
2. Relatively small aneurysms in the presence of concerning symptoms should still be taken seriously.
3. Aneurysms between 3 and 5 cm need follow-up with a vascular surgeon.
4. Aneurysms greater than 5 cm need immediate vascular consultation.

Summary

AAA is a potentially devastating disease process that carries high mortality in the presence of rupture. Prompt evaluation and diagnosis, particularly in an unstable patient who may not be appropriate for a computed tomography scan, is paramount to the patient's survival.

IVC
Clinical Problem/Statistics

Evaluation of the IVC may be useful in the evaluation of a critically ill patient, and multiple algorithms (such as the RUSH [rapid ultrasonography for shock and hypotension] protocol[37]) have incorporated it. The size of the IVC has been shown to significantly change relative to intravascular volume status, with increased accuracy at particularly low or high collapsibility ranges.[38,39] In critically ill patients, those suffering from severe sepsis or septic shock, goal-directed therapy includes achieving a central venous pressure (CVP) of 8 to 12 mm Hg, as recommended by the Surviving Sepsis Campaign.[40] Emergent placement of a central venous catheter in the ED is not always feasible, and there are associated risks to the procedure. Central venous access may be avoided in patients not requiring pressors by monitoring appropriate fluid resuscitation via large-bore intravenous catheters with serial evaluation of the IVC with bedside ultrasonography.

Size and collapsibility may be extrapolated to estimate CVP, intravascular volume status, and fluid responsiveness. The IVC shows respiratory variation, expanding with inspiration and

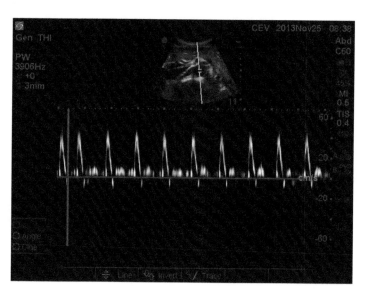

Fig. 12. When diagnosing an AAA, color or pulse wave Doppler can be used to help identify the aorta.

contracting with expiration in a positive-pressure–ventilated patient as a result of the changes in intrathoracic pressure. In an unventilated patient, those relationships are reversed, and the IVC expands with expiration (positive intrathoracic pressure) and contracts with inspiration (negative intrathoracic pressure). Evaluating the size and collapsibility of the IVC has been shown to be a reliable surrogate for CVP, fluid responsiveness in ventilated patients,[41] and volume status.

The caval index is a measure of the respiratory variation of the size of the IVC. A caval index greater than 50% has been shown to be a sensitive and specific surrogate for CVP less than 8 mm Hg, a critical measurement in the evaluation and resuscitation of patient's suffering from severe sepsis or septic shock.[42]

tilting the transducer back toward the patient's feet. One may also locate the IVC by starting in a sagittal plane, rocking the ultrasound beam toward the head, and viewing its origin at the right atrium (Videos 10–12).

Although the aorta is typically evaluated in a traverse plane, the sagittal plane is typically most useful in evaluating the IVC. If the IVC is located in a transverse plane, center it in the ultrasonographic image and then rotate the transducer 90° so the indicator is pointing toward the patient's head for a sagittal view.

The IVC should be measured perpendicular to the vessel wall approximately 2 cm from the convergence of the hepatic veins and the IVC. Although respiratory variation has been shown to be equivalent 2 cm from the atrium with locations occurring

$$\text{Caval index (\%)} = [(\text{IVC diameter}_{expiration} - \text{IVC diameter}_{inspiration})/\text{IVC diameter}_{expiration}] \times 100$$

Anatomy

Proximally to distally
The inferior vena cava originates at the right atrium and passes through the aortic hiatus just to the right of the aorta and terminates distally as it bifurcates into the common iliac veins. Compared with the aorta, it is relatively thin walled and compressible, larger, and varies with respiration.

Imaging Protocols

Transducer
A phased array or curvilinear transducer ranging from 3.5 to 5 MHz.

Positioning
When evaluating the IVC, the patient should be placed in the same supine position as when evaluating the abdominal aorta. The sonologist and ultrasound machine are again positioned at the patient's right.

Technique
The IVC may be located by starting in a transverse plain perpendicular to the abdominal wall in a subxiphoid position in the same manner as locating the aorta. Again, the IVC may range in appearance depending on the patient's intravascular volume, and a small amount of pressure may be enough to cause collapse. If unable to view the IVC, it may be advantageous to apply as little pressure as possible. It may also help to tilt the transducer toward the head, obtain a subxiphoid view, locate the right atrium, and trace it down into the IVC by

distally, measurements taken at the junction of the right atrium and IVC have been shown not to be equivalent and should be avoided (**Fig. 13**).[43]

Pathology

A severely compressed IVC or a large amount of respiratory variation may indicate low intravascular volume in an ill patient. A caval index greater than 50% correlates to a CVP less than 8 mm Hg. In ventilated patients, percent change in IVC diameter has been shown to be a reliable predictor of fluid responsiveness (**Fig. 14**, Video 13).[41]

Pearls, Pitfalls, and Variants

Pearls
- Tracing the IVC from the right atrium is a good way to locate the IVC.
- Severe intravascular volume depletion may lead to difficulty localizing the IVC secondary to significant effacement.
- Make sure to view findings with an appropriate clinical context.

Pitfalls
- The IVC may appear enlarged or noncompliant in the setting of increased right-sided heart pressure secondary to causes such as congestive heart failure,[44] pulmonary hypertension, cardiac tamponade (pericardial effusion), and tension pneumothorax.[45]
- As with visualizing the aorta, bowel gas may impede imaging; using the liver as an ultrasonographic window may aid in visualization.

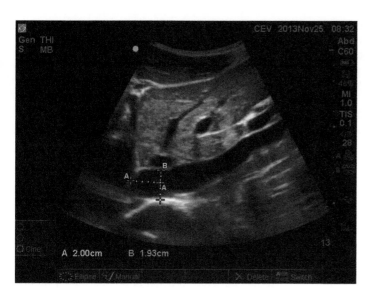

Fig. 13. The IVC should be measured perpendicularly to vessel wall and approximately 2 cm from the convergence of the hepatic vein into the IVC. Although respiratory variation has been shown to be equivalent 2 cm from the atrium with locations occurring distally, measurement taken at the junction of the right atrium and IVC have been shown to not be equivalent and should be avoided.

Variants
- Variants include rare anatomic abnormalities, such as situs inversus, in which the aorta and IVC are on the patient's right and left, respectively.

What the Treating Physician Needs to Know

1. Prompt evaluation of the IVC in a critically ill patient may help delineate therapy early in the resuscitative process and may help in avoiding unnecessary placement of a central venous catheter.
2. IVC change is reversed when comparing appearance in positive-pressure–ventilated patients with unventilated patients.
3. Although IVC may add critical data while a patient is being diagnosed and treated, findings should be considered within the clinical context and in light of additional data.

FURTHER VASCULAR APPLICATIONS

The following vascular applications may be beneficial when evaluating specific types of patients in the ED, although further research is needed to establish their specific role and accuracy in the setting of the ED when performed by emergency medicine physicians.

Septic Thrombophlebitis

Clinical problem
Septic (or suppurative) thrombophlebitis is concurrent bacteremia in the presence of an infected intravascular thrombus. Although most commonly

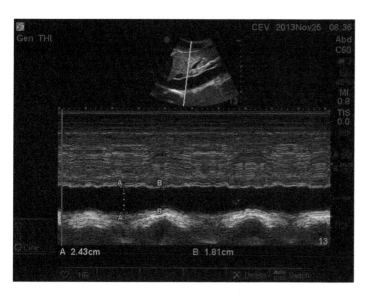

Fig. 14. A severely compressed IVC or a large amount of respiratory variation may indicate low intravascular volume in an ill patient. A caval index greater than 50% correlates to a CVP less than 8 mm Hg. In ventilated patients, percent change in IVC diameter has been shown to a reliable predictor of fluid responsiveness.

associated with peripheral or central venous catheters, other manifestations of septic thrombophlebitis exist as well.[46] Lemierre's syndrome is a prominent example, in which an infected thrombus forms within the internal jugular vein, most commonly seeded by a peritonsillar abscess.[47] Other examples include association with the pelvic veins secondary to obstetric or gynecologic causes or procedures, the portal vein, and most frequently, the femoral veins.[48,49]

Septic thrombophlebitis can occur anywhere in the venous system. Lemierre syndrome is associated with the internal jugular vein, but septic thrombophlebitis does not have to occur there and at times is a diagnosis of exclusion. Most commonly, it is seen involving the femoral veins or associated with central venous catheter placement.

Imaging

Although some vessels are more easily assessed with ultrasonography than others, it is important to be familiar with the anatomy, variants, and pitfalls when evaluating for thrombus in a specific part of the venous system. The choice of transducer depends on the area of the patient's body being imaged and the patient's body habitus. Generally, a high-frequency, linear transducer should be adequate for evaluating peripheral vascular structures. Diagnostic criteria consist of the presence of an infected intravascular thrombus indicated by a noncompressible vein,[50] bacteremia systemic inflammatory response syndrome, and presumed sepsis. Treatment consists of removing the inciting factor (such as a central venous catheter) and starting parenteral antibiotics. Anticoagulation remains controversial despite potential for septic emboli.[46]

Carotid Artery Intima-Media Thickness

Clinical problem/statistics

Heart disease is the leading cause of death worldwide and responsible for 600,000 deaths in the United States annually; 385,000 of those deaths are secondary to coronary artery disease (CAD).[51] The cost of CAD in the United States is approximately $108.9 billion when considering the associated expense of medications, health care services, and lost productivity.[52,53] Given the morbidity, mortality, and overall cost secondary to CAD, new and innovative ways aimed at improving prevention, diagnosis and treatment are being pursued. Ultrasonographic evaluation of the carotid intima-media thickness (CIMT) is one such method that may hold promise in improving risk stratification. A meta-analysis performed in 2007 reported CIMT as a strong independent predictor of future vascular events such as myocardial infarction and stroke, with increased risk per 0.1 mm of increased CIMT.[54,55]

Imaging and measurement

From intraluminal to extraluminal, the intima and media are the 2 innermost layers of the carotid artery. Imaging the intraluminal surface of the vessel allows for assessment of atherosclerosis earlier in the disease process.[56] Three different 1-cm areas are evaluated with a linear high-frequency probe ranging from 7.5 MHz to 10 MHz: the common carotid artery, the carotid bulb (just distal to the carotid artery and the beginning of the bifurcation), and the internal carotid artery. Generally, the common carotid artery is most amenable to imaging, and the intima-media thickness of the far wall is measured, with increased cardiovascular risk believed to begin at greater than 1 mm in thickness.[56,57]

SUMMARY

Although some authorities remain dubious about the usefulness of CIMT measures in addition to other risk factors predictive of CAD,[57] measurement of CIMT is a relatively noninvasive, inexpensive test to help with risk stratification. Further research is needed to provide standardized protocols, given that studies have shown varying cardiovascular risks associated with thickening in different areas of the carotid artery.[58] Further research is also needed to delineate its role in the evaluation of CAD, particularly in ED patients presenting with acute chest pain.

SUPPLEMENTARY DATA

Videos related to this article can be found online at http://dx.doi.org/10.1016/j.cult.2014.01.007.

REFERENCES

1. American College of Emergency Physicians. Emergency ultrasound guidelines. Ann Emerg Med 2009;53:550–70.
2. Grosse SD. Incidence-based cost estimates require population-based incidence data. A critique of Mahan et al. Thromb Haemost 2012; 107:192–3.
3. Barnes GD, Gafoor SM, Wakefield T, et al. National trends in venous disease. J Vasc Surg 2010;51(6): 1467–73.
4. Deep vein thrombosis (DVT)/pulmonary embolism (PE)–blood clot forming in a vein. Centers for Disease Control and Prevention; 2013. Available at: http://www.cdc.gov/ncbddd/dvt/data.html. Accessed December 4, 2013.

5. Pomero F, Brignone C, Serraino C, et al. Venous lower-limb evaluation in patient with acute pulmonary embolism. South Med J 2011;104(6): 405–11.
6. Frazee BW, Snoey ER, Levitt A. Emergency department compression ultrasound to diagnose proximal deep vein thrombosis. J Emerg Med 2001; 20(2):107–12.
7. Bernardi E, Camporese G, Büller HR, et al. Serial 2-point ultrasonography for diagnosing suspected symptomatic deep vein thrombosis: a randomized controlled trial. JAMA 2008;300(14):1653–9.
8. Kline JA, O'Malley PM, Tayal VS, et al. Emergency clinician-performed compression ultrasonography for deep venous thrombosis of the lower extremity. Ann Emerg Med 2008;52(4):437–45.
9. Rios M, Lewiss R, Saul T. Focus on: emergency ultrasound for deep vein thrombosis. 2009. Available at: http://www.acep.org/content.aspx?id=44490. Accessed November 18, 2013.
10. Caronia J, Sarzynski A, Tofighi B, et al. Resident performed two-point compression ultrasound is inadequate for diagnosis of deep vein thrombosis in the critically ill. J Thromb Thrombolysis 2013. [Epub ahead of print].
11. Blaivas M, Lamber MJ, Harwood RA, et al. Lower-extremity Doppler for deep venous thrombosis–can emergency physicians be accurate and fast? Acad Emerg Med 2000;7(2):120–6.
12. Theodoro D, Blaivas M, Duggal S, et al. Real-time B-mode ultrasound in the ED saves time in the diagnosis of deep vein thrombosis (DVT). Am J Emerg Med 2004;22(3):197–200.
13. Lockhart ME, Sheldon HI, Robbin ML. Augmentation in lower extremity sonography for detection of deep venous thrombosis. AJR Am J Roentgenol 2005;184:419–22.
14. Lensing AW, Doris CI, McGrath FP, et al. A comparison of compression ultrasound with color Doppler ultrasound for the diagnosis of symptomless postoperative deep vein thrombosis. Arch Intern Med 1997;156:765–8.
15. Dona E, Fletcher JP, Hughes TM, et al. Duplicate popliteal and superficial femoral veins: incidence and potential significance. Aust N Z J Surg 2000; 70:438–40.
16. Mustafa S, Stein PD, Patel KC, et al. Upper extremity deep venous thrombosis. Chest 2003;123:1953–6.
17. Lee JA, Zierler BK, Zierler RE. The risk factors and clinical outcomes of upper extremity deep vein thrombosis. Vasc Endovascular Surg 2012;46: 139–44.
18. Blaivas M. Ultrasound in the detection of venous thromboembolism. Crit Care Med 2007;35: S224–34.
19. Rosen T, Chang B, Kaufman M, et al. Emergency department diagnosis of upper extremity deep venous thrombosis using bedside ultrasonography. Crit Ultrasound J 2012;4(1):4.
20. Schleyer AM, Jarman KM, Calver P, et al. Upper extremity deep vein thrombosis in hospitalized patients: a descriptive study. J Hosp Med 2014;9(1): 48–53.
21. Joffe HV, Goldhaber SZ. Upper-extremity deep vein thrombosis. Circulation 2002;106:1874–80.
22. Di Nisio M, Van Sluis GL, Bossuyt PM, et al. Accuracy of diagnostic tests for clinically suspected upper extremity deep vein thrombosis: a systematic review. J Thromb Haemost 2010;8:684–92.
23. Sajid MS, Ahmed N, Desai M, et al. Upper limb deep vein thrombosis: a literature review to streamline the protocol for management. Acta Haematol 2007;118:10–8.
24. Aortic aneurysm fact sheet. In: Centers for Disease Control and Prevention: Division of Heart Disease and Stroke Prevention. 2013. Available at: http://www.cdc.gov/dhdsp/data_statistics/fact_sheets/fs_aortic_aneurysm.htm. Accessed November 13, 2013.
25. Akkersdijk GJ, van Bockel JH. Ruptured abdominal aortic aneurysm: initial misdiagnosis and the effect on treatment. Eur J Surg 1998;164:29–34.
26. Marston WA, Ahlquist R, Johnson G Jr, et al. Misdiagnosis of ruptured abdominal aortic aneurysms. J Vasc Surg 1992;16:17–22.
27. Lyon C, Clark D. Diagnosis of acute abdominal pain in older patients. Am Fam Physician 2006; 74:1537–44. Available at: http://www.aafp.org/afp/2006/1101/p1537.html. Accessed December 1, 2013.
28. Kuhn M, Bonnin RL, Davey MJ, et al. Emergency department ultrasound scanning for abdominal aortic aneurysm: accessible, accurate, and advantageous. Ann Emerg Med 2000;36:219–23.
29. Tayal VS, Graf CD, Gibbs MA. Prospective study of accuracy and outcome of emergency ultrasound for abdominal aortic aneurysm over two years. Acad Emerg Med 2003;10:867–71.
30. Knaut AL, Kendall JL, Patten R, et al. Ultrasonographic measurement of aortic diameter by emergency physicians approximates results obtained by commuted tomography. J Emerg Med 2005; 28:119–26.
31. Rubano E, Mehta N, Caputo W, et al. Systematic review: emergency department bedside ultrasonography for diagnosing suspected abdominal aortic aneurysm. Acad Emerg Med 2013;20:128–38.
32. Salen P, Melanson S, Buro D. ED screening to identify abdominal aortic aneurysms in asymptomatic geriatric patients. Am J Emerg Med 2003;21:133–5.
33. Moore CL, Holliday RS, Hwang JQ, et al. Screening for abdominal aortic aneurysm in asymptomatic at-risk patients using emergency ultrasound. Am J Emerg Med 2008;26:883–7.

34. Rowland JL, Kuhn M, Bonnin RL, et al. Accuracy of emergency department bedside ultrasonography. Emerg Med (Fremantle) 2001;13:305–13.

35. Lyon M, Brannam L, Ciamillo L, et al. False positive abdominal aortic aneurysm on bedside emergency ultrasound. J Emerg Med 2004;26:193–6.

36. Blaivas M, Theodoro D. Frequency of incomplete abdominal aorta visualization by emergency department bedside ultrasound. Acad Emerg Med 2004;11:103–5.

37. Weingart S. Rapid ultrasound for shock and hypotension. In: EMCrit Blog. A discussion of the practice of ED critical care. 2009. Available at: http://emcrit.org/rush-exam/original-rush-article/. Accessed December 5, 2013.

38. Lyon M, Blaivas M, Brannam L. Sonographic measurement of the inferior vena cava as a marker of blood loss. Am J Emerg Med 2005;23:45–50.

39. Stawicki SP, Braslow BM, Panebianco NL, et al. Intensivist use of hand-carried ultrasonography to measure IVC collapsibility in estimating intravascular volume status: correlations with CVP. J Am Coll Surg 2009;209(1):55–61.

40. Dellinger RP, Levy MM, Rhodes A, et al. Surviving sepsis campaign: international guidelines for management of severe sepsis and septic shock: 2012. Crit Care Med 2013;41:580–637.

41. Barbier C, Loubières, Schmit C, et al. Respiratory changes in inferior vena cava diameter are helpful in predicting fluid responsiveness in ventilated septic patients. Intensive Care Med 2004;30:1740–6.

42. Nagdev AD, Merchant RC, Tirado-Gonzalez A, et al. Emergency department bedside ultrasonographic measurement of the caval index for noninvasive determination of low central venous pressure. Ann Emerg Med 2010;55:290–5.

43. Wallace DJ, Allison M, Stone MB. Inferior vena cava percentage collapse during respiration is affected by the sampling location: an ultrasound study in health volunteers. Acad Emerg Med 2010;17:96–9.

44. Blehar DJ, Dickman E, Gaspari R. Identification of congestive heart failure via respiratory variation of inferior vena cava diameter. Am J Emerg Med 2009;27:71–5.

45. Goldflam K, Saul T, Lewiss R. Focus on: inferior vena cava ultrasound. 2011. Available at: http://www.acep.org/Content.aspx?id=80791. Accessed November 18, 2013.

46. Dimitropoulou D, Lagadinou M, Papayiannis T, et al. Septic thrombophlebitis caused by Fusobacterium necrophorum in an intravenous drug use. Case Rep Infect Dis 2013;2013:870846.

47. David H. A 21-year-old man with fever and abdominal pain after recent peritonsillar abscess drainage. Am J Emerg Med 2009;27:515.e3–4.

48. Jaiyeoba O. Postoperative infections in obstetrics and gynecology. Clin Obstet Gynecol 2012;55:904–13.

49. Levine DP, Brown PD. Infections in injection drug users. In: Mandell GL, Bennett JE, Dolin R, editors. Douglas and Bennett's principles and practice of infectious diseases. 7th edition. Philadelphia: Churchill Livingstone Elsevier; 2009. p. 3875–90.

50. Adhikari S. Point-of-care ultrasound diagnosis of peripheral vein septic thrombophlebitis in the emergency department. J Emerg Med 2013;44:183–4.

51. Kochanek KD, Xu JQ, Murphy SL, et al. Deaths: final data for 2009. Natl Vital Stat Rep 2011;60:1–116.

52. Heidenreich PA, Trogdon JG, Khavjou OA, et al. Forecasting the future of cardiovascular disease in the United States: a policy statement from the American Heart Association. Circulation 2011;123:933–44.

53. Heart disease. In: Centers for Disease Control and Prevention. 2013. Available at: http://www.cdc.gov/heartdisease/index.htm. Accessed November 22, 2013.

54. Lorenz MW, Markus HS, Bots ML, et al. Prediction of clinical cardiovascular events with carotid intima-media thickness: a systemic review and meta-analysis. Circulation 2007;115:459–67.

55. Zielinski T, Dzielinska Z, Januszewicz A, et al. Carotid intima-media thickness as a marker of cardiovascular risk in hypertensive patients with coronary artery disease. Am J Hypertens 2007;20:1058–64.

56. O'Leary DH, Bots ML. Imaging of atherosclerosis: carotid intima media thickness. Eur Heart J 2010;3:1682–9.

57. Simon A, Megnien JL, Chironi G. The value of carotid intima-media thickness for predicting cardiovascular risk. Arterioscler Thromb Vasc Biol 2010;30:182–5.

58. Polak JF, Person SD, Wei GS, et al. Segment-specific associations of carotid intima-media thickness with cardiovascular risk factors: the Coronary Artery Risk Development in Young Adults (CARDIA) study. Stroke 2010;41:9–15.

Pediatric Emergency Ultrasound

Lorraine Ng, MD[a],*, Jennifer R. Marin, MD, MSc[b]

KEYWORDS

- Pediatric • Emergency medicine • Point-of-care ultrasound • Pyloric stenosis • Intussusception
- Skull fractures • Hip effusion

KEY POINTS

- Pyloric stenosis should be considered in infants 2 to 6 weeks of age with projectile emesis, and is diagnosed sonographically if muscle thickness exceeds 3 mm and pyloric channel length exceeds 15 mm.
- Intussusception is seen in young children with emesis and colicky abdominal pain, and can be diagnosed sonographically based on the presence of a target sign (transverse) and/or pseudokidney sign (longitudinal) most commonly seen in the right abdomen.
- Infants with head trauma and scalp swelling should be evaluated for an underlying skull fracture, which can be seen sonographically as a disruption in the hyperechoic linear bony cortex.
- Children with a limp or knee pain should be evaluated with ultrasound for a hip effusion, which is diagnosed sonographically if more than a 2 mm difference is seen in the anterior synovial space thickness between the symptomatic and contralateral hip, or if the thickness on the affected side exceeds 5 mm.

 Videos of picture frame and lawnmower scanning of the abdomen for intussusception accompany this article at http://www.ultrasound.theclinics.com/

INTRODUCTION

The importance of point-of-care ultrasound (POCUS) in the daily practice of emergency medicine physicians is established and underscored by the comprehensive and well-cited guidelines from various emergency medicine organizations. The American Board of Emergency Medicine, American College of Emergency Physicians, Emergency Medicine Residency Review Committee, and Society of Academic Emergency Medicine have deemed POCUS a required core component for training emergency medicine residents.[1,2] That curriculum encompasses core applications that focus primarily on adult disease states, such as focused abdominal sonography in trauma, imaging in early pregnancy, aortic imaging, emergent cardiac imaging, and procedural imaging.[3]

POCUS is rapidly expanding to include pediatric-specific applications that aid in the diagnosis of pediatric clinical conditions and guidance of invasive procedures. Most pediatric emergency visits in the United States occur in hospitals that do no have a full spectrum of specialized pediatric

The authors have nothing to disclose.
a Division of Pediatric Emergency Medicine, Columbia University Medical Center (CUMC), New York Presbyterian - Morgan Stanley Children's Hospital of New York, 622 West 168th Street, PH - 137, New York, NY 10032, USA;
b Division of Pediatric Emergency Medicine, Children's Hospital of Pittsburgh, 4401 Penn Avenue, AOB Suite 2400, Pittsburgh, PA 15224, USA
* Corresponding author.
E-mail address: ln2136@columbia.edu

Box 1
Clinical features of hypertrophic pyloric stenosis

- Infant aged 4 ± 2 weeks
- Nonbilious emesis immediately after feeding
- Interested in eating
- Palpable "olive-like" mass in epigastrium
- Hypokalemic hypochloremic metabolic alkalosis

services.[4] POCUS by emergency physicians has the potential for earlier diagnosis and expedited transfer to a facility that has specialized pediatric radiology and pediatric surgical services. This article highlights novel POCUS applications that focus on pediatric emergency care.

APPLICATIONS OF POCUS
Hypertrophic Pyloric Stenosis

Anatomy
The clinical features of hypertrophic pyloric stenosis are outlined in **Box 1**; however, the anatomy of the pylorus relative to other structures must be understood before the sonographic evaluation is performed.

The pylorus is located in the epigastrium, right (lateral) of midline at the end of the gastric outlet, posterior to the liver, and adjacent to or posterior to the gallbladder (**Fig. 1**).

Imaging protocols The superficial pylorus is best visualized with a high-frequency linear transducer. The examination may be performed with the

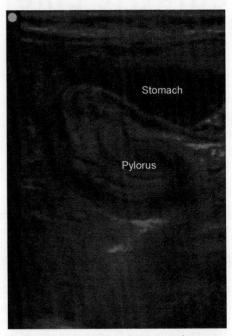
Fig. 2. Gastric antrum emptying into pylorus.

patient in the supine or right lateral decubitus position. Placement in the decubitus position will allow fluid to fall toward the most dependent area against the pylorus, which will provide a better sonographic window to visualize the pylorus and moves gas out of the way to the left side of the abdomen or stomach fundus.

If the stomach is too distended, the pylorus may be positioned posterior to the stomach. If the stomach is empty, the infant may be permitted to drink a small amount, which will allow the physician performing the POCUS to follow the flow of

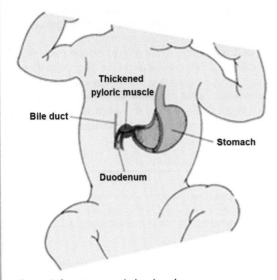
Fig. 1. Pylorus anatomic landmarks.

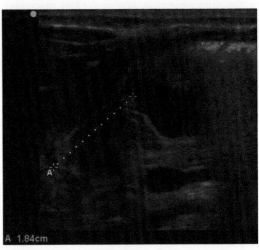
Fig. 3. Pyloric channel length measurement (A).

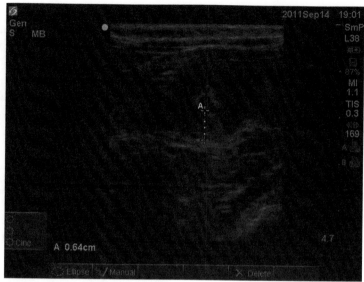

Fig. 4. Pyloric muscle wall thickness measurement (A).

fluid from the stomach toward the pylorus. Ideally, the infant will have nothing in the stomach before beginning the examination. If the infant has fed before the examination, further feeding may lead to overdistention of the gastric antrum and false-negative measurements of the pylorus.

The landmarks that should be identified include the gastric antrum, liver, and gallbladder.

Once the gastric antrum is identified, it should be traced toward the patient's right side until the stomach is seen emptying into the pylorus (**Fig. 2**). If visualization of structures is impaired because of gas, gentle graded compression with the ultrasound probe will aid in displacing bowel gas.

Diagnostic criteria Once the pylorus is identified it should be measured in both the transverse and longitudinal planes. The pyloric channel length is measured in the longitudinal plane, and measurements exceeding 15 mm indicate hypertrophic pyloric stenosis (**Fig. 3**). In the transverse plane, the pylorus will appear as a "donut" or "target," with the central echogenic mucosa surrounded by hypoechoic thickened muscle (**Fig. 4**). In this view, a muscle thickness exceeding 3 mm is

---

Box 2
Sonographic features of hypertrophic pyloric stenosis

- Muscle wall thickness exceeding 3 mm
- Channel length exceeding 15 mm
- Pylorus in longitudinal plane
  - Shoulder sign: hypertrophied muscle bulging into the gastric antrum (**Fig. 5**)
  - Nipple sign: redundant pyloric mucosa protruding into the gastric antrum (**Fig. 6**)
- Pylorus in transverse plane
  - Donut sign: thickened hypoechoic muscular layer (**Fig. 7**)

Box 3
Pearls and pitfalls of POCUS for hypertrophic pyloric stenosis

Pearls

- Nothing by mouth before ultrasound
- Feed during ultrasound to follow flow of fluid from stomach toward pylorus
- Right lateral decubitus aids in gravitational flow of gastric contents and ability to use contents as a sonographic window
- Graded compression to displace bowel gas air

Pitfalls

- False-positive findings on ultrasound for pyloric stenosis
  - Pylorospasm
  - Gastric decompression
- False-negative findings on ultrasound for pyloric stenosis
  - Gastric distention
  - Premature infants

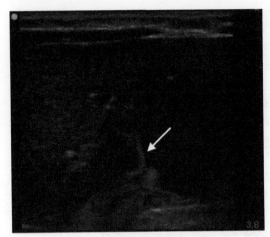

Fig. 5. Shoulder sign of pyloric stenosis (*arrow*).

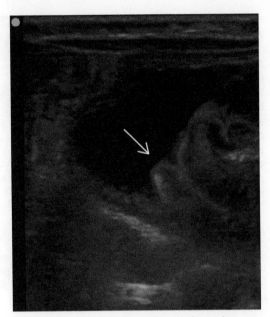

Fig. 6. Nipple sign of pyloric stenosis (*arrow*).

considered to be hypertrophic. If borderline measurements are obtained, the physician should consider repeating the examination in a few minutes, because pylorospasm can mimic that of hypertrophic pyloric stenosis sonographically, but can be distinguished by the resolution of sonographic abnormalities. Additionally, dehydration can affect the thickness of the pylorus, and a severely dehydrated child should be scanned again after intravenous hydration if pylorus measurements were borderline. It is also important to visualize the passing of gastric contents through the pyloric channel in real time to rule out the diagnosis of hypertrophic pyloric stenosis.

Several secondary signs of hypertrophic pyloric stenosis should be noted, which are listed in **Box 2**. **Box 3** presents the pearls and pitfalls associated with POCUS for hypertrophic pyloric stenosis.

The evidence

Although ultrasound has long been the preferred diagnostic modality for pyloric stenosis,[5–8] only

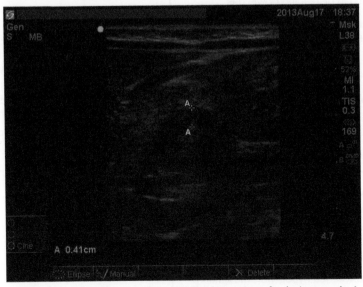

Fig. 7. Measurement of the pyloric muscle thickness, with the donut sign of pyloric stenosis. A denotes the muscle wall thickness measurement.

a couple of case reports have delineated its role within emergency medicine and POCUS.[9–11]

A recent study by Sivitz and colleagues[12] showed that trained pediatric emergency medicine (PEM) physicians were able to accurately assess the pylorus with ultrasound after a 45-minute training session. When compared with radiology studies, PEM physicians were able to identify the pylorus and accurately diagnose pyloric stenosis with a sensitivity of 100% and specificity of 100%. In addition, no statistical difference in pylorus measurements were seen compared with those of radiology staff.

Intussusception

Anatomy

Intussusception occurs when a bowel segment telescopes onto itself, resulting in bowel obstruction (**Fig. 8**). An ileocolic intussusception is the most common type of intussusception seen in children and is most commonly identified on the right side of the abdomen. **Box 4** outlines the clinical features of intussusception.

Imaging protocols The pediatric bowel is best visualized with a high-frequency linear transducer. The patient should be placed in the supine position, and scanning may occur in 1 of 2 ways:

1. Picture frame format (Video 1): beginning with the transducer in the right lower quadrant (visualizing the psoas muscle) in transverse, the ascending bowel is scanned up toward the

---

Box 4
Clinical features of intussusception

- Children aged 3 months to 6 years
- Vomiting (bilious or nonbilious)
- Colicky abdominal pain
- Irritability or lethargy
- Right upper quadrant mass
- Bloody stool (may only be hemoccult-positive) is a late sign

---

right upper quadrant. The transducer is then rotated clockwise to the longitudinal plane and the transverse colon is scanned toward the left upper quadrant. Then, the transducer should be rotated counterclockwise back to the transverse plane and the descending colon should be scanned toward the rectum.

2. Lawnmower or zigzag format (Video 2): beginning with the transducer in the right lower quadrant (visualizing the psoas muscle) in transverse plane with respect to the patient, the ascending bowel is scanned up toward the right upper quadrant. The transducer is then moved medially and scanned caudally down to the pelvis just medial the segment that was just scanned. This technique is repeated in repeating sagittal sections of the abdomen until the entire abdomen has been scanned.

Diagnostic criteria Sonographically, intussusception will appear as alternating layers of hyperechoic compressed mucosa with hypoechoic muscle. In its transverse plane (cross-section), an

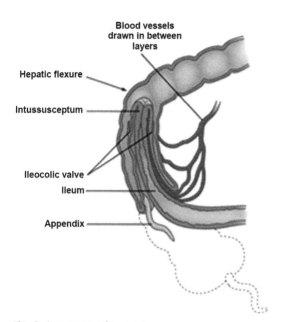

Fig. 8. Intussusception anatomy.

Blood vessels drawn in between layers

Hepatic flexure

Intussusceptum

Ileocolic valve

Ileum

Appendix

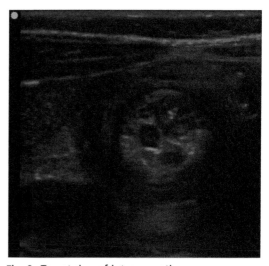

Fig. 9. Target sign of intussusception.

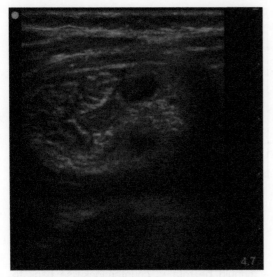

Fig. 10. Pseudokidney sign of intussusception.

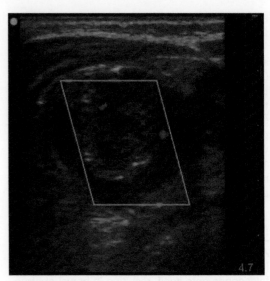

Fig. 12. Hyperemia seen with intussusception.

intussusception it is often described as a "donut" or "target" sign (**Fig. 9**) and in longitudinal plane, it may appear as a "pseudokidney" (**Fig. 10**). Intussusception can be distinguished from normal bowel based on its diameter, which should exceed 3 cm, and the lack of peristalsis. As a result of the obstruction, the proximal bowel may appear dilated and fluid-filled with thickened walls (**Fig. 11**). Color Doppler may show hyperemia initially (**Fig. 12**), but decreased or absent flow may be present, suggesting ischemia/infarction. **Box 5** summarizes several sonographic features, and **Box 6** presents the pearls and pitfalls associated with POCUS for intussusception.

The evidence

Although ultrasound has been used as a diagnostic tool for intussusception since the 1980s with a high sensitivity and specificity in the hands of resident radiologists,[13] until recently only single case reports have described the use of POCUS to diagnose intussusception in pediatric patients.[14–16]

In 2012, Riera and colleagues[17] published the first prospective observational study evaluating PEM physician–performed POCUS for the evaluation of intussusception. In this study, PEM physicians underwent a 1-hour training session conducted by a senior radiology attending that

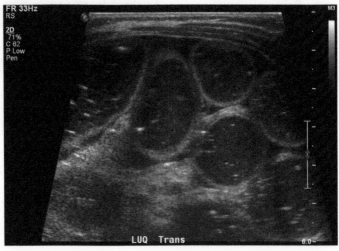

Fig. 11. Proximal dilated loop of bowel of intussusception.

consisted of a didactic component and a hands-on scanning technique component. A total of 82 patients were enrolled in the study, of whom 16% were diagnosed with ileocolic intussusception through ultrasound examination in the radiology department. Test characteristics of PEM physician–performed POCUS had a sensitivity of 85%, specificity of 97%, positive predictive value of 85%, and negative predictive value of 97%. These findings suggest that POCUS can be used as a "rule in" test, whereby negative findings may warrant further imaging or observation.

Skull Fractures

Anatomy

Key anatomic considerations when imaging for skull fractures include the skin, dura, and periosteum.

Imaging protocols The superficial skull bone is best visualized with a high-frequency linear transducer. The examination should begin over the area of trauma, as indicated by tenderness, scalp hematoma, or ecchymosis. Copious gel should be used as a stand-off to minimize pain and better visualize structures in the focal zone. Contralateral imaging is helpful to determine normal versus abnormal findings. The area should be imaged in 2 orthogonal planes. A list of clinical features found in skull fractures is provided in **Box 7**.

Diagnostic criteria Normal bone will appear as a bright, hyperechoic curvilinear structure with posterior acoustic shadowing (**Fig. 13**). If significant soft tissue swelling is present, this can also be appreciated sonographically, with the superficial tissues appearing thicker than adjacent normal scalp (**Fig. 14**). A fracture will appear as a hypoechoic disruption in the echogenic bone and may reveal cortical displacement, which is suggestive of a depressed skull fracture (**Fig. 15**). Hypoechoic collections around the periosteum suggest subperiosteal hematomas, and heterogeneous echodensities are suggestive of lipoma. The dura can occasionally be visualized posterior to the fracture. Normal dura will appear as a bright hyperechoic structure, and its absence confirms a dural tear.

Because cranial suture lines can appear similar to fractures sonographically, it is important to have an understanding of suture anatomy (**Fig. 16**). Imaging of the contralateral scalp can help differentiate skull fractures from sutures, particularly the bilateral

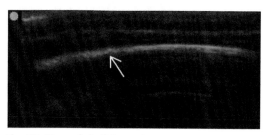

Fig. 13. Normal skull (*arrow*).

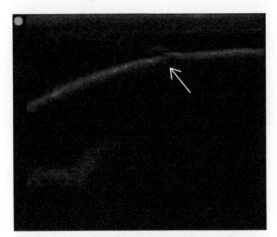

Fig. 14. Skull with soft tissue swelling (*arrow*).

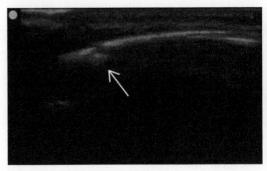

Fig. 15. Skull fracture (*arrow*).

coronal and lambdoid sutures. Key sonographic features of skull fractures are highlighted in **Box 8**, pearls and pitfalls associated with POCUS for skull fractures are provided in **Box 9**, and additional tips on performing POCUS for skull fractures are listed in **Box 10**. In addition, sutures can be traced back to the fontanelle and should not show cortical displacement, which is seen in depressed skull fractures.

The evidence
Ultrasound has shown superior sensitivity compared with radiographs in detecting long bone skeletal fractures, with an ability to detect certain types of fractures up to 1 mm.[18,19] A few small studies have demonstrated the utility of POCUS for the evaluation skull fractures.[20–23]

Rabiner and colleagues[24] conducted a prospective study to determine the accuracy of PEM physician–performed POCUS for this indication. Of the 69 patients evaluated, 12% had a computed tomography–confirmed diagnosis of skull fracture. As part of the study, the authors pooled their data with 3 other studies[20,22,23] and found that for the 185 total patients, POCUS had a sensitivity of 94%, specificity of 96%, positive likelihood ratio of 25.4, and negative likelihood ratio of 0.06. These findings suggest that a positive finding should be used to "rule in" the diagnosis, whereas negative ultrasound findings should prompt further evaluation.

Hip Effusions

Anatomy
The anatomic landmarks important to recognize when evaluating hip effusions include (**Fig. 17**) the femoral head, femoral neck, anterior synovial

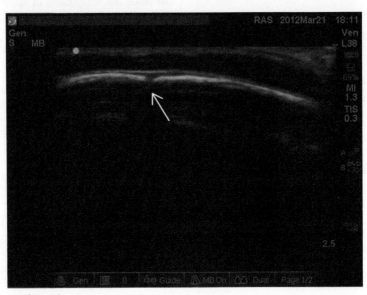

Fig. 16. Cranial suture (*arrow*).

Box 8
Sonographic features of skull fractures

- Disruption of the typically smooth, linear bony cortex
- Soft tissue swelling
- Subperiosteal hematomas
- Hematomas or lipomas
- Bony fragments

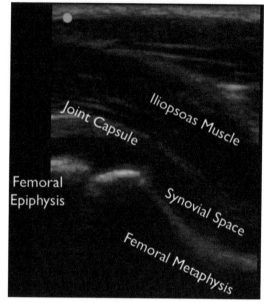

Fig. 17. Hip anatomic landmarks.

Box 9
Pearls and pitfalls of POCUS for skull fractures

Pearls

- Suture lines and skull fractures can be differentiated
  - Suture lines can be traced back to a fontanelle
- Contralateral skull can be scanned for comparison to further delineate a suture line

Pitfalls

- A suture line can be mistaken for a fracture (false-positive)
- A fracture can be mistaken for a suture line (false-negative)
- A skull fracture may not be considered because of a lack of signs or symptoms in a patient with blunt head trauma
- Skull ultrasound has no role in ruling out intracranial injuries

capsule, iliopsoas muscle, and appearance of normal physiologic fluid in the joint space.

The femoral head, neck, and shaft will appear as hyperechoic structures with posterior acoustic shadowing. The joint capsule is bordered anteriorly by the anterior synovial joint capsule (which lies just posterior to the iliopsoas muscle), and posteriorly by the anterior surface of the femoral neck. The normal joint space will have a concave shape, and fluid within the joint will appear hypoechoic. Clinical features of hip effusions are listed in **Box 11**.

Imaging protocols The superficial pediatric hip joint is best visualized with the high-frequency linear transducer. With the patient in the supine position, the hip should be placed in a slightly abducted position. The transducer should be placed in a longitudinal plane parallel to the femoral neck (**Fig. 18**). The anterior synovial space should be measured from the anterior concavity of the femoral neck to the posterior surface of the iliopsoas muscle (**Fig. 19**). The contralateral unaffected

Box 10
Tips on performing POCUS for skull fractures

- Copious amounts of gel should be used to minimize transducer pressure and increase visualization
- Disruption of bony cortex and secondary signs of injury should be sought
- The contralateral side should be scanned for comparison
- Suture lines and fractures should be differentiated

Box 11
Clinical features of hip effusions

- Hip pain, limp, or refusal to bear weight
- Possible knee pain (referred from the hip)
- Hip classically held in external rotation
- Fever, depending on the origin

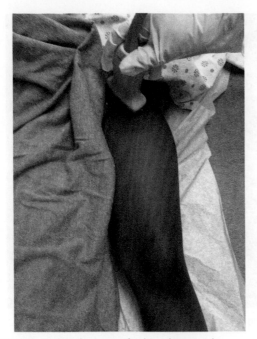

Fig. 18. Probe placement for hip ultrasound.

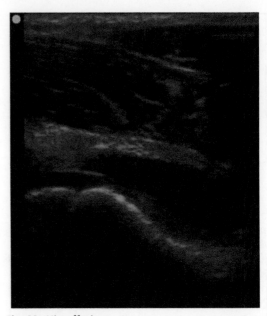

Fig. 20. Hip effusion.

side must be visualized for comparison. The split screen function is useful for real-time comparison. Contrary to most other examinations, the joint space is only imaged in one plane.

Diagnostic criteria The joint space should be measured from the anterior surface of the femoral neck to the posterior surface of the iliopsoas muscle. Fluid within the joint space will usually appear hypoechoic. However, when pus is present in the joint space, the effusion can have a relatively hyperchoic appearance compared with the typical anechoic effusion. A significant effusion is defined as either a joint space measurement exceeding 5 mm or more than a 2 mm difference between the affected and unaffected joints. With an increase in fluid within the joint space, the normally concave space becomes convex (**Fig. 20**) because of distention and bulging of the anterior

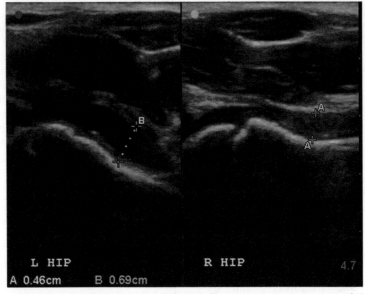

Fig. 19. Hip effusion measurements demonstrating left hip effusion. A, is measurement of the right joint space and B, is the measurement of the left joint space.

joint capsule. Ultrasound cannot reliably determine the type of effusion present (ie, infectious vs reactive), and if a septic arthritis is a concern, fluid should be aspirated for further evaluation. Sonographic features of hip effusions are listed in **Box 12**, pearls and pitfalls associated with POCUS for hip effusions are provided in **Box 13**, and key points regarding hip effusions are listed in **Box 14**.

The evidence

Several case reports demonstrate the ability of PEM physicians to use POCUS to detect hip effusions, diagnose transient synovitis and septic arthritis,[25–27] and guide arthrocentesis to obtain synovial fluid for analysis.[27,28]

Most recently, a prospective study evaluating 28 children who required hip ultrasound as part of their PED management showed that PEM physicians with focused training in hip POCUS were able to detect hip effusions with a sensitivity of 85% and specificity of 93%, suggesting that positive findings may be used to rule in the diagnosis of hip effusion, and negative findings may prompt further evaluation or observation.[29]

SUMMARY

POCUS has a range of applications in emergency medicine. As the armamentarium of applications expands, the development of pediatric-specific applications can help diagnose common pediatric clinical conditions.

SUPPLEMENTARY DATA

Videos related to this article can be found online at http://dx.doi.org/10.1016/j.cult.2014.01.012.

REFERENCES

1. Hockberger RS, Binder LS, Graber MA, et al. The model of the clinical practice of emergency medicine. Ann Emerg Med 2001;37(6):745–70.
2. Heller MB, Mandavia D, Tayal VS, et al. Residency training in emergency ultrasound: fulfilling the mandate. Acad Emerg Med 2002;9(8):835–9.
3. Akhtar S, Theodoro D, Gaspari R, et al. Resident training in emergency ultrasound: consensus recommendations from the 2008 Council of Emergency Medicine Residency Directors Conference. Acad Emerg Med 2009;16:S32–6.
4. Gausche-Hill M, Schmitz C, Lewis RJ. Pediatric preparedness of US emergency departments: a 2003 survey. Pediatrics 2007;120:1229–37.
5. Hunter AK, Liascouras CA. Hypertrophic pylori stenosis. In: Kliegman R, Nelson WE, editors. Nelson textbook of pediatrics. 19th edition. Philadelphia: Elsevier/Saunders; 2011. p. 1274.
6. Siegel MJ. Pediatric sonography. 4th edition. Philadelphia: Lippincott Williams & Wilkins; 2011. p. 342–5.
7. Forster N, Haddad RL, Choroomi S, et al. Use of ultrasound in 187 infants with suspected infantile hypertrophic pyloric stenosis. Australas Radiol 2007; 51:560–3.
8. Maheshwari P, Abograra A, Shamam O. Sonographic evaluation of gastrointestinal obstruction in

infants: a pictorial essay. J Pediatr Surg 2009;44: 2037–42.

9. Niedzielski J, Kobielski A, Sokal J, et al. Accuracy of sonographic criteria in the decision for surgical treatment in infantile hypertrophic pyloric stenosis. Arch Med Sci 2011;7(3):508–11.

10. Pathak TD, Pollock AN. Clinical impression: intussusception. An abdominal ultrasound is obtained: surprise. Pediatr Emerg Care 2010;26(8):611–2.

11. Malcolm GE, Raio CC, Del Rios M, et al. Feasibility of emergency physician diagnosis of hypertrophic pyloric stenosis using point-of-care ultrasound: a multicenter case series. J Emerg Med 2009;37(3):283–6.

12. Sivitz AB, Tejani C, Cohen SG. Evaluation of hypertrophic pyloric stenosis by pediatric emergency physician sonography. Acad Emerg Med 2013; 20(7):646–51.

13. Henderson AA, Anupindi SA, Servaes S, et al. Comparison of 2-view abdominal radiographs with ultrasound in children with suspected intussusception. Pediatr Emerg Care 2013;29:145–50.

14. Shad I, Gorenstein A, Serour F, et al. Intussusception in children: can we rely on screening sonography performed by junior residents? Pediatr Radiol 2004;34:134–7.

15. Karma N, Kaiafis C, Shih R. Diagnosis of pediatric intussusception by an emergency physician-performed bedside ultrasound: a case report. Pediatr Emerg Care 2009;25:177–80.

16. Helm BM, Boychuk RB, Franke AA. Diagnosis of intussusception using point-of-care ultrasound in the pediatric ED: a case report. Am J Emerg Med 2011;29:354.e1–3.

17. Riera A, Hsiao AL, Langhan ML, et al. Diagnosis of intussusception by physician novice sonographers in the emergency department. Ann Emerg Med 2012;60(3):264–8.

18. Cho KH, Lee SM, Lee YH, et al. Ultrasound diagnosis of either an occult or missed fracture of an extremity in pediatric-aged children. Korean J Radiol 2010;11(1):84–94.

19. Grechenig W, Clement HG, Fellinger M, et al. Scope and limitations of ultrasonography in the documentation of fractures—an experimental study. Arch Orthop Trauma Surg 1998;117(6–7):368–71.

20. Weinberg ER, Tunik MG, Tsung JW. Accuracy of clinician-performed point-of-care ultrasound for the diagnosis of fractures in children and young adults. Injury 2010;41(8):862–8.

21. Ramirez-Schrempp D, Vinci RJ, Liteplo AS. Bedside ultrasound in the diagnosis of skull fractures in the pediatric emergency department. Pediatr Emerg Care 2011;27:312–4.

22. Parri N, Crosby BJ, Glass C, et al. Ability of emergency ultrasonography to detect pediatric skull fractures in children: unnecessary harassment or useful addition to X-ray? Ultraschall Med 2008; 29(3):267–74.

23. Riera A, Chen L. Ultrasound evaluation of skull fractures in children: a feasibility study. Pediatr Emerg Care 2012;28(5):420–5.

24. Rabiner JE, Friedman LM, Khine H, et al. Accuracy of point-of-care ultrasound for diagnosis of skull fractures in children. Pediatrics 2013;131(6): e1757–64.

25. Miralles M, Gonzalez G, Pulpeiro JR, et al. Sonography of the painful hip in children: 500 consecutive cases. AJR Am J Roentgenol 1989;152:579–82.

26. Shavit I, Eidelman M, Galbraith R. Sonography of the hip joint by the emergency physician: its role in the evaluation of children presenting with acute limp. Pediatr Emerg Care 2006;22(8):570–3.

27. Minardi JJ, Lander OM. Septic hip arthritis: diagnosis and arthrocentesis using bedside ultrasound. J Emerg Med 2012;43(2):316–8.

28. Tsung JW, Blaivas M. Emergency department diagnosis of pediatric hip effusion and guided arthrocentesis using point-of-care ultrasound. J Emerg Med 2008;35(4):393–9.

29. Vieira RL, Levy JA. Bedside ultrasonography to identify hip effusions in pediatric patients. Ann Emerg Med 2010;55(3):284–9.

Airway and Thoracic Ultrasound

Jared T. Marx, MD[a],*, Michael Blaivas, MD[b],
Srikar Adhikari, MD, MS[c]

KEYWORDS

- Airway ultrasound • Thoracic ultrasound • Resucitation • Emergency department
- Critical care ultrasound

KEY POINTS

- Ultrasound continues to grow in use for rapid diagnosis and assessment within the emergency department.
- Ultrasound aids the physician in early diagnosis for resuscitation of the critical patient.
- With new emerging research, airway ultrasound shows promise as not only diagnostic but also therapeutic adjunct to a patient's care.
- Thoracic ultrasound allows for evaluation of insults to the breathing component of resuscitation and also can diagnostically direct therapy earlier than previously available in critical care areas.

 Videos of the sonographic airway extending from the oropharynx through thoracic cavity to the level of the diaphragm accompany this article at http://www.ultrasound.theclinics.com/

INTRODUCTION

A patent airway and respiration are central to the resuscitation of any critical patient within the emergency department and frequently when a critical patient presents, there is little medical information available to supplement care. Often these patients are unable to provide history to their illness or cooperate with a physical examination. Ultrasound has shown to be useful in immediate resuscitation of critical patients with such applications as the focused assessment with sonography in trauma or multiple other protocols developed for assessment of shock. Prior studies typically addressed circulation in the critical patient. However, recently ultrasound is showing promise as a rapid diagnostic bedside adjunct for evaluation of the airway and breathing (thoracic) in these critical patients.

AIRWAY ULTRASOUND ANATOMY

As emergency ultrasound continues to develop, one area of interest is as a novel tool for airway assessment. In the last several years, there have been many techniques developed for airway assessment from intraoral to external cutaneous examinations.[1–3] Each examination offers a different vantage point for evaluation of the structures of the airway but all with limitations because of orientation of osseous and cartilaginous structures and air interference within the airway itself.

SUBLINGUAL (INTRAORAL) SCANNING WINDOW

Tsui and colleagues[2,3] in a letter to the editor in the Canadian Journal of Anesthesia proposed an

The authors have nothing to disclose.
[a] Emergency Medicine, University of Kansas Hospital, 3901 Rainbow Boulevard, Kansas City, KS 66160, USA;
[b] Department of Emergency Medicine, St Francis Hospital, 2122 Manchester Expy, Columbus, GA 31904, USA; [c] Department of Emergency Medicine, University of Arizona Medical Center, 1501 North Campbell Avenue, Tucson, AZ 85724, USA
* Corresponding author.
E-mail address: jaredtmarx@gmail.com

Ultrasound Clin 9 (2014) 211–216
http://dx.doi.org/10.1016/j.cult.2014.01.011
1556-858X/14/$ – see front matter © 2014 Elsevier Inc. All rights reserved.

alternative route to external scanning by placing a curved high-frequency probe in the sublingual fossa. There is limited research to its use at this point but in the position the oropharynx can be evaluated by avoiding the gagging reflex of the soft palate. Further definition of sonographic anatomy and research is needed before this becomes a common scanning window when evaluating the airway.

EXTERNAL ULTRASOUND WINDOW

The hyoid bone separates the neck anatomy into two separate sonographic windows when performing external ultrasound. This landmark splits the airway into suprahyoid and infrahyoid scanning windows.[1,4] With the ultrasound transducer in a transverse orientation to the patient's body the hyoid bone can be identified in its long axis as a hyperechoic inverted U-shape with posterior acoustic shadowing (Video 1). In the sagittal or parasagittal orientation the hyoid bone can be visualized in cross-section as a superficial hyperechoic curved structure with posterior acoustic shadowing (Video 2).

Suprahyoid

Using either a linear high-frequency or curved low-frequency probe the floor of the mouth, tongue, and salivary glands can be visualized in transverse, sagittal, and parasagittal views (Video 3).[1,5]

Infrahyoid

Sonography of the infrahyoid region is ideal with use of a linear high-frequency probe because of the superficial structures of the neck. In this position the epiglottis can be partially visualized, as can the thyroid membrane, vocal cords, cricoid, trachea, and esophagus (**Figs. 1** and **2**, Videos 4–7).

CLINICAL USE

There has been little research performed in the emergency department for the clinical use of airway ultrasound. The more promising studies so far have been assessment of airway for difficult intubation,[6] evaluating the differentiation of trachea intubation versus esophageal intubation,[7–12] identification of anatomy for surgical airway,[1,5,13,14] and evaluation of the epiglottis.[15,16] Yet much of the clinical use in the emergency department is ill defined at this time. There is promise with further research.

Assessment of the Airway for Difficult Intubation

Difficult laryngoscopy occurs frequently in elective and emergent intubations. Evaluation of the airway is most commonly done using Mallampati test, which initially identified difficulty intubation with a high amount of accuracy. However, subsequent studies have showed mixed results of the Mallampati test to predict a difficulty airway in individuals undergoing elective intubation.[17] This can prove

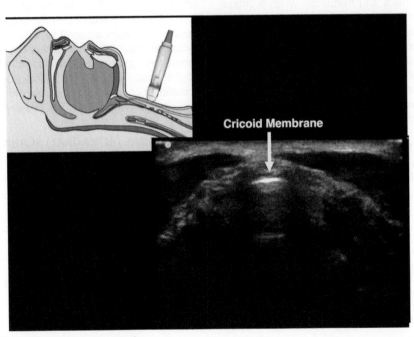

Cricoid Membrane

Fig. 1. Cricoid membrane transverse neck.

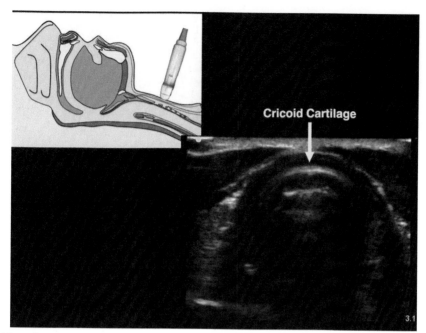

Fig. 2. Cricoid cartilage transverse neck.

particularly difficult in the emergency department because the Mallampati test requires an awake and cooperative patient.

Adhikari and colleagues[6] showed in individuals undergoing elective intubation for surgical procedures that an increased measurement of the soft tissue of the neck and tongue at the level of the hyoid was predictive of difficult intubation. Further clinical research in the emergency department is needed to determine its clinical use and validity in patients undergoing emergent intubation.

Endotracheal Tube Verification

Misidentification of an esophageal intubation as an endotracheal intubation can be disastrous and leads to increased morbidity and mortality. Capnography is becoming the gold standard for endotracheal tube placement verification but is not always available.

Different methods have been described in using ultrasound for identifying endotracheal tube location by filling the endotracheal balloon with saline versus air.[7–12] Recently, Chou and colleagues[9] and Adi and colleagues[7] have shown in the emergent setting that endotracheal intubation can be correctly identified with similar accuracy to wave capnography in the emergency setting. Adi and colleagues were able to show that an endotracheal tube location demonstrated the presence of two hyperechoic parallel lines within the trachea. In the presence of an esophageal intubation the hyperechoic parallel lines were absent in the trachea

but instead found in the esophagus when the probe was moved from the midline to left of midline showing a normally unidentifiable esophagus with the two parallel hyperechoic parallel lines. Chou and colleagues described the esophageal intubation as double tract sign with both the trachea and intubated esophagus showing comet tail artifact because of the air-mucosa interface (**Fig. 3**, Video 8).

Identification of Anatomy for Surgical Airway

When direct laryngoscopy cannot result in a definitive airway for the critical patient a surgical airway may be needed. Unfortunately, surface landmarks may not be as useful in identifying correct anatomy for cricothorotomy.[18] Ultrasonography is highly accurate in correctly identifying the cricothyroid membrane for successful cricothyroidotomy (see **Fig. 1**).[13,14]

Evaluation of the Epiglottis

Evaluation of the epiglottis is a novel ultrasound application that is noninvasive and holds considerable promise. Using ultrasound to identify epiglottitis needs further research to validate its application clinically. Limited research performed on evaluation of the epiglottis has shown success, and increased measurement of the epiglottis may be diagnostic for epiglottitis[15,16] but is limited because of the overlap between normal measured values of the epiglottis and measured values in patients with epiglottitis. Because of this overlap

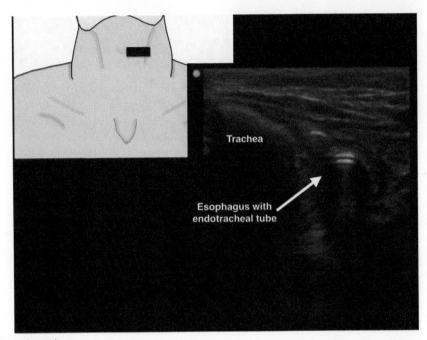

Fig. 3. Intubated esophagus.

further studies are needed to better qualify the measurements of normal compared with abnormal and also examine findings of other oropharynx infectious etiologies and their effect on measurements of the epiglottis.

Hung and colleagues[19] describe the presence of epiglottitis as an "alphabet P sign" for the hyperechoic appearance of the thickened epiglottis in relation to the acoustic shadowing with the hyoid bone.

Clinician-performed ultrasound shows initial signs of being an effective tool for evaluating epiglottitis but further research is needed to validate clinical use as a mainstay when compared with the gold standard of indirect laryngoscopy.

THORACIC ULTRASOUND

Thoracic ultrasound offers a noninvasive diagnostic study at the bedside for evaluation of breathing in critical patients. It has long been studied and used clinically for evaluation of pneumothorax, thoracic free fluid, pulmonary edema, and diagnosis of pneumonia. It has routinely been added to such protocols as the e-focused assessment with sonography in trauma evaluating for free thoracic fluid and also pneumothorax and BLUE protocol for evaluation of acute respiratory failure (**Figs. 4** and **5**, Videos 9 and 10).[20,21]

THORACIC ULTRASOUND ANATOMY

Many different viewing windows have been described for thoracic ultrasound and vary by

publication. However, sensitivity of thoracic ultrasound increases when larger areas of the thorax are evaluated. Most protocols include evaluation of the anterior, lateral, posterior, and bases of the thoraces bilaterally and ultrasound evaluation includes visualizing the pleural interface through the intercostal windows.[22]

PNEUMOTHORAX

Diagnosis of pneumothorax by radiograph has variable low sensitivity especially in the supine patient. Sonography of the least gravitationally dependent areas increases sensitivity of pneumothorax detection and has a high specificity for ruling out pneumothorax.[22–27]

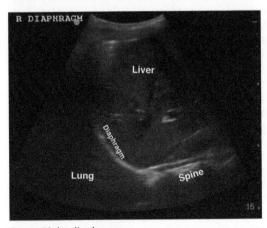

Fig. 4. Right diaphragm.

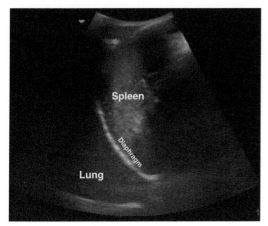

Fig. 5. Left diaphragm.

Evaluation includes assessment of the intercostal spaces anteriorly in the supine patient with movement inferior and laterally as more intercostal spaces are evaluated. In normal lung the parietal and visceral pleural are in contact with each other and ultrasound is able to demonstrate the presence of movement along this pleural interface, which has been described as lung sliding. The presence of lung sliding rules out the presence of pneumothorax at that intercostal space and sensitivity and specificity improve with increasing number of rib spaces evaluated. If air were to be present between the two pleural layers, as in the case of a pneumothorax, no sliding would be seen. Medical ultrasound does not penetrate air and the visceral pleura would not be visualized, thus eliminating lung sliding.

The presence of pneumothorax is associated with the presence of a lung point (area at which the pneumothorax begins) (Video 11), absence of lung sliding, absence of sonographic B-lines, and absence of lung pulse (movement of the lung caused by beating heart).

INTERSTITIAL SYNDROME

Interstitial syndrome can include extravascular fluid as in pulmonary edema, interstitial pneumonia, pneumonitis, or diffuse parenchymal lung disease. Its presence can be diagnosed by ultrasound by the presence of B-lines also known as comet tails (Video 12).[20,28–31]

B-lines are sonographic artifacts that begin at the pleural line and vertical hyperechoic reverberation artifacts that continue to the bottom of the ultrasound screen without loss of intensity and move with the lung sliding.

Three or more B-lines in an intercostal space represent a positive finding. Two or more positive intercostal spaces bilaterally represent diffuse interstitial disease, whereas focal B-lines may represent other entities, such as atelectasis, pulmonary contusion, or infarction.

LUNG CONSOLIDATION

Consolidated lung can be differentiated from other thoracic disease by loss of the normal sonographic appearance of aerated lung with lung that appears to be tissue-like in appearance by sonographic evaluation.[32,33] For a consolidation to be recognized by ultrasound the consolidation must come in contact with the outer thoracic wall.

PLEURAL FREE FLUID

Pleural free fluid can be visualized by sonography as an anechoic region and at times may have internal echoes. Thoracic free fluid may represent transudative, exudative, or even traumatic fluid. The examination is performed by evaluating the most gravity-dependent regions of the lung for anechoic regions consistent with fluid (Video 13).[20–22,34]

SUMMARY

Ultrasound continues to grow in use for rapid diagnosis and assessment within the emergency department. This diagnostic tool aids the physician in early diagnosis for resuscitation of the critical patient. With new emerging research airway ultrasound shows promise as not only a diagnostic but also a therapeutic adjunct to a patient's care. In addition, thoracic ultrasound allows for evaluation of insults to the breathing component of resuscitation and also can diagnostically direct therapy earlier than previously available in critical care areas.

SUPPLEMENTARY DATA

Supplementary data related to this article can be found online at http://dx.doi.org/10.1016/j.cult.2014.01.011.

REFERENCES

1. Singh M, Chin KJ, Chan VW, et al. Use of sonography for airway assessment: an observational study. J Ultrasound Med 2010;29(1):79–85.
2. Tsui BC, Hui CM. Sublingual airway ultrasound imaging. Can J Anaesth 2008;55(11):790–1.
3. Tsui BC, Hui CM. Challenges in sublingual airway ultrasound interpretation. Can J Anaesth 2009;56(5):393–4.
4. Prasad A, Singh M, Chan VW. Ultrasound imaging of the airway. Can J Anaesth 2009;56(11):868–9 [author reply: 869–70].

5. Kundra P, Mishra SK, Ramesh A. Ultrasound of the airway. Indian J Anaesth 2011;55(5):456–62.

6. Adhikari S, Zeger W, Schmier C, et al. Pilot study to determine the utility of point-of-care ultrasound in the assessment of difficult laryngoscopy. Acad Emerg Med 2011;18(7):754–8.

7. Adi O, Chuan TW, Rishya M. A feasibility study on bedside upper airway ultrasonography compared to waveform capnography for verifying endotracheal tube location after intubation. Crit Ultrasound J 2013;5(1):7.

8. Werner SL, Smith CE, Goldstein JR, et al. Pilot study to evaluate the accuracy of ultrasonography in confirming endotracheal tube placement. Ann Emerg Med 2007;49(1):75–80.

9. Chou HC, Tseng WP, Wang CH, et al. Tracheal rapid ultrasound exam (T.R.U.E.) for confirming endotracheal tube placement during emergency intubation. Resuscitation 2011;82(10):1279–84.

10. Uya A, Spear D, Patel K, et al. Can novice sonographers accurately locate an endotracheal tube with a saline-filled cuff in a cadaver model? A pilot study. Acad Emerg Med 2012;19(3):361–4.

11. Weaver B, Lyon M, Blaivas M. Confirmation of endotracheal tube placement after intubation using the ultrasound sliding lung sign. Acad Emerg Med 2006;13(3):239–44.

12. Drescher MJ, Conard FU, Schamban NE. Identification and description of esophageal intubation using ultrasound. Acad Emerg Med 2000;7(6):722–5.

13. Curtis K, Ahern M, Dawson M, et al. Ultrasound-guided, bougie-assisted cricothyroidotomy: a description of a novel technique in cadaveric models. Acad Emerg Med 2012;19(7):876–9.

14. Nicholls SE, Sweeney TW, Ferre RM, et al. Bedside sonography by emergency physicians for the rapid identification of landmarks relevant to cricothyrotomy. Am J Emerg Med 2008;26(8):852–6.

15. Ko DR, Chung YE, Park I, et al. Use of bedside sonography for diagnosing acute epiglottitis in the emergency department: a preliminary study. J Ultrasound Med 2012;31(1):19–22.

16. Werner SL, Jones RA, Emerman CL. Sonographic assessment of the epiglottis. Acad Emerg Med 2004;11(12):1358–60.

17. Lee A, Fan LT, Gin T, et al. A systematic review (meta-analysis) of the accuracy of the Mallampati tests to predict the difficult airway. Anesth Analg 2006;102(6):1867–78.

18. Elliott DS, Baker PA, Scott MR, et al. Accuracy of surface landmark identification for cannula cricothyroidotomy. Anaesthesia 2010;65(9):889–94.

19. Hung TY, Li S, Chen PS, et al. Bedside ultrasonography as a safe and effective tool to diagnose acute epiglottitis. Am J Emerg Med 2011;29(3):359.e1–3.

20. Lichtenstein DA, Meziere GA. Relevance of lung ultrasound in the diagnosis of acute respiratory failure: the BLUE protocol. Chest 2008;134(1):117–25.

21. Bouhemad B, Zhang M, Lu Q, et al. Clinical review: bedside lung ultrasound in critical care practice. Crit Care 2007;11(1):205.

22. Volpicelli G, Elbarbary M, Blaivas M, et al. International evidence-based recommendations for point-of-care lung ultrasound. Intensive Care Med 2012;38(4):577–91.

23. Ouellet JF, Ball CG, Panebianco NL, et al. The sonographic diagnosis of pneumothorax. J Emerg Trauma Shock 2011;4(4):504–7.

24. Nagarsheth K, Kurek S. Ultrasound detection of pneumothorax compared with chest X-ray and computed tomography scan. Am Surg 2011;77(4):480–4.

25. Rowan KR, Kirkpatrick AW, Liu D, et al. Traumatic pneumothorax detection with thoracic US: correlation with chest radiography and CT–initial experience. Radiology 2002;225(1):210–4.

26. Raja AS, Jacobus CH. How accurate is ultrasonography for excluding pneumothorax? Ann Emerg Med 2013;61(2):207–8.

27. Blaivas M, Lyon M, Duggal S. A prospective comparison of supine chest radiography and bedside ultrasound for the diagnosis of traumatic pneumothorax. Acad Emerg Med 2005;12(9):844–9.

28. Agricola E, Bove T, Oppizzi M, et al. "Ultrasound comet-tail images": a marker of pulmonary edema: a comparative study with wedge pressure and extravascular lung water. Chest 2005;127(5):1690–5.

29. Lichtenstein D, Meziere G. A lung ultrasound sign allowing bedside distinction between pulmonary edema and COPD: the comet-tail artifact. Intensive Care Med 1998;24(12):1331–4.

30. Liteplo AS, Marill KA, Villen T, et al. Emergency thoracic ultrasound in the differentiation of the etiology of shortness of breath (ETUDES): sonographic B-lines and N-terminal pro-brain-type natriuretic peptide in diagnosing congestive heart failure. Acad Emerg Med 2009;16(3):201–10.

31. Picano E, Frassi F, Agricola E, et al. Ultrasound lung comets: a clinically useful sign of extravascular lung water. J Am Soc Echocardiogr 2006;19(3):356–63.

32. Parlamento S, Copetti R, Di Bartolomeo S. Evaluation of lung ultrasound for the diagnosis of pneumonia in the ED. Am J Emerg Med 2009;27(4):379–84.

33. Blaivas M. Lung ultrasound in evaluation of pneumonia. J Ultrasound Med 2012;31(6):823–6.

34. Reissig A, Copetti R, Kroegel C. Current role of emergency ultrasound of the chest. Crit Care Med 2011;39(4):839–45.

Procedural Guidance with Ultrasound in the Emergency Patient

Richard Amini, MD

KEYWORDS

• Paracentesis • Lumbar puncture • Thoracentesis • Pericardiocentesis • Transvenous pacemaker

KEY POINTS

- The anatomic landmark approach for procedures is being replaced with ultrasound-aided techniques.
- Ultrasound-assisted or ultrasound-guided paracentesis has been shown to decrease adverse events (1.4% vs 5%) and increase success rates (95% vs 61%) when compared with the anatomic landmark approach.
- The complication rate of landmark-based thoracentesis ranges from 20% to 50%. The use of ultrasound-assisted protocols demonstrated a decrease in complications such as pneumothorax from 9% to 1%.
- Ultrasound-assisted lumbar puncture in obese patients decreases difficulty and can reach a success rate of 100%.
- Ultrasound-assisted pericardiocentesis has a success rate of 97%.

 Videos pertinent to paracentesis, thoracentesis, pericardiocentesis, and transvenous pacing accompany this article at http://www.ultrasound.theclinics.com/

DISCUSSION OF PROBLEM/CLINICAL PRESENTATION

Successful performance of emergent procedures relies on the experience, competence, and skills of the operator.[1] An ultrasound-aided approach to emergency procedures has been demonstrated to increase patient safety and operator confidence and is frequently replacing the anatomic landmark approach as the new standard. From the most mundane and simple procedure, such as intravenous catheter placement, to the most complex and technically challenging procedure, such as transvenous pacing, ultrasound provides a means for success. The use of ultrasound reduces the number of attempts, the complication rates, and the amount of anesthetic used.

Ultrasound enhancement of emergent procedures involves 2 techniques: ultrasound guidance and ultrasound assistance. Ultrasound-guided techniques use real-time ultrasound imaging to direct needle placement, whereas the ultrasound-assisted technique uses ultrasound to evaluate patient anatomy, identifying the most accurate location or effective approach for the procedure. In this article, the authors aim to discuss how ultrasound enhances intravenous catheter placement, paracentesis, thoracentesis, lumbar puncture (LP), peritonsillar abscess drainage, pericardiocentesis, and transvenous

The authors have nothing to disclose.
Department of Emergency Medicine, University of Arizona, 1609 North Warren, FOB 122C, Tucson, AZ 85719, USA
E-mail address: ramini@aemrc.arizona.edu

Ultrasound Clin 9 (2014) 217–226
http://dx.doi.org/10.1016/j.cult.2014.01.001
1556-858X/14/$ – see front matter © 2014 Elsevier Inc. All rights reserved.

pacing in the emergency and critical care settings.

GENERAL APPROACH

Ultrasound guidance is often used for aspiration of fluid or catheter placement. To accomplish this successfully, a skilled clinician uses ultrasound to evaluate patient anatomy, determine the safest location for needle insertion, and direct needle placement. There is a certain level of dexterity that is required for ultrasound-guided procedures that can be achieved through practice. Real-time ultrasound guidance with visualization of the needle path is the best and safest approach. In certain situations, a skin marker can be used to define the ideal location for needle insertion. As with any procedure, the use of sterile probe covers, sterile gel, and sterile gloves is recommended to minimize the risk of infection. When appropriate, the superficial region is infiltrated with a wheal of local anesthetic before accessing deeper structures. Attention should be given to avoiding neurovascular structures while inserting needle under ultrasound guidance.

TRANSDUCERS

The choice of ultrasound probe depends on the type of procedure. High-frequency linear probes are ideal to assess for musculoskeletal and superficial soft tissue structures. The benefits of high-frequency transducers are improved axial resolution; however, the primary limitation to high-frequency transducers is that it can only image superficial structures. Curvilinear transducers are lower frequency probes that are better suited for deeper structures. These transducers are ideal for obese patients and procedures with depths greater than 6 cm. Last, endocavitary transducers are higher frequency probes with excellent axial resolution and overall imaging quality. Unique to this probe is the ability to image nearly 180°.

PARACENTESIS
Background

Paracentesis is a common emergency procedure, which for decades has been performed with the direction of physical examination findings. Paracentesis is a relatively safe procedure that carries a 1% to 5% complication rate.[2–4] The incorporation of point-of-care ultrasound for paracentesis not only allows for a more rapid diagnosis of peritoneal fluid but also provides a more accurate assessment for ideal procedure site. Ultrasound assessment can identify as little as 250 mL of free intraperitoneal fluid and has been show to increase success rates when compared with landmark techniques (95% vs 65%).[5,6]

A common concern among clinicians regarding paracentesis is the time required to aspirate what can be a staggering quantity of fluid. Another potential barrier is physician comfort and experience with this procedure. Despite these concerns, studies have shown that clinician-performed ultrasound-guided or ultrasound-assisted paracentesis is equally successful to the interventional radiologist. Furthermore, studies have shown a smaller number of adverse events when ultrasound was used (1.4% vs 4.7%).[4] In addition, sonographic evaluation can identify patients who do not have peritoneal fluid or whose quantity is so small that performing a procedure would be dangerous.[5] Clinicians are encouraged to become facile at this procedure to improve patient safety.[7]

Indications

Paracentesis is generally performed to evaluate patients for peritoneal infections such as spontaneous bacterial peritonitis. In addition, a large amount of ascites may lead to respiratory compromise secondary to a mass effect on the diaphragm, where drainage may prove more prudent than mechanical ventilation. In situations where the type of peritoneal fluid is in question, paracentesis can help to distinguish ascites from blood. In less emergent situations, paracentesis can help diagnose malignancy by performing cytology on aspirated fluid.

Imaging and Technique

A curvilinear transducer is ideal for abdominal imaging. Intraperitoneal fluid serves as an excellent conductor of ultrasound waves. As with a focused assessment with sonography in trauma examination, the right upper quadrant should be assessed for hepatomegaly and right kidney location. This examination is performed in the coronal plane with the transducer indicator directed toward the patient's head. If the rib shadow creates difficulty, the transducer should be angled so as to follow the external oblique muscles (slightly rotate the indicator counterclockwise). Enlarged organs can create a mass effect and lead to inadvertent organ biopsy when performing this procedure blind. In addition, renal cysts can mimic free fluid when enlarged and if accidentally punctured may lead to hemorrhagic complications. In the left upper quadrant, splenomegaly and left kidney abnormalities can create similar complications if not evaluated with ultrasound. Imaging is performed in the coronal plane using the same approach discussed above. In the pelvis, it is important to evaluate for an enlarged bladder. This imaging can be performed in the transverse or longitudinal plane and must be addressed before continuing with the procedure. Ultrasound of the peritoneal fluid may indicate the type of fluid present; fluid from abscesses or hemoperitoneum may contain echoes from blood cells, fecal material, purulent fluid, or fibrinous tissue (which may also create complex septations).

The sonographic evaluation of the abdomen will reveal the largest pocket of fluid (which is usually in the lower quadrants) and its identification is paramount to a successful procedure. To maximize success, the patient may be placed in the left lateral decubitus position. The position of bowel, mesentery, and bladder should be noted. The distance from the skin surface to the fluid pocket should be noticed (**Fig. 1**). Once the largest pocket of free fluid is identified and skin is marked with a surgical marker, the patient's positioning must not be altered. Before the insertion of the needle, an evaluation of the superficial structures with a high-frequency transducer should be performed to assess superficial vessels such as the epigastric artery (Video 1). Although superficial and relatively small, when punctured, these vessels may bleed into the peritoneum and create complications.

Using sterile precautions, the patient should be prepared and draped for the procedure. For the ultrasound-guided approach, the transducer should be covered with a sterile sheath. At the desired location, a superficial wheal should be created with anesthetic solution (lidocaine with epinephrine) using a small-gauge needle. With a scalpel, a small incision should be made in the skin, large enough for the peritoneal catheter to advance. When performing the ultrasound-guided technique, the needle entry should be guided in real-time. The needle will appear echogenic with a ring-down artifact in the ascitic fluid, which appears as numerous "copies" of the needle echoing down into the fluid. Depending on the thickness of the catheter, it may be imaged to confirm the location or to evaluate when troubleshooting. To prevent the complication of a fistula, the skin and soft tissue should be moved laterally before the needle is inserted, thereby creating a tunneled path between the skin and peritoneum. This technique will help tamponade the wound after the procedure. Not uncommon, the negative pressure created by the vacuum containers may cause mesenteric fat or bowel to become stuck to the catheter. If necessary, a saline flush may be used to disengage the catheter to resume aspiration.

Pearls and Pitfalls

- Ultrasound can identify as little as 250 mL of intraperitoneal fluid.[6]
- Ultrasound-assisted paracentesis has a 95% success rate.[5]
- Sonographic evaluation of the peritoneum before paracentesis can reduce failed attempts in patients with minimal or no intraperitoneal fluid.[5]
- Placing the patient in the reverse Trendelenburg or in the lateral decubitus position can maximize the pocket of fluid.
- Ovarian cysts, renal cysts, distended bowel, or a distended bladder may be misinterpreted for free fluid.

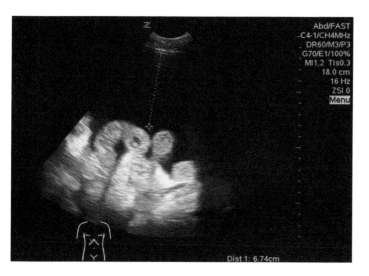

Fig. 1. B-mode image showing free fluid in abdomen and bowel. The distance from the skin surface to the fluid pocket is measured.

- Failure to identify epigastric vessels can lead to puncture and significant bleeding.
- Before performing the bedside paracentesis, appropriate laboratory tests such as platelet count and coagulation factors should be reviewed.

LP
Background

Perhaps one of the most routine procedures encountered by the emergency physician, the LP, is used to evaluate patient cerebral spinal fluid for certain disease processes, such as sepsis, meningitis, or subarachnoid bleed. This procedure requires precision, because an accurate angle of needle entry can result in saved time, decreased patient/practitioner stress, and decreased post-LP complications.[8] In an era where nearly 70% of the U.S. population is overweight or obese, the use of ultrasound to determine anatomic landmarks can be extremely useful to an emergency physician.[9] Numerous studies have demonstrated that the use of ultrasound can decrease the number of attempts as well as the number of complications.[10–14] Furthermore, a randomized controlled trial performed in 2007 demonstrated an overall success rate of 96% and a 100% success rate in obese patients. This study also demonstrated an overall decrease in difficulty appreciated by the operator.[10]

Indications

In this procedure, ultrasound is generally used for assistance, not guidance. The technique for LP is a static approach whereby anatomic landmarks are evaluated and delineated. The use of ultrasound for this procedure is not routine; it is generally used for patients with difficult or sensitive anatomy. When used, the primary purpose is to establish the midline, locate the appropriate interspinous space, and demonstrate the depth necessary to reach the subarachnoid space. A recent study performed in 2010 demonstrates ultrasound assistance in LPs to be superior in any body mass index range.[15]

Imaging and Technique

As mentioned above, ultrasound assistance for LP is ideal for obese patients, infants, and patients who have had failed LPs. If unsure, a good rule of thumb comes from a recent study that demonstrated that patients who lack a visible spine on physical examination may prove to be difficult LPs or traumatic LPs.[16] Ultrasound imaging can help locate the spinous process and evaluate for

the ideal interspinous space for needle insertion. Imaging is performed with the patient in either upright or lateral decubitus position. Once imaged and marked, the patient should not be moved because this can distort the patient anatomy. The curvilinear probe is ideal for obese patients, because it uses lower frequencies, which improves tissue penetration. The linear array probe is generally used for thin and pediatric patients.

The first step in the ultrasound-assisted technique is to establish the midline. To do this, the probe is placed on the patient in the transverse plane at the lumbar region (**Fig. 2**). In this plane, the paraspinal muscles appear as circular bundles on either side of the spinous process (**Fig. 3**). The spinous process will appear as a hyperechoic crescent with posterior shadow. A common mistake seen with novice practitioners is an attempt at an LP below the L4/L5 interspace; this can be avoided with ultrasound assistance, because the sacral bones are more prominent and do not have a crescent shape. Once the spinous process is centered, a skin marker is used to mark above and below the transducer, thereby establishing the midline.

Next, the sagittal plane is scanned by rotating the probe 90°, searching for the interspinous spaces (**Fig. 4**). In the long axis, one can visualize

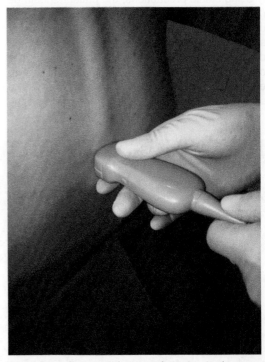

Fig. 2. B-mode image showing the spine in the transverse plane (using a low-frequency curvilinear transducer).

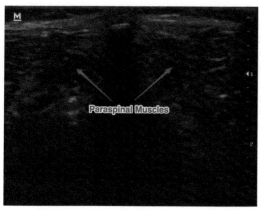

Fig. 3. Transverse plane imaging demonstrates bilateral paraspinal muscles with a central hyperechoic line and subsequent shadowing of the spinous process.

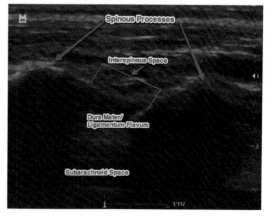

Fig. 5. Sagittal plane imaging demonstrates the spinous processes as well as the interspinous space. In children and thin adults, the subarachnoid space may be visualized.

multiple spinous processes and their interspaces simultaneously (**Fig. 5**). The interspinous space is centered in the middle of the screen and the interspinous space is marked.[17] The point at which the sagittal and transverse plane markings intersect is the best location for needle insertion. It is recommended to mark at least 2 interspinous spaces so as to maximize success.

A seasoned practitioner knows that the angle of approach is critical to successful completion of an

LP and ultrasound can aid in demonstrating the best angle. One way to do this is to mirror the angle of the spinous process. Remember also to measure the depth required to enter the subarachnoid space. Doing so can help determine the length of the spinal needle to be chosen as well as relieve operator stress when using longer spinal needles in obese patients. Real-time ultrasound guidance is rarely used in emergency department settings for this procedure.

Pearls and Pitfalls

- To maximize success, the patient is placed in a position of comfort before the bedside ultrasound to prevent repositioning until the procedure is complete.
- Ultrasound transducer selection is critical and is largely directed by body habitus.
- One must measure the depth required to enter the subarachnoid space. An inappropriately chosen needle length may lead to a failed procedure.

THORACENTESIS
Background

Thoracentesis has evolved since its first mention as a surgical procedure in the medical literature in the early 1800s. Despite becoming less invasive, thoracentesis carries complication rates as high as 20% to 50% when performed using the anatomic landmark technique.[18–20] With the incorporation of ultrasound assistance, one study found that the pneumothorax incidence decreased to 0%.[21] In an era where the number of moderately overweight and obese patients is on the rise, ultrasound-assisted thoracentesis has proven its usefulness.[22] It can demonstrate the best location

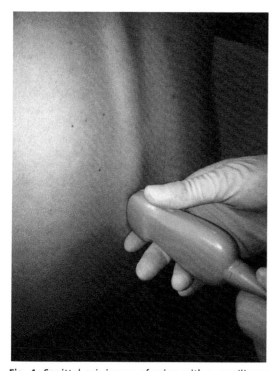

Fig. 4. Sagittal axis image of spine with a curvilinear transducer.

for needle insertion and it can locate thoracic organs and other landmarks to help avoid complications.

Indications

Ultrasound-assisted thoracentesis is ideal for patients who are slightly overweight, for patients whose anatomic landmarks are difficult to assess, and in patients with only a small or unknown sized pleural effusion.

Imaging and Technique

A phased array low-frequency probe is ideal for the ultrasound-guided thoracentesis. First the patient should be positioned upright and seated to allow fluid to collect at the costophrenic sulci. The phased array probe should be used to identify the liver, spleen, lung, and diaphragm to avoid accidental injury during the procedure. Once the size and location of the pleural effusion is evaluated, the diaphragmatic excursion should be watched and the superior and inferior portions of the fluid collection should be assessed (**Fig. 6**). The pleural effusion will appear as anechoic fluid above the echogenic diaphragm (**Fig. 7**). The lung is seen as a mobile hyperechoic structure within the pleural fluid with its position varying with respiratory cycle (Video 2).

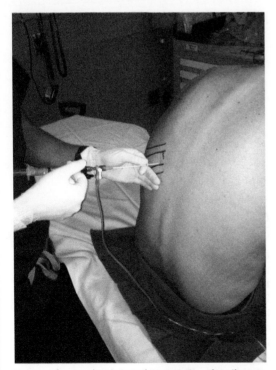

Fig. 6. After evaluating and annotating the ribs posteriorly, the needle should be directed superior to a rib so as to avoid the neurovascular bundle.

Once imaging is complete, 2 sequential ribs should be outlined by marking the thoracic wall. The chosen interspace corresponds to an area that, on ultrasound, consistently demonstrates a fluid collection. The patient should not move after this point. Next, the distance between surface of the skin and visceral pleura should be measured to minimize the risk to parietal pleura. Using sterile precautions, the patient should be prepared and draped for the procedure.

At the site marked for puncture, a small-gauge needle is used to create a superficial wheal of anesthetic solution such as lidocaine with epinephrine. With a scalpel, a small incision is made in the skin large enough for the thoracentesis catheter to advance. For the ultrasound-guided approach, the transducer should be covered with a sterile sheath and the needle should be directed into the space of interest.

Pearls and Pitfalls

- Morbid obesity and subcutaneous emphysema can limit ultrasonography.
- The thoracic anatomy should be surveyed for vital organs before performing a thoracentesis.
- The interspace chosen for thoracentesis should be evaluated during the entire respiratory cycle.
- It should be remembered to guide the needle above a rib because the neurovascular bundle runs below ribs.

PERICARDIOCENTESIS
Background

The average patient has approximately 10 to 50 cc of pericardial fluid.[23] This fluid is an ultrafiltrate of plasma and is a lubricant between the tough outer parietal pericardium and the inner layer, visceral pericardium. The tough pericardium can dilate over time; however, it is acutely inelastic. If an effusion develops quickly, it can create tamponade physiology. Bedside sonography is the modality of choice for the diagnosis of pericardial effusions and can help evaluate for signs of impending tamponade physiology. If present, emergency pericardiocentesis should be performed.

Pericardiocentesis was first performed in 1890 and was described using an anatomic landmark approach.[24] This technique involves inserting a needle at the subxyphoid location, aiming for the patient's left nipple. This procedure requires penetration of skin, soft tissue, liver, and pericardial space. The landmark technique carries inherent risks, such as liver injury, pneumothorax and ventricle injury, and coronary laceration. On the

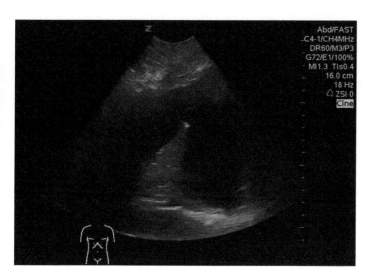

Fig. 7. B-mode image of a pleural effusion and decompressed lung. When a patient takes a deep breath, the compressed lung may resemble the tail of a fish in water, sometimes referred to as the "goldfish sign."

other hand, the ultrasound-guided technique provides the operator with immediate feedback regarding the location of the needle, wire, and catheter. In addition, it can help minimize complications as well as demonstrate resolution of tamponade physiology.

Indications

Pericardiocentesis is an emergency procedure and should be performed when a patient has sonographic evidence of a pericardial effusion with signs of tamponade physiology. Ultrasound-assisted pericardiocentesis has proven to be an effective procedure with a success rate of 97%.[25]

Imaging and Technique

To maximize success, a bedside echocardiogram should be performed with a low-frequency phased array transducer. Imaging the subxyphoid, apical, and parasternal locations will demonstrate the optimal acoustic window and identify the largest fluid pocket and therefore safest location for the insertion of the needle. The distance to effusion should be measured to determine the angle of approach required for successful instrumentation. Each approach carries its own risks and benefits: the parasternal approach creates a potential risk of lacerating the mammary artery or the left anterior descending coronary artery; the subxyphoid approach may require penetration of the liver before pericardium. As a result, some experts prefer the para-apical approach when used in combination with bedside ultrasound.

Subxyphoid approach
The transducer should be placed just below the xyphoid process directing the indicator and

footprint of the transducer toward the patient's left shoulder (**Fig. 8**). The needle should be inserted lateral to the probe on the patient's right side. It will enter in a 30-degree axis, through the liver and into the pericardium (Video 3). The needle should be directed toward the patient's left nipple or shoulder.

Parasternal approach
The transducer should be placed to the left of the sternum with the indicator and footprint aimed toward the patient's right shoulder and the 3rd or 4th intercostal space should be scanned obliquely. The probe should be directed so as to obtain a long-axis view of the heart. The needle should be inserted lateral to the probe and directed toward the patient's spine.

Para-apical approach
The transducer should be placed over the apical impulse of the patient's chest. In men, this is just lateral and inferior to the left nipple. In women,

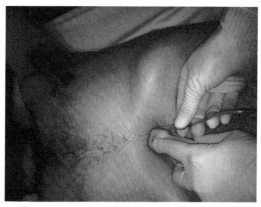

Fig. 8. Subxyphoid approach to pericardiocentesis.

this is generally under the left breast. The indicator is aimed at the patient's left hip and the footprint is aimed toward the base of the heart (**Fig. 9**). Once a 4-chamber view is obtained and the pericardial effusion is visualized, the needle is inserted lateral to the probe (Video 4). This technique is best performed where the pericardial effusion can be best imaged. Once this view is obtained, the needle is directed in the same angle as the probe is used to visualize the space.

Pearls and Pitfalls

- The speed at which pericardial fluid accumulates is vastly more important than the quantity of fluid present.
- Ultrasound-assisted pericardiocentesis has proven to be an effective procedure with a success rate of 97%.[25]
- Hemodynamically stable patients with large effusions may require a pericardial window and should be taken to the operating room for either the pericardiocentesis or the pericardial window.
- Although there are 3 favored locations to perform the pericardiocentesis, they are not absolute. The patient should be thoroughly evaluated with ultrasound to establish the best location for needle insertion.
- Placing the patient in left lateral decubitus position can bring forward a posterior effusion.

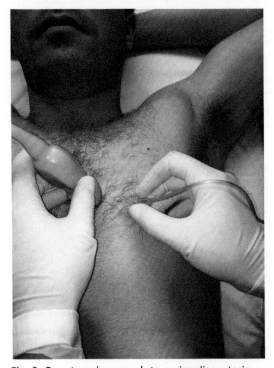

Fig. 9. Parasternal approach to pericardiocentesis.

TRANSVENOUS CARDIAC PACING
Background

Emergent cardiac pacing is a procedure that emergency physicians encounter on rare occasions but must be completed with rapid execution. The traditional approach involves blindly passing the pacing wire through a central line until capture is seen on electrocardiogram. Although this procedure has been documented to have success rate rates as low as 10%, recent studies demonstrate much higher success rates when performed with ultrasound guidance.[26]

Indications

There are various indications for emergency cardiac pacing; however, the most common indication is the patient who is bradycardic and unstable.

Imaging and Technique

Similar to the imaging required to perform a pericardiocentesis, the patient should be evaluated using ultrasound to establish the best sonographic window to view the right side of the heart. Different cardiac windows can be used for pacemaker wire visualization, including the subcostal, apical, and parasternal approaches. Generally speaking, the subxyphoid approach is the most useful and is most easily obtained on a supine patient.[27] The subxyphoid approach is obtained by placing the probe below the xyphoid process with the indicator aimed toward the patient's left shoulder. The transducer footprint should be aimed at the left posterior shoulder and adjusted to obtain a long-axis view of the heart. In this position, the right ventricle should appear on the left side of the screen and is where the operator's attention should be placed.

The pacemaker wire is easily seen on ultrasound because it creates a hyperechoic linear echo (Video 5). As the operator advances the wire through the sheath (subclavian or internal jugular), the wire can be seen in real-time as it enters through the superior vena cava into the right atrium and then through the tricuspid valves into the right ventricle. As compared with the traditional approach where the practitioner looks at an electrocardiogram monitor for secondary signs of correct pacer placement, the ultrasound-guided technique provides immediate feedback.

When patients require emergency transvenous pacing secondary to an unstable situation, rapid placement and immediate adjustments are necessary. The ultrasound-guided approach can demonstrate incorrect pacer wire trajectories (passage into inferior vena cava, coiling into right atrium, passage into pulmonary vasculature) more quickly than a blind approach.[27] Although limited by obesity or poor sonographic windows, the ultrasound-guided approach may soon become the new standard for emergency transvenous pacer placement.

Pearls and Pitfalls

- Success rates for transvenous pacer capture ranges from 10% to 90%.[26,27]
- The ultrasound-guided approach provides immediate feedback and can help troubleshoot inadequate pacer wire trajectories.
- In obese patients or patients with chronic obstructive pulmonary disease, visualization of pacemaker wire can be difficult. The linear echoes produced by pacemaker wire look similar to normal anatomic structures such as valves. Scanning in different angles and using additional cardiac windows can be helpful to locate the pacemaker wire.

SUMMARY

Bedside ultrasound is a useful tool to provide needle guidance for many emergent procedures. It increases operator confidence and helps to determine the ideal location for needle insertion. The use of ultrasound has been shown to increase success rates, decrease complication rates, and reduce health care costs. With practice, physicians can obtain the skills and competence required to incorporate ultrasound into their daily practice while performing procedures.

SUPPLEMENTARY DATA

Videos related to this article can be found online at http://dx.doi.org/6.1016/j.cult.2014.01.001.

REFERENCES

1. Costantino TG, Satz WA, Dehnkamp W, et al. Randomized trial comparing intraoral ultrasound to landmark-based needle aspiration in patients with suspected peritonsillar abscess. Acad Emerg Med 2012;19(6):626–31. http://dx.doi.org/10.1111/j.1553-2712.2012.01380.x.
2. Runyon BA. Paracentesis of ascitic fluid. A safe procedure. Arch Intern Med 1986;146(11):2259–61.
3. Banimahd F, Spinello IM. Large-volume paracentesis: a fast, convenient, and safe technique. J Emerg Med 2009;37(4):409–10. http://dx.doi.org/10.1016/j.jemermed.2008.09.022.
4. Branney SW, Wolfe RE, Moore EE, et al. Quantitative sensitivity of ultrasound in detecting free intraperitoneal fluid. J Trauma 1995;39(2):375–80.
5. Nazeer SR, Dewbre H, Miller AH. Ultrasound-assisted paracentesis performed by emergency physicians vs the traditional technique: a prospective, randomized study. Am J Emerg Med 2005;23(3):363–7.
6. Rose JS. Ultrasound in abdominal trauma. Emerg Med Clin North Am 2004;22(3):581–99. http://dx.doi.org/10.1016/j.emc.2004.04.007, vii.
7. Barsuk JH, Cohen ER, Feinglass J, et al. Clinical outcomes after bedside and interventional radiology paracentesis procedures. Am J Med 2013;126(4):349–56. http://dx.doi.org/10.1016/j.amjmed.2012.09.016.
8. Bruccoleri RE, Chen L. Needle-entry angle for lumbar puncture in children as determined by using ultrasonography. Pediatrics 2011;127(4):e921–6. http://dx.doi.org/10.1542/peds.2010-2511.
9. Flegal KM, Carroll MD, Kit BK, et al. Prevalence of obesity and trends in the distribution of body mass index among US adults, 1999-2010. JAMA 2012;307(5):491–7. http://dx.doi.org/10.1001/jama.2012.39.
10. Nomura JT, Leech SJ, Shenbagamurthi S, et al. A randomized controlled trial of ultrasound-assisted lumbar puncture. J Ultrasound Med 2007;26(10):1341–8.
11. Ferre RM, Sweeney TW, Strout TD. Ultrasound identification of landmarks preceding lumbar puncture: a pilot study. Emerg Med J 2009;26(4):276–7. http://dx.doi.org/10.1136/emj.2007.057455.
12. Peterson MA, Abele J. Bedside ultrasound for difficult lumbar puncture. J Emerg Med 2005;28(2):197–200. http://dx.doi.org/10.1016/j.jemermed.2004.09.008.
13. Ferre RM, Sweeney TW. Emergency physicians can easily obtain ultrasound images of anatomical landmarks relevant to lumbar puncture. Am J Emerg Med 2007;25(3):291–6. http://dx.doi.org/10.1016/j.ajem.2006.08.013.
14. Stiffler KA, Jwayyed S, Wilber ST, et al. The use of ultrasound to identify pertinent landmarks for lumbar puncture. Am J Emerg Med 2007;25(3):331–4. http://dx.doi.org/10.1016/j.ajem.2006.07.010.
15. Mofidi M, Mohammadi M, Saidi H, et al. Ultrasound guided lumbar puncture in emergency department: time saving and less complications. J Res Med Sci 2013;18(4):303–7.
16. Shah KH, McGillicuddy D, Spear J, et al. Predicting difficult and traumatic lumbar punctures. Am J Emerg Med 2007;25(6):608–11. http://dx.doi.org/10.1016/j.ajem.2006.11.025.
17. John Ma O, Mateer JR, Blaivas M. Emergency ultrasound. New York: McGraw-Hill; 2008.
18. Duncan DR, Morgenthaler TI, Ryu JH, et al. Reducing iatrogenic risk in thoracentesis: establishing best practice via experiential training in a zero-risk environment. Chest 2009;135(5):1315–20. http://dx.doi.org/10.1378/chest.08-1227.

19. Jones PW, Moyers JP, Rogers JT, et al. Ultrasound-guided thoracentesis: is it a safer method? Chest 2003;123(2):418–23.

20. Hibbert RM, Atwell TD, Lekah A, et al. Safety of ultrasound-guided thoracentesis in patients with abnormal preprocedural coagulation parameters. Chest 2013;144(2):456–63. http://dx.doi.org/10.1378/chest.12-2374.

21. Grogan DR, Irwin RS, Channick R, et al. Complications associated with thoracentesis. A prospective, randomized study comparing three different methods. Arch Intern Med 1990;150(4):873–7.

22. Mercaldi CJ, Lanes SF. Ultrasound guidance decreases complications and improves the cost of care among patients undergoing thoracentesis and paracentesis. Chest 2013;143(2):532–8.

23. Jung HO. Pericardial effusion and pericardiocentesis: role of echocardiography. Korean Circ J 2012;42(11): 725–34. http://dx.doi.org/10.4070/kcj.2012.42.11.725.

24. L'Italien AJ. Critical cardiovascular skills and procedures in the emergency department. Emerg Med Clin North Am 2013;31(1):151–206. http://dx.doi.org/10.1016/j.emc.2012.09.011.

25. Tsang TS, Enriquez-Sarano M, Freeman WK, et al. Consecutive 1127 therapeutic echocardiographically guided pericardiocenteses: clinical profile, practice patterns, and outcomes spanning 21 years. Mayo Clin Proc 2002;77(5):429–36. http://dx.doi.org/10.4065/77.5.429.

26. Aguilera PA, Durham BA, Riley DA. Emergency transvenous cardiac pacing placement using ultrasound guidance. Ann Emerg Med 2000;36(3): 224–7. http://dx.doi.org/10.1067/mem.2000.108654.

27. Pinneri F, Mazza A, Garzaro L, et al. Temporary emergency cardiac pacing under continuous echocardiographic control. Feasibility and safety of the procedure without using fluoroscopy. Ital Heart J Suppl 2003;4(7):581–6 [in Italian].

Symptom-Based Ultrasonography

Jehangir Meer, MD, RDMS*, Sierra Beck, MD, RDMS, RDCS,
Karim Ali, MD

KEYWORDS

- Ultrasonography • Symptom-based • Emergency department • Point of care

KEY POINTS

- Point-of-care (POC) ultrasonography can be used to rapidly aid in working up patients presenting with chest pain, dyspnea, and abdominal pain.
- To evaluate patients with chest pain or dyspnea, the clinician sonologist should scan the heart, pleura, lung bases, and inferior vena cava.
- POC ultrasonography can assist with unstable patients with chest pain or dyspnea by evaluating for pericardial tamponade, evidence of right ventricular strain/massive pulmonary embolism, tension pneumothorax, aortic dissection, and acute severe mitral regurgitation in the setting of ST-elevation myocardial infarction (suggestive of acute papillary muscle rupture).
- Unstable trauma patients with chest pain or dyspnea can be examined for hemopericardium, hemothorax, and tension pneumothorax.
- Patients with unstable vital signs and abdominal pain can be rapidly evaluated by examining the Morrison pouch to look for presence of free fluid/intraperitoneal bleeding, and other life-threatening conditions as directed by history, physical examination, and clinical context.

 Videos showing heart with large pericardial effusion and tamponade physiology, McConnell's Sign with RV strain, thrombus in RA/RV, severe mitral regurgitation with color doppler imaging, pleural effusion, severely reduced LV systolic function, inferior wall motion hypokinesia, calcified aortic valve and absence of pleural sliding accompany this article at http://www.ultrasound.theclinics.com/

INTRODUCTION

The use of point-of-care (POC) ultrasonography as a rapid assessment tool has been adopted in emergency departments (EDs), inpatient units, critical care bays, and outpatient settings. Ultrasonography has numerous advantages: it is noninvasive, portable, does not carry the risk of ionizing radiation, and can be performed rapidly at a patient's bedside. In this article, algorithms are proposed for a symptom-based approach to the use of ultrasonography in the evaluation of patients presenting with dyspnea, chest pain, and abdominal pain.

CHEST PAIN AND DYSPNEA SYMPTOM COMPLEX

Undifferentiated chest pain and dyspnea are common complaints in emergency medicine, and patients frequently present with both symptoms. Emergency physicians often perform a battery of tests to help differentiate the varied causes of chest pain or dyspnea and rule out life-threatening causes. Often, these patients are admitted for further workup.

Dyspnea and chest pain are in the top 5 complaints of patients presenting to the ED.[1] However,

Funding Sources: None.
Conflicts of Interest: None.
Department of Emergency Medicine, Department Administration, Emory University School of Medicine, 531 Asbury Circle, Annex Building, Suite N340, Atlanta, GA 30322, USA
* Corresponding author. Department of Emergency Medicine, Emory University, 68 Armstrong Street, Suite 334, Atlanta, GA 30303.
E-mail address: jehangir.meer@emory.edu

the diagnostic differential for each is complex and often cumbersome to investigate.[2] In addition, the patient history may be misleading. POC ultrasonography may guide the clinical investigation and facilitate bedside diagnosis of emergent conditions. Chest pain and dyspnea may be provoked by both acute and chronic diseases. Although it may not be possible to diagnose every cause in the ED, the role of the emergency physician is to diagnose conditions that may be life-threatening if missed. Although additional tests may be required to confirm certain diagnoses, the portability, clinical applicability, and simplicity make POC ultrasonography an indispensable bedside tool for rapidly ruling in critical diagnoses.

POC ultrasonography can help to reduce the time to diagnosis and disposition in certain situations. There is considerable overlap between evaluating chest pain and dyspnea, because they share some of the same pathologic conditions. Our proposed unified algorithm when evaluating patients with a chief complaint of chest pain or dyspnea with POC ultrasonography is shown in **Fig. 1**.

The approach to assessment for patients with dyspnea in the ED has already been published using the RADiUS (rapid assessment of dyspnea with ultrasonography) approach outlined by Manson and Hafez.[3] We propose extending that approach

to patients with chest pain as well. Using the RADiUS approach, one can sequentially look at the heart, pleura/lungs, and the inferior vena cava (IVC) in these patients to obtain clinically relevant information on patients. Look at the heart through 3 windows if possible (subcostal, parasternal long/short axis, and apical 4-chamber [A4C]) to maximize the information you can gather. Next, examine the lungs by looking at the pleura line, dividing each lung into 4 quadrants. After that examination, move the transducer to the supradiaphragmatic window to look for pleural effusions (similar to FAST [focused assessment with sonography for trauma] examination). Examine the IVC for caliber and variability with respiration.

CHEST PAIN AND DYSPNEA IN THE HEMODYNAMICALLY UNSTABLE PATIENT

Patients with hemodynamic instability presenting with chief complaints of chest pain or dyspnea represent unique challenges. They require concurrent resuscitation and stabilization, while a diagnostic workup is performed. The history may be limited because of the patient's clinical status, physical examination has limited usefulness, and ancillary tests can take time to perform and can put the patient at risk, because they require the patient to be sent out of the ED for further testing.

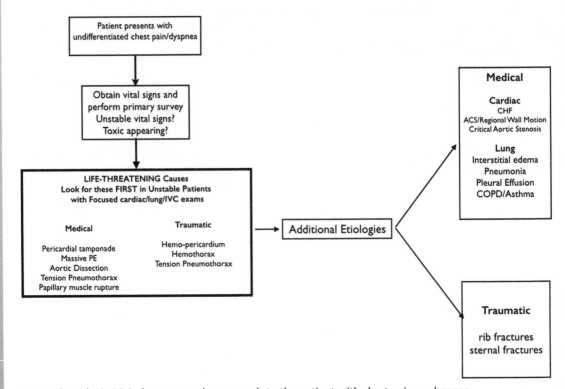

Fig. 1. Algorithmic POC ultrasonography approach to the patient with chest pain or dyspnea.

Many of these conditions require emergent surgery or procedural interventions, and POC ultrasonography can cut down on time to definitive management. Nontraumatic causes of chest pain (and dyspnea), depending on the clinical scenario, may also require an emergent 12-lead electrocardiogram (ECG) in addition to an immediate POC echocardiogram to evaluate for the possibility of an ST-elevation myocardial infarction (STEMI), which in most clinical settings, necessitates immediate activation of a cardiac catheterization laboratory or administration of thrombolytic therapy.

The following causes should be actively sought out first in the unstable patient with chest pain or dyspnea: pericardial effusion with tamponade, massive pulmonary embolism (PE), aortic dissection, tension pneumothorax, and severe mitral regurgitation in the setting of a STEMI. Hemopericardium, hemothorax, and tension pneumothorax should be actively sought after in the unstable trauma patient.

Pericardial Effusion with Tamponade

Unstable patients with pericardial effusion with a variety of causes often present with chest pain and dyspnea and are likely to have a large pericardial effusion. High-risk populations for pericardial effusions include patients who have cancer, patients with congestive heart failure (CHF) or uremia, pericarditis, and lupus.[4] The classic Beck triad of muffled heart sounds, hypotension, and jugular venous distension is not often seen in ED patients.[5] Pericardial effusion can be picked up by the emergency physician (EP) at the bedside, when looking for circumferential black or anechoic fluid surrounding the heart within the pericardium (Video 1).

Although tamponade should be a clinical diagnosis, echocardiographic signs suggestive of tamponade include right atrial systolic collapse and right ventricular (RV) diastolic collapse.[6] In addition, a swinging heart may be seen in a large pericardial effusion, the ultrasonographic equivalent of electrical alternans. The IVC would show a plethoric vessel with no respirophasic variation (Video 2).[7]

Massive PE

These patients may also have a massive PE, which can be identified on POC echocardiogram by noting evidence of right heart strain: a dilated RV compared with the left ventricle (LV). Normally, the RV/LV ratio should be 0.5:1.[8] With acute right heart strain, as seen with massive PE, the RV is commonly rounder and the same size or larger than the LV. This finding can be best seen on the

A4C view, which allows direct comparison of right and left heart chambers (**Fig. 2**).

However, RV dilatation can be seen on the other echocardiographic windows. Tricuspid regurgitation can be found when color Doppler gate is applied over tricuspid valve on A4C view (**Fig. 3**).[8] Ventricular septal flattening resulting in a D-shaped LV in PSSX window can also be seen (**Fig. 4**).[9]

The McConnell sign, which is 94% specific for PE, describes the echocardiographic findings of RV free wall akinesia with RV apical wall motion sparing, secondary to increased right heart pressures. However, it does not distinguish acute PE from acute RV infarction.[10] The IVC should also be examined, because it is dilated. Other causes of right heart strain include chronic lung disease, pulmonary hypertension, and pulmonic stenosis and are usually chronic. Acute right heart strain can be differentiated from chronic right heart strain by noting the thickness of the RV free wall. Normal RV free wall thickness is usually 2 to 3 mm and is considered hypertrophied when it is greater than 5 mm from chronic causes.[11] The clinical situation is of considerable importance in deciding the possible cause of right heart strain.

POC echo can also sometimes visualize echogenic thrombus in either the RA or RV, providing further evidence of a PE (Videos 3 and 4).

Acute Aortic Dissection

Patients with severe chest pain and acutely increased blood pressure, particularly if the chest pain radiates to the back or below the diaphragm, or involves neurologic symptoms, can be a presentation of acute aortic dissection. Bedside echocardiogram and POC aorta examination can be valuable in ruling in this clinical entity. However, it is not so useful in ruling out aortic dissection. Echo clues include looking for aortic root dilatation (>3.8 cm) on the parasternal long axis window or dissection flap in the descending aorta, seen in

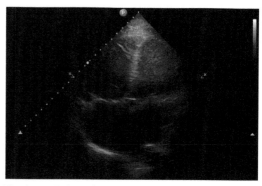

Fig. 2. A4C view showing dilated RV equal in size to LV, which indicates RV strain.

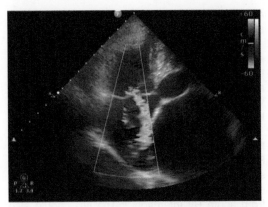

Fig. 3. A4C view showing tricuspid regurgitation jet in the setting of RV dilatation when viewed with color Doppler imaging.

cross-section below the posterior pericardium (**Fig. 5**).[8]

A pericardial effusion may also be found if the dissection propagates proximally. In addition, placing the probe in the suprasternal notch, with the transducer pointing down into the chest, can allow for examination of the arch of the aorta, looking for a dissection flap in that area (**Fig. 6**).[8]

For abdominal aortic dissections, a POC aorta scan could show a dissection flap in the lumen of the aorta. Although type A aortic dissections require cardiothoracic surgical intervention, having clinical suspicion confirmed by bedside ultrasonography would allow immediate control of hypertension with titratable antihypertensives, such as esmolol and nitroprusside, and earlier consultation with cardiothoracic surgery (**Fig. 7**).

Tension Pneumothorax

Patients can also present with pleuritic chest pain and dyspnea when having a pneumothorax. The classic triad of hypotension, decreased breath

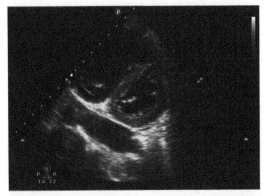

Fig. 4. PSSX window showing ventricular septal bowing resulting in a D-shaped LV, also suggestive of RV strain.

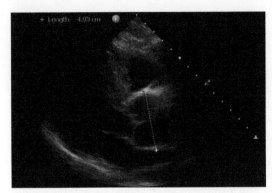

Fig. 5. Dilated aortic root on PSLX window.

sounds, and tracheal deviation is not always seen in tension pneumothorax.

One of the basic premises of lung sonography is the concept of lung sliding. It represents a layer of visceral pleura sliding on parietal pleura lubricated by a small amount of pleural fluid. During breathing (spontaneous or mechanic), lung expansion creates a sliding movement between layers of pleura. Lung sliding is noted as a shimmering motion of the pleura with respiration. Lung sliding can be seen all over the lung surface where visceral pleura

A

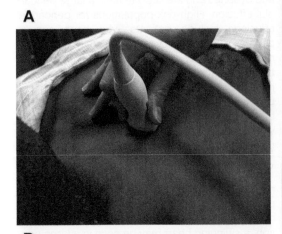

B

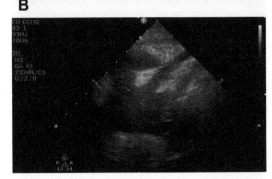

Fig. 6. (A) Transducer positioning to obtain suprasternal notch view. (B) Suprasternal notch ultrasonographic image.

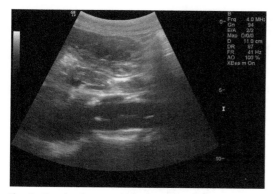

Fig. 7. Proximal aorta with dissection flap.

is directly adherent to the chest wall. Normal healthy lung without pleural injury shows pleural sliding. Clear identification of lung sliding excludes pneumothorax at that specific point.[12]

M-mode may be used to document pneumothorax; healthy pleura with sliding shows a difference in motion artifact posterior to the pleura, which is known as the seashore sign. In a patient with pneumothorax, no sliding motion is present at the pleural interface. Therefore, the M-mode image appears static and there is no difference in the appearance of the soft tissue layers compared with the pleural interface. This finding is sometimes referred to as the stratosphere sign, given its stillness, or the barcode sign.[13] Modern equipment obviates using M-mode to diagnose pneumothorax, however, it may still be useful to document absence of lung sliding if a still image is being used (most practitioners do not use M-mode to diagnose pneumothorax with modern equipment; some still use it for documentation in cases of a still image) (Figs. 8 and 9).

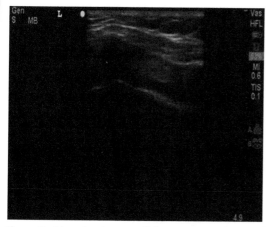

Fig. 8. Absent lung sliding suggestive of pneumothorax.

Bedside ultrasonography can quickly confirm the absence of lung sliding, which is suggestive of pneumothorax. The visualization of a lung point is pathognomic for a pneumothorax and increases sensitivity to 100%. In addition, the location of the lung point roughly correlates with the radiographic size of the pneumothorax.[12] This sign appears as pleural sliding that intermittently slides into view with respiration and is the anatomic point at which the collapsed lung meets normal expanded lung.

Acute Papillary Muscle Rupture/Severe Mitral Regurgitation

Patients presenting with acute papillary muscle rupture have chest pain and dyspnea and are usually in cardiogenic shock with a STEMI. One may or may not hear a holosystolic murmur in a busy, noisy ED. These are a very sick group of patients who have close to 80% mortality, unless they are recognized and referred for cardiothoracic surgery for repair of their mitral valve.[14]

Acute mitral regurgitation causes acute increase in LV filling pressures, increased pulmonary pressures, and cardiogenic shock. Although there are a variety of causes of acute severe mitral regurgitation, including leaflet perforation from endocarditis, in the setting of an acute STEMI, strong consideration must be given to acute papillary muscle rupture. On ED echo, papillary muscle rupture can sometimes be seen when viewing the mitral valve in various cardiac windows. It is usually the posteromedial papillary muscle that is involved, because it has a single coronary artery supplying it (in contrast to the anterolateral papillary muscle, which has a dual supply) (Fig. 10).[15]

What is not variable, and is consistently present, is severe mitral regurgitation, which is represented as a large blue regurgitant jet filling the entire LA on color Doppler imaging (Video 5).

These patients will not do well if simply sent to the catheterization laboratory for percutaneous transluminal coronary angioplasty. If severe acute heart failure is present a rapid bedside echo can expedite referral to cardiothoracic surgery for coronary artery bypass graft and repair of mitral valve.

Hemopericardium

Patients with blunt or penetrating chest trauma may develop a hemopericardium. Although an anechoic fluid stripe may be seen in the pericardium surrounding the heart, another likely finding is an echogenic layer in the pericardium caused by presence of clotted blood in the pericardium. This finding can be easily missed by a novice sonologist and is a potential pitfall of the FAST examination. These patients can also

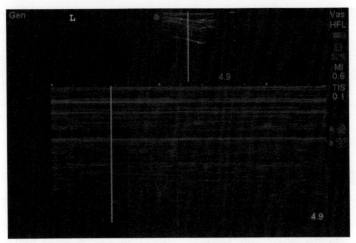

Fig. 9. M-mode without pleural artifact motion (barcode sign) suggestive of pneumothorax.

show echocardiographic signs of tamponade, as detailed in the cardiac tamponade section (**Fig. 11**).

Hemothorax

Patients with chest wall trauma may also manifest ipsilateral or bilateral hemothoraces. These clinical entities are difficult to pick up on supine chest radiographs, which are commonly ordered in multisystem trauma. Bedside ultrasonography, on the other hand, has a very high sensitivity for picking up pleural fluid/hemothorax and can visualize as little as 25 to 50 mL of fluid.[16] The clinician should look for black anechoic fluid above the diaphragm, or the presence of the spine sign to indicate a pleural effusion (Video 6).

CHEST PAIN AND DYSPNEA IN THE STABLE NONTRAUMATIC PATIENT

Additional causes that should be elicited in nontraumatic patients include CHF, regional wall motion abnormalities, and critical aortic stenosis when looking at the heart. During pleural/lung examination, one should look for evidence of interstitial edema, pleural effusion, and pneumonia.

CHF

Patients with exacerbation of CHF inevitably present with dyspnea. Moore and colleagues[17] in 2002 showed that EPs with limited training could visually estimate with accuracy normal or depressed LV function when compared with formal echocardiography. Systolic dysfunction is noted as lack of significant myocardial thickening and inward wall motion of LV during systole. In addition, poor excursion of the mitral valve anterior leaflet to the interventricular septum in diastole can be a useful marker of systolic dysfunction. This distance from the tip of the anterior leaflet of the mitral valve to the interventricular septum is known as E-point septal separation, and when greater than 7 mm, it can be used to mark systolic dysfunction.[18] A sequela of poor forward blood flow, pulmonary edema contributing to dyspnea, may be detected earlier and with higher sensitivity than plain film radiography using ultrasound. One can also see LV free wall thickening or dilated LV in patients with systolic heart dysfunction. Evaluation of pleura can show evidence of interstitial

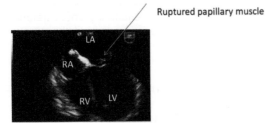

Ruptured papillary muscle

Fig. 10. Image of papillary muscle rupture.

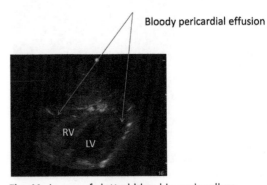

Bloody pericardial effusion

Fig. 11. Image of clotted blood in pericardium.

edema in support of CHF (see section on pulmonary interstitial edema) (**Fig. 12**, Video 7).

In concert with cardiac and pulmonary ultrasonography assessments, IVC assessment clues the clinician in the right diagnostic direction. Decreased ejection fraction leads to backup of blood flow and subsequently increased volume in the venous system. IVC caliber appears plethoric and has minimal respiratory variation (**Fig. 13**).

Regional Wall Motion Abnormalities

Patients with a clinical history concerning for acute coronary syndrome or ischemic chest pain can have an ED echo evaluation for regional wall motion abnormalities, in addition to the usual diagnostic tests (ECG, cardiac troponins, chest radiograph). This evaluation requires more advanced skill, and may be beyond the scope of the average EP sonologist. However, for simplification, one can obtain a fairly good idea if there is reduced contractility in a segment of the LV using the PSSX window. Normally, all areas of the LV in the PSSX window should contract equally, resulting in concentric thickening of the LV wall circumferentially. If a certain segment of the LV wall has reduced contractility in relation to the rest of the LV, then that suggests evidence of either acute cardiac ischemia or old infarct (**Fig. 14**, Video 8).[8]

Critical Aortic Stenosis

Diagnosis of aortic stenosis by ED echo is an advanced technique and is technically challenging. Chest pain, dyspnea/CHF, and syncope can be a manifestation of severe/critical aortic

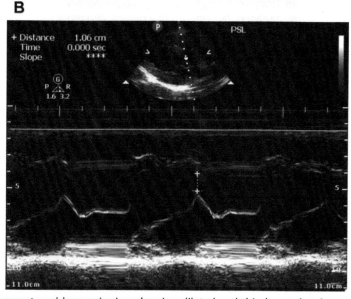

Fig. 12. (A) Cardiac parasternal long axis view showing dilated and thin heart chambers suggestive of dilated cardiomyopathy. (B) M-mode showing E-point septal separation in patient with reduced systolic LV function.

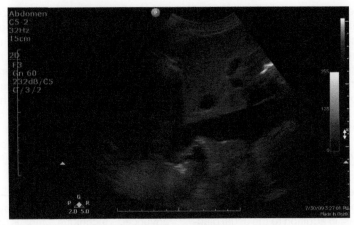

Fig. 13. Note the plethoric IVC, suggestive of volume overload.

stenosis. This diagnosis is important, because the treatment is surgical repair of the valve. Syncope occurs because these patients have a fixed cardiac output, and when demand increases, they cannot meet it, develop hypotension, and syncope. The typical patient is older, usually older than 75 years, but younger patients can develop aortic stenosis if they have bicuspid valves. On physical examination, they should have a systolic crescendo-decrescendo murmur at the right sternal border, although with critical stenosis the murmur may not be loud. On ED echo, the sonologist can visualize a stenotic calcified aortic valve that does not open well during systole. Although there are multiple formal echo criteria for diagnosing severe aortic stenosis,[19] ED echo can be a good screening tool to suspect the diagnosis by placing a continuous wave Doppler through the aortic valve. Critical aortic stenosis is suggested when peak aortic valve velocities are greater than 450 cm/s. Formal echocardiography should be obtained to confirm these findings (**Fig. 15**, Video 9).

Pulmonary Interstitial Edema

Acute lung interstitial edema is noted by the presence of B-line artifact on lung ultrasonography. B-lines, which are vertical hyperechoic lines starting at the pleura, are caused by any process that increases the normal size of the interlobular pulmonary septae, including fluid, fibrosis, or infection.[20,21]

Multiple bilateral B-lines are consistent with a patient with the alveolar-interstitial syndrome: CHF exacerbation, acute respiratory distress syndrome, diffuse interstitial lung disease, or noncardiogenic pulmonary edema.[3] In the clinical setting of a patient with reduced systolic function, as seen on ED bedside echo, with bilateral multiple B-lines

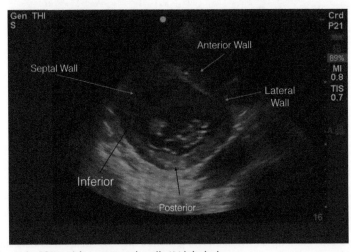

Fig. 14. Image of heart in PSSX with segmental walls LV labeled.

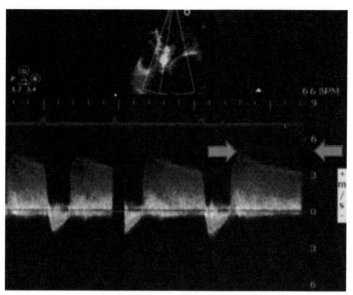

Fig. 15. Apical 5-chamber view showing very high continuous wave velocities through the aortic valve.

on pleural examination, acute pulmonary edema secondary to systolic heart failure is highly suggested (**Fig. 16**).

Pneumonia

Alveolar consolidation is a basic concern in critically ill patients. Radiography is not a precise tool, and referral to computed tomography (CT) raises problems with transport, irradiation, and cost. Ultrasonography provides a reliable noninvasive, bedside method for accurate detection and location of alveolar consolidation in critically ill patients.[22]

Although aerated lung obstructs the ultrasound beam, alveolar consolidation improves transmission in patients with pneumonia, allowing delineation of lung parenchyma, which resembles the sonographic appearance of liver tissue. This process is

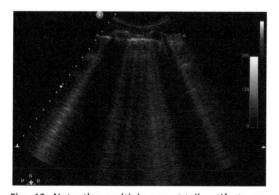

Fig. 16. Note the multiple comet-tail artifacts per lung field. In the appropriate clinical context, these artifacts are highly sensitive for pulmonary edema.

known as lung hepatization.[23] Within the consolidation, hyperechoic punctiform images can be seen, corresponding to air bronchograms (air-filled bronchi). Penetration of gas into the bronchial tree of the consolidation during inspiration produces an inspiratory reinforcement of these hyperechoic punctiform images.[24] In addition, presence of infectious fluid in the lung may result in B-line artifact, which, unlike CHF exacerbations, is usually present only unilaterally in focal pneumonia (**Fig. 17**).

Pleural Effusion

Pleural effusion, in either lung, may be easily located using ultrasonography, and views are usually easy to acquire, because it requires a small modification to hepatorenal and splenorenal windows for the FAST scan. Ultrasonography can aid in determining size of the pleural effusion, as well as assisting in thoracentesis if drainage is required.[25,26] Unilateral effusions are commonly associated with pneumonia, PE, aortic dissection, and traumatic hemothorax. Bilateral effusions are associated with volume overload, noncardiogenic pulmonary edema, and CHF (**Figs. 18** and **19**).[25]

Chronic Obstructive Pulmonary Disease/Asthma

The accurate diagnosis and reversal of reactive airway disease such as asthma and chronic obstructive pulmonary disease (COPD), through rapid bronchodilation treatments, result in favorable patient outcomes.[27] Frequently, ED physicians struggle to delineate reactive airway disease from CHF exacerbations, because both

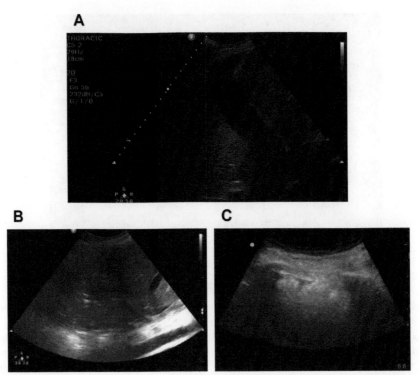

Fig. 17. Various manifestations of pneumonia on ultrasound. (*A*) Pleural effusion with appearance of lung "hepatization". (*B*) Consolidated lung with hyper echoic "air bronchograms". (*C*) Sub pleural consolidations.

diseases are present in many patients. Lung ultrasonography differentiates these diseases adeptly. In a study conducted by Lichtenstein and Meziere,[25] predominant A-lines plus lung sliding in the absence of B-lines indicated asthma or COPD with 89% sensitivity and 97% specificity (**Fig. 20**).

TRAUMATIC CAUSES OF CHEST PAIN IN THE STABLE PATIENT
Rib Fractures

Patients with chest trauma can have rib fractures, but plain film chest radiographs have low

sensitivity for picking them up. Ultrasonography allows for the detection of radiographically occult rib fractures, having a sensitivity of 78% compared with 11% for plain chest radiographs.[28–30] Using a high-frequency transducer, a clinician can target the rib cage of interest by having the patient point to the area of pain, if the patient is cooperative. Scanning in the longitudinal axis, rib cage fractures on ultrasonography appear as a break in the bony cortex of the rib, allowing for assessment of degree of displacement. In addition, if rib fractures are found, the clinician can perform a pleural

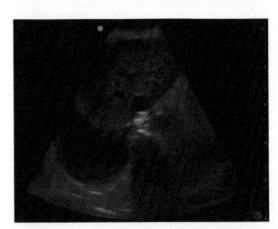

Fig. 18. Left lung with pleural effusion noted.

Fig. 19. Right lung with pleural effusion noted.

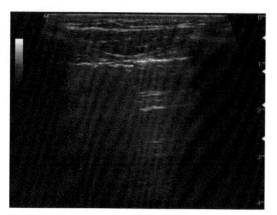

Fig. 20. Accentuated reverberation artifact (A-lines), suggestive of COPD/asthma.

examination to look for an associated pneumothorax (**Fig. 21**).

Sternal Fractures

Patients with sternal fractures are usually the victims of high-speed motor vehicle collisions. They complain of significant midsternal chest pain and have tenderness to palpation over the sternum. Bedside ultrasonography can show a disruption of the bony cortex of the sternum and has been found to be almost 100% sensitive in a small case series.[31] These patients should also have an ED echocardiogram performed to evaluate for pericardial effusion, or echocardiographic evidence of thoracic aortic dissection. A common pitfall is to mistake the sternomanubrial joint for a sternal fracture. Some ways to recognize the sternomanubrial joint include lack of tenderness when the transducer makes contact over the area; the expected location of that joint is in the proximal portion of the sternum.

ABDOMINAL PAIN

Undifferentiated acute abdominal pain is a common symptom prompting patients to seek emergent care. Both benign self-limited conditions and life-threatening diseases can present similarly. It is imperative that clinicians are able to narrow a broad differential rapidly. In patients with acute abdominal pain, ultrasonography leads to increased diagnostic confidence and can help to rule in or out leading differential diagnoses or offer new diagnoses in cases in which the clinical picture is uncertain.[32] Our proposed algorithm for the use of ultrasonography in the assessment of patients with undifferentiated abdominal pain is shown in **Fig. 22**.

Abdominal Pain in the Unstable Patient

In hemodynamically unstable patients, abdominal pain may be accompanied by altered mental status, dyspnea, or other factors limiting history and physical examination. In addition, in the critically ill patient, resuscitation and diagnostic workup must occur simultaneously. Evaluation with ultrasonography should focus on the rapid identification of reversible causes of hemodynamic instability and triage of patients with surgical disease to operative care.

Intraperitoneal hemorrhage

Focused assessment for intraperitoneal free fluid is a rapid first step in the evaluation of hemodynamically unstable patients. We propose quickly performing a single right upper quadrant FAST view of the Morrison pouch (hepatorenal recess) to identify large volume intraperitoneal fluid, which in the appropriate clinical context may represent hemorrhage. In patients receiving normal saline infusion via diagnostic peritoneal lavage, an

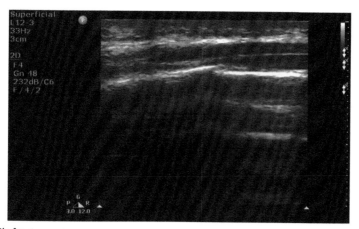

Fig. 21. Image of rib fracture.

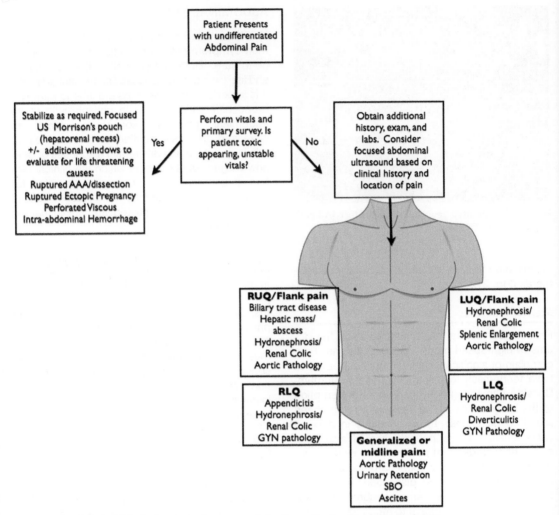

Fig. 22. Algorithmic POC ultrasonography approach to the patient with abdominal pain.

average of 668 mL ± 194 mL is required for the detection of free fluid in the Morrison pouch (**Box 1**).[33]

Although less sensitive than a 4-view FAST examination, a single view saves time and may rapidly identify patients with hemodynamically significant quantities of intraperitoneal hemorrhage. If the diagnosis of smaller quantities of free fluid is indicated, a more exhaustive search can be performed. Not all intraperitoneal fluid represents blood; ultrasonographic findings must be interpreted in the clinical context (**Fig. 23**).

Ectopic pregnancy

Studies of ectopic pregnancy have also shown that a positive single right upper quadrant, Morrison pouch view predicts the need for operative intervention.[34,35] Regardless of the quantity of fluid seen, in pregnant patients without evidence of

definitive intrauterine pregnancy, ectopic pregnancy must be considered (**Fig. 24**).

In elderly patients presenting with back, flank, or generalized abdominal pain, the diagnosis of ruptured abdominal aortic aneurysm (AAA) must be considered.[36] AAAs tend to be infrarenal. A diagnostic study must evaluate the entire length of the aorta. Most AAAs (87%) rupture into the left retroperitoneum.[37] Hemoperitoneum may not be seen if there is contained retroperitoneal bleeding (**Fig. 25**).

Bowel perforation

In toxic appearing patients who present with peritoneal signs, bowel perforation should be considered. Peritoneal free air, suggesting bowel perforation, can be detected on ultrasonography as enhancement of the peritoneal stripe with comet-tail artifacts at the interface of the ventral

Box 1
Causes of large intraperitoneal free fluid

Ascites (infectious, malignant, heart failure, end stage renal disease, liver disease)

AAA with intraperitoneal rupture

Bowel perforation

Peritoneal dialysis

Post-operative hemorrhage

Ruptured ectopic pregnancy

Ruptured ovarian cyst

Splenic rupture

Unreported trauma

liver and the diaphragm.[38] However, this ultrasonographic examination is operator dependent; interposed colon, lung, subcutaneous emphysema, and rib shadows can all appear similar to peritoneal free air.[39,40]

Assessment of the Hemodynamically Stable Patient

In hemodynamically stable patients, a more focused ultrasonographic examination should be performed based on the pretest probability of specific diseases and the location of the patient's pain.

Midline/generalized abdominal pain

In patients with generalized or midline abdominal pain, ultrasonography may be used to assess aortic

A

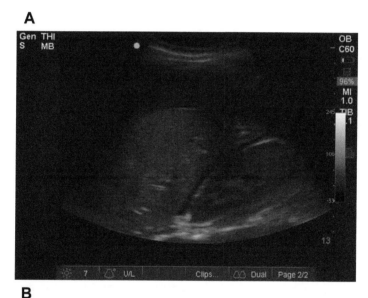

B

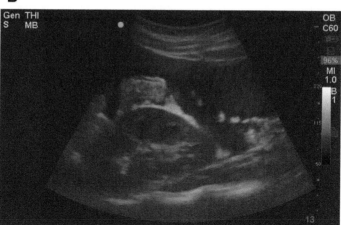

Fig. 23. (*A*) A 31-year-old woman presented hypotensive, with abdominal pain and altered mental status; a pregnancy test was negative. Bedside ultrasonography showed large volume intraperitoneal free fluid. (*B*) A further view showed that fluid was complex, with internal echoes, suggesting hemorrhage. The patient was subsequently diagnosed with phrenic artery rupture after a recent surgical procedure.

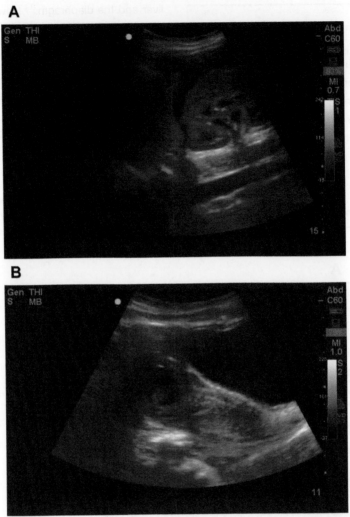

Fig. 24. Ruptured cornual ectopic: pregnant woman presented hypotensive with abdominal pain. (*A*) Ultrasonography showed large intraperitoneal free fluid. (*B*) Extrauterine pregnancy was identified on transabdominal pelvic views.

disease, acute urinary retention, bowel obstruction, ascites, abdominal masses, or early appendicitis. When evaluating a patient with generalized pain, it may be helpful to have the patient identify their point of maximal tenderness and perform a focused examination of this area (**Fig. 26**).

Small bowel obstruction In patients with generalized or midline abdominal pain, ultrasonography is an ideal initial test to evaluate for possible small bowel obstruction. Dilated loops of bowel on ultrasonography (>25 mm) outperform plain film radiography with a sensitivity of 91% and specificity of 84% for small bowel obstruction (**Fig. 27**).[41]

Urinary retention Given wide variations in the bladder shape,[42] bladder volumes can be difficult

to calculate exactly using two-dimensional ultrasonography, but bladder distention and gross assessment of urinary retention are easy to diagnose and can be used to rapidly screen patients before catheterization (**Fig. 28**).

Right upper quadrant/left upper quadrant pain
Patient with right upper quadrant pain may benefit from evaluation of the biliary tree, hepatic parenchyma, right kidney, or the aorta. In the left upper quadrant, splenic, left renal, or aortic evaluations may be considered.

Hepatobiliary disease Ultrasonography is the initial test of choice in patients with suspected biliary disease. Identification of a positive sonographic

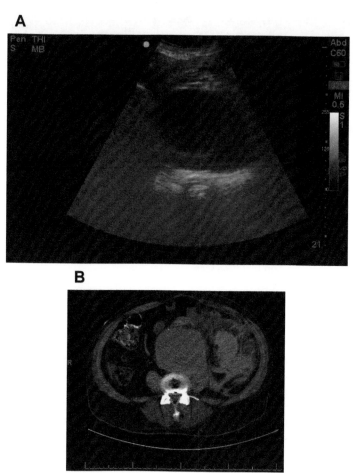

Fig. 25. (*A*) A 73-year-old man presented with hypotension and abdominal pain; ultrasonography with 10-cm infrarenal AAA. CT showed contained retroperitoneal rupture. (*B*) CT scan obtained with evidence of contained retroperitoneal rupture.

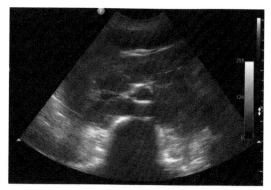

Fig. 26. Large retroperitoneal mass (chronic lympho-cytic leukemia) encasing the aorta and IVC in a patient presenting with 1 week of generalized abdominal pain. Patient asked to identify location of his pain and this image was obtained.

Murphy's sign and gallstones is most suggestive of a diagnosis of acute cholecystitis.[43,44] Wall thickening and pericholecystic fluid may also be seen but are less specific. Ultrasonography may also detect choledocolithiasis, hepatic abscess, or masses (**Figs. 29** and **30**).

Renal disease Renal ultrasonography is an important alternative to CT imaging for evaluation of renal colic. Although this modality is less sensitive and specific than CT for diagnosis of stones, the presence of hydronephrosis is fairly sensitive and specific for the detection of large stones larger than 5 mm.[45] With a negative predictive value of 98%, it may be an appropriate screening tool to expedite care and determine which patients do not require additional imaging. Renal

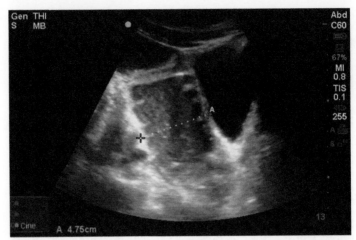

Fig. 27. Patient with small bowel obstruction; note dilated loops of bowel with prominent plicae circularis; dysfunctional peristalsis was noted on real-time scan.

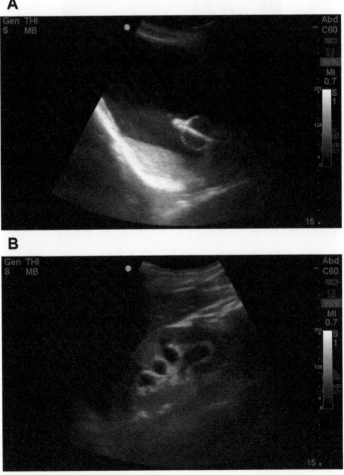

Fig. 28. (*A*) Patient with Foley malfunction and acute urinary retention, Sediment seen layering in the bladder. (*B*) Renal scan showed associated moderate hydronephrosis.

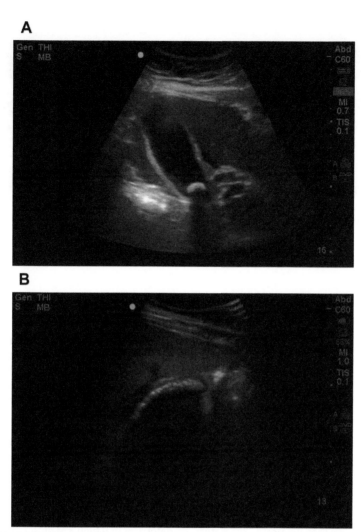

Fig. 29. Cholecystitis: (*A*) impacted stone at the gall bladder neck with wall thickening and pericholecystic fluid. (*B*) Wall echo shadow sign in a patient with acute cholecystitis.

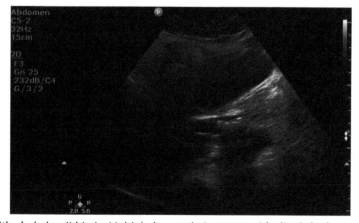

Fig. 30. Patient with choledocolithiasis. Multiple hyperechoic stones with distal shadowing are seen within a dilated common bile duct.

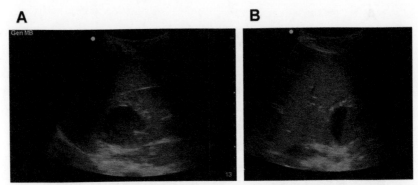

Fig. 31. Renal abscess: otherwise healthy 25-year-old man presented with several weeks of fever and right flank pain despite recent treatment of urinary tract infection, Ultrasonography showed a complex cystic structure in the right kidney (*A*) with fluid-fluid layering (*B*). Aspirate was positive for *Escherichia coli*.

ultrasonography can identify renal masses, cysts, or evidence of infection (**Fig. 31**).

Right lower quadrant/left lower quadrant

Evaluation of the lower abdomen includes consideration of female pelvic disease, renal disease, and, in the right lower quadrant, evaluation for appendicitis. Ultrasonography may have a role in the evaluation of patients presenting with a history suggestive of diverticulitis.

Appendicitis Ultrasonography is the initial imaging study of choice for evaluation of acute appendicitis in children. Evaluation may be nondiagnostic in obese adults. Appendicitis on ultrasonography is diagnosed when noncompressible appendix is found measuring more than 6 mm in diameter. Complications including periappendiceal fluid,

abscess, or fat stranding may also be visualized (**Fig. 32**).[46,47]

Diverticulitis In some parts of the world, ultrasonography is the initial study of choice for the evaluation of suspected diverticulitis. Identification of thickened colonic wall, surrounding fat enhancement, and complications such as abscess formation may be seen on ultrasonography.[48] This examination is highly operator dependent and may be less successful in obese patients (**Fig. 33**).

In patients with undifferentiated abdominal pain, ultrasonography can help to rapidly rule in or out key diagnoses, and may be a valuable first step in triaging patients to the operating room, guiding early treatment and resuscitation, and determining which patients require additional imaging studies.

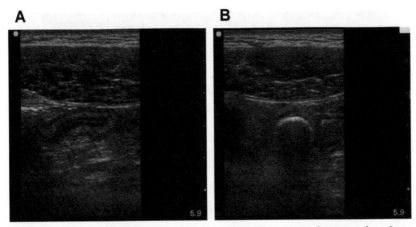

Fig. 32. Acute appendicitis: blind ending noncompressible appendix measured greater than 6 mm across (*A*); in second image (*B*), appendicolith was identified.

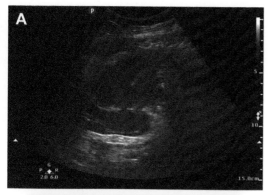

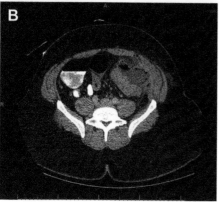

Fig. 33. (*A*) Left lower quadrant ultrasound in a patient with diverticulitis, micro perforation and abscess formation; note thickened colonic wall enhancement of surrounding fat and overlying abscess. (*B*) Confirmatory CT.

SUMMARY

POC ultrasonography is a useful tool to rapidly evaluate patients with chest pain, dyspnea, and abdominal pain, especially if they are hemodynamically unstable. It can provide answers to key clinical questions and rule out critical conditions at the bedside. In conjunction with the history, physical examination, and ancillary tests, bedside ultrasonography allows for rapid disposition and life-saving treatment to be initiated and minimizes delays.

SUPPLEMENTARY DATA

Video related to this article can be found online at http://dx.doi.org/10.1016/j.cult.2014.01.003.

REFERENCES

1. Pitts S, Niska R, Xu J, et al. National Hospital Ambulatory Medical Care Survey: 2006 emergency department summary. Natl Health Stat Report 2008;(7):1–38.
2. Lansing R, Gracely R, Banzett R. The multiple dimensions of dyspnea: review and hypotheses. Respir Physiol Neurobiol 2009;30(167):53–60.
3. Manson W, Hafez NM. The rapid assessment of dyspnea with ultrasound: RADiUS, ultrasound. Clinics 2011;6(2):261–76.
4. Mandavia D, Hoffner R, Mahaney K, et al. Bedside echocardiography by emergency physicians. Ann Emerg Med 2001;38(4):377–82.
5. Beck CS. Acute and chronic compression of the heart. Am Heart J 1937;14:515.
6. Tsang T, Oh J, Seward J. Diagnosis and management of cardiac tamponade in the era of echocardiography. Clin Cardiol 1999;22:446–52.
7. Oh J, Seward J, Tajik A. Pericardial diseases. In: The echo manual. 3rd edition. Philadelphia: Lippincott Williams & Wilkins; 2006. p. 289–309.
8. Reardon R, Joing S. Cardiac. In: Ma O, Mateer J, Blaivas M, editors. Emergency ultrasound. 2nd edition. New York: McGraw-Hill; 2008. p. 109–48.
9. Jardin F, Dubourg O, Gueret P, et al. Quantitative two-dimensional echocardiography in massive pulmonary embolism: emphasis on ventricular interdependence and leftward septal displacement. J Am Coll Cardiol 1987;10:1201–6.
10. Lopez-Candalez A, Edelman K, Candales MD. Right ventricular apical contractility in acute pulmonary embolism: the McConnell sign revisited. Echocardiography 2010;27(6):614–20.
11. Stein J. Opinions regarding the diagnosis and management of venous thromboembolic disease. ACCP Consensus Committee on Pulmonary Embolism. Chest 1996;109:233–7.
12. Lichtenstein D, Meziere G, Biderman P, et al. The "lung point": an ultrasound sign specific to pneumothorax. Intensive Care Med 2000;26(10):1434–40.
13. Chan S. Emergency bedside ultrasound to detect pneumothorax. Acad Emerg Med 2003;10(1):91–4.
14. Stout K, Verrier E. Acute valvular regurgitation. Circulation 2009;119:3232–41.
15. Oh J, Seward J, Tajik A. Coronary artery disease and acute myocardial infarction. In: The echo manual. 3rd edition. Philadelphia: Lippincott Williams & Wilkins; 2006. p. 154–74.
16. Rose JS. Ultrasound in abdominal trauma. Emerg Med Clin North Am 2004;22(3):581–99, vii.
17. Moore C, Rose G, Tayal V, et al. Determination of left ventricular function by emergency physician echocardiography of hypotensive patients. Acad Emerg Med 2002;9(3):186–93.
18. Secko M, Lazar J, Salciccioli L, et al. Can junior emergency physicians use E-point septal separation to accurately estimate left ventricular function in acutely dyspneic patients? Acad Emerg Med 2011;18(11):1223–6.

19. Oh J, Seward J, Tajik A. Valvular heart disease. In: The echo manual. 3rd edition. Philadelphia: Lippincott Williams & Wilkins; 2006. p. 289–309.

20. Agricola E, Bove T, Oppizzi M, et al. Ultrasound comet-tail images: a marker of pulmonary edema: a comparative study with wedge pressure and extra-vascular lung water. Chest 2005;127(5):1690–5.

21. Noble V, Murray A, Capp R, et al. Ultrasound assessment for extravascular lung water in patients undergoing hemodialysis: time course for resolution. Chest 2009;135(6):1433–9.

22. Lichtenstein D, Lascols N, Meziere G, et al. Ultrasound diagnosis of alveolar consolidation in the critically ill. Intensive Care Med 2004;30(2):276–81.

23. Andrea D, Nagdev A. Ultrasound detection of lung hepatization. West J Emerg Med 2010;11(4):322–3.

24. Bouhemad B, Zhang M, Lu Q, et al. Clinical review: bedside lung ultrasound in critical care practice. Crit Care 2007;11:205.

25. Lichtenstein DA, Meziere GA. Relevance of lung ultrasound in the diagnosis of acute respiratory failure: the BLUE protocol. Chest 2008;134(1):117–25.

26. Tayal VS, Nicks BA, Norton HJ. Emergency ultrasound evaluation of symptomatic nontraumatic pleural effusions. Am J Emerg Med 2006;24(7):782–6.

27. Snow V, Lascher S, Mottur-Pilson C. Evidence base for management of acute exacerbations of chronic obstructive pulmonary disease. Ann Intern Med 2001;134(7):595.

28. Turk F, Kurt A, Saglam S. Evaluation by ultrasound of traumatic rib fractures missed by radiography. Emerg Radiol 2010;17(6):473–7.

29. Chan S. Emergency bedside ultrasound for the diagnosis of rib fractures. Am J Emerg Med 2009;27(5):617–20.

30. Rainer T, Griffith J, Lam E, et al. Comparison of thoracic ultrasound, clinical acumen, and radiography in patients with minor chest injury. J Trauma 2004;56:1211–3.

31. You J, Chung Y, Kim D, et al. Role of sonography in the emergency room to diagnose sternal fractures. J Clin Ultrasound 2010;38(3):135–7.

32. Dhillon S, Halligan S, Goh V, et al. The therapeutic impact of abdominal ultrasound in patients with acute abdominal symptoms. Clin Radiol 2002;57:268–71.

33. Barbara J, Sukumvanich P, Seibel R, et al. Ultrasound for the detection of intraperitoneal fluid: the role of Trendelenburg positioning. Am J Emerg Med 1999;17:117–20.

34. Rodgerson J, Heegaard W, Plummer D, et al. Emergency department right upper quadrant ultrasound is associated with a reduced time to diagnosis and treatment of ruptured ectopic pregnancies. Acad Emerg Med 2001;8:331–6.

35. Moore C, Todd WM, O'Brien E, et al. Free fluid in Morison's pouch on bedside ultrasound predicts need for operative intervention in suspected ectopic pregnancy. Acad Emerg Med 2007;14(8):755–8.

36. Golledge J, Abrokwah J, Shenoy KN, et al. Morphology of ruptured abdominal aortic aneurysms. Eur J Vasc Endovasc Surg 1999;18:96–104.

37. Burger T, Meyer F, Tautenhahn J, et al. Ruptured infrarenal aortic aneurysm–a critical evaluation. Vasa 1990;28:30–3.

38. Hoffmann B, Nürnberg D, Westergaard MC. Focus on abnormal air: diagnostic ultrasonography for the acute abdomen. Eur J Emerg Med 2012;19(5):284–91.

39. Moriwaki Y, Sugiyama M, Toyoda H, et al. Ultrasonography for the diagnosis of intraperitoneal free air in chest-abdominal-pelvic blunt trauma and critical acute abdominal pain. Arch Surg 2009;144(2):137–41.

40. Chen S, Wang H, Chen W, et al. Selective use of ultrasonography for the detection of pneumoperitoneum. Acad Emerg Med 2002;9(6):643–5.

41. Jang T, Schindler D, Kaji A. Bedside ultrasonography for the detection of small bowel obstruction in the emergency department. Emerg Med J 2011;28(8):676–8.

42. Hwang J, Byun S, Oh S, et al. Novel algorithm for improving accuracy of ultrasound measurement of residual urine volume according to bladder shape. Urology 2004;64(5):887–91.

43. Ralls P, Colletti P, Lapin S, et al. Real-time sonography in suspected acute cholecystitis: prospective evaluation of primary and secondary signs. Radiology 1985;155:767–71.

44. Laing F, Federle M, Jeffrey R, et al. Ultrasonic evaluation of patients with acute right upper quadrant pain. Radiology 1981;5(2):449–55.

45. Moak J, Lyons M, Lindsell C. Bedside renal ultrasound in the evaluation of suspected ureterolithiasis. Am J Emerg Med 2012;30(1):218–21.

46. Jeffrey R, Laing F, Townsend R. Acute appendicitis: sonographic criteria based on 250 cases. Radiology 1988;167:327–9.

47. Rao P, Boland G. Imaging of acute right lower abdominal quadrant pain. Clin Radiol 1998;53:639–49.

48. Helou N, Abdalkader M, Abu-Rustum R. Sonography: first-line modality in the diagnosis of acute colonic diverticulitis? J Ultrasound Med 2013;32(10):1689–94.

Head and Neck Sonography in the Emergency Setting

Shannon B. Snyder, MD*, Robinson M. Ferre, MD,
Jeremy S. Boyd, MD

KEYWORDS

- Head and neck • Ear/nose/throat • Ultrasonography • Emergency • Clinician-performed
- Point-of-care • Bedside

KEY POINTS

- High-resolution sonography is ideal for the evaluation of many oropharyngeal and neck structures because of their superficial nature.
- Clinicians can use point-of-care ultrasonography to evaluate for different types of infectious and inflammatory conditions in this area.
- Some of these infectious and inflammatory conditions include cellulitis and/or abscess formation of the superficial soft tissues, peritonsillar abscess, cervical lymphadenitis, salivary gland inflammation and sialolithiasis, dental abscess, inflammation of the thyroid gland, internal jugular thrombosis and thrombophlebitis, and sinusitis.

 This articles is accompanied by supplemental videos demonstrating both the normal anatomy and pathology illustrated by still ultrasound images, available at http://www.ultrasound. theclinics.com/

HEAD AND NECK SONOGRAPHY IN THE EMERGENCY SETTING

Sonography of the head and neck has traditionally been used by radiologists, primarily for the evaluation of benign and malignant lesions, and in real-time procedural guidance for fine-needle aspiration and core biopsies. Recent improvements in the resolution and capabilities of portable ultrasound technology have made the use of sonography in evaluating head and neck disorders more accessible to office-based and emergency department (ED) clinicians.

High-resolution sonography is ideal for the evaluation of many oropharyngeal and neck structures because of their superficial nature. Clinicians can use point-of-care sonography to evaluate for different types of infectious and inflammatory conditions in this area, including cellulitis and/or abscess formation of superficial soft tissues, peritonsillar abscess (PTA), cervical lymphadenitis, salivary gland inflammation and sialolithiasis, dental abscess, inflammation of the thyroid gland, internal jugular thrombosis and thrombophlebitis, and sinusitis.

SONOGRAPHY OF THE HEAD AND NECK: SCANNING TECHNIQUE AND NORMAL ANATOMY
Scanning Technique

The extracranial structures of the head and neck are best visualized using a linear array, high-frequency transducer. Frequencies higher than

Disclosures: R.M. Ferre: Soma Access Systems: Industry Sponsored Research.
Division of Emergency Ultrasound, Department of Emergency Medicine, Vanderbilt University Medical Center, 703 Oxford House, 1313 21st Avenue South, Nashville, TN 37232, USA
* Corresponding author.
E-mail address: snyder20@icloud.com

10 MHz are ideal for superior resolution of the most superficial structures, especially in thinner patients. A standoff pad can be used for better visualization of lesions that lie immediately beneath the dermis. Ideally when performing sonographic studies, the patient should be in the supine position with the neck in mild hyperextension.

For intraoral studies of the peritonsillar area a high-frequency, endocavitary transducer is used. The patient should be pretreated with an anesthetic, and the probe covered with a glove or other appropriate nonsterile barrier after placing gel on the transducer footprint.

For both superficial and intraoral imaging all structures should be imaged in at least two orthogonal planes, and color Doppler should be used to aid in the identification of vascular structures.

Anatomic Overview

A basic understanding of head and neck anatomy and the structures most commonly visualized with sonography will aid the clinician in distinguishing between normal anatomy and pathologic conditions. **Fig. 1** provides an anterior and lateral overview of basic superficial anatomy encountered during head and neck sonography.

Major Vascular Structures

Anteriorly, the carotid arteries and internal jugular veins run in the cranial-caudal direction and can be easily visualized from just below the angle of the mandible to the clavicle. For the clinician sonographer (sonologist), a good starting point is to locate these vessels in the axial plane in the midportion of the neck at the level of the thyroid gland. Having the patient rotate the neck 30° to 45° toward the contralateral side aids in visualization of the side of interest.

At this level, the right and left carotid arteries can be visualized immediately deep to the sternocleidomastoid and just lateral to the thyroid gland on each side. The common carotid arteries appear as circular structures with hyperechoic, pulsatile walls. Lateral and usually more superficial relative to the carotid arteries, the internal jugular veins can be identified as thinner-walled structures with a triangular or ovoid shape. The internal jugular veins are easily compressible; thus, in upright patients as well as those with volume depletion, they may not always be apparent. However, if the sonologist ensures gentle pressure with the transducer and repositions the patient into a supine or Trendelenburg position, the internal jugular veins are usually visualized without difficulty. Having the patient perform a Valsalva maneuver will also make the internal jugular vein more

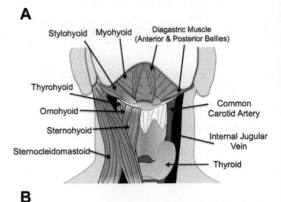

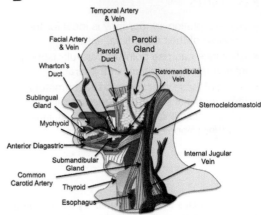

Fig. 1. Overview of head and neck anatomy encountered during sonographic evaluation. (*A*) Anterior. (*B*) Lateral.

pronounced, and aid in its identification. The astute sonologist will notice that at this level the vagus nerve completes this neurovascular bundle, and appears as a small structure in the triangular space between the posterior border of the carotid and internal jugular vessels (**Fig. 2**).

If one follows the major vessels from the midcervical region cranially to the angle of the mandible, the common carotid artery bifurcates into the internal and external carotid arteries, the internal carotid lying deep to the external carotid artery. The first branch of the external carotid artery is the facial artery, and can be seen arising anteriorly to the external carotid artery. At this same level, the facial vein and retromandibular vein join the internal jugular vein through the short trunk of the common facial vein.

Cervical Lymph Nodes

When evaluating any area of pain or swelling involving the superficial structures of the neck, it is essential to have a basic understanding of both the distribution of cervical lymph nodes and

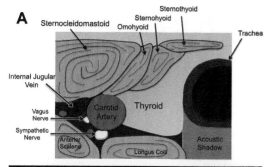

A

Sternothyroid
Sternohyoid
Sternocleidomastoid Omohyoid
Trachea
Internal Jugular Vein
Vagus Nerve
Carotid Artery   Thyroid
Sympathetic Nerve
Anterior Scalene
Acoustic Shadow
Longus Coli

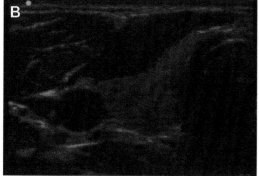

B

Fig. 2. Major vascular structures and surrounding anatomy. (*A*) Regional anatomy. (*B*) Axial image at C6 level.

the sonographic appearance of normal cervical nodes. Of the approximately 800 lymph nodes in the human body, approximately 300 are in the neck.[1] The location of the superficial cervical lymph nodes is fairly consistent and can be organized into several major groupings, illustrated in **Fig. 3**. Whereas radiologists and surgeons classify the distribution of cervical nodes using a more complex system for the purposes of cancer staging,[2] a simplified version is sufficient for the emergency clinician.

Normal and benign reactive cervical lymph nodes typically range in size from 3 to 25 mm.[1] These nodes usually appear as solitary, ovoid nodules with a hypoechoic cortex peripherally and an echogenic medulla that includes the vascular hilum (**Fig. 4**).[3] Reactive lymph nodes are common in the neck, and usually represent a benign response to a systemic or local infection. The more experienced sonologist will notice that they resemble atrophic kidneys. The vascular supply, which coalesces in the hilum, can sometimes be visualized with color or power Doppler, especially in reactive nodes. However, in smaller, nonreactive nodes both the echogenic hilum and flow on Doppler can be difficult to detect. **Fig. 5** and Video 1 show the classic sonographic and Doppler appearance of reactive submandibular nodes.

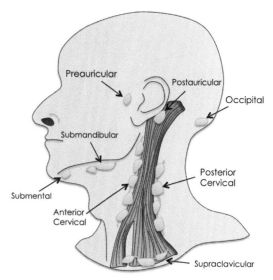

Preauricular
Postauricular
Occipital
Submandibular
Posterior Cervical
Submental
Anterior Cervical
Supraclavicular

Fig. 3. Distribution of commonly visualized superficial cervical lymph nodes.

Salivary Glands

Sonography can be used to visualize the entire submandibular and sublingual salivary glands, and most of the parotid gland. The posteromedial aspect of the parotid lies deep to the mandible, which prevents ultrasonographic examination of this portion. **Fig. 6** illustrates an anatomic overview of the major salivary glands.

The submandibular gland can be readily identified as a well-encapsulated structure in the submandibular fossa. Its parenchyma appears relatively homogeneous and hyperechoic relative to surrounding adipose and muscle tissue. The facial artery and vein can be visualized crossing the parenchyma of this gland. **Fig. 7** shows a normal submandibular gland.

The submandibular duct (Wharton's duct) appears as a hypoechoic, linear structure emerging medially from the gland and coursing deep between the mylohyoid and the hyoglossus muscles toward the sublingual region (**Fig. 8**). It is usually

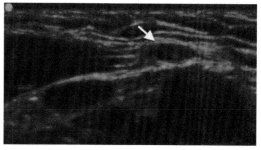

Fig. 4. Normal cervical lymph node (*arrow*) anterior to carotid artery.

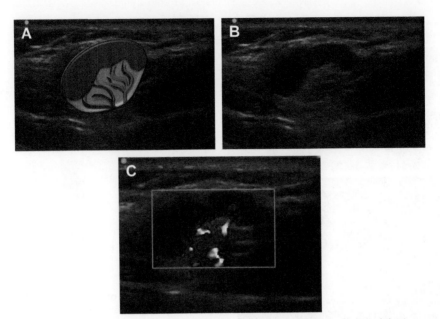

Fig. 5. Reactive submandibular lymph nodes in a patient with ipsilateral facial cellulitis. (*A*) Diagram of reactive submandibular lymph node showing cortex (*dark purple*), medulla (*light purple*), and vascular hilum. (*B*) Coronal image of reactive submandibular node measuring 17 mm in the long axis. (*C*) Color Doppler image showing increased hilar blood flow in this lymph node.

visualized easily in normal individuals, and is best seen in an oblique plane.[4,5]

The parotid gland is located in the retromandibular fossa, wrapping around the ascending ramus of the mandible. It extends from the angle of the mandible superiorly to the external auditory canal, which also serves as its posterior border. The gland projects anteriorly over the mandibular ramus covering the posterior aspect of the masseter muscle. The deep portion of the parotid, which

lies under the mandibular ramus, is obscured by acoustic shadowing from the overlying bone. The parotid is similar in appearance to the submandibular gland with its hyperechoic, uniform texture. The external carotid and retromandibular vein can normally be visualized as vascular structures within the parotid. Small (5–6 mm) lymph nodes within this gland are a normal finding (**Fig. 9**).

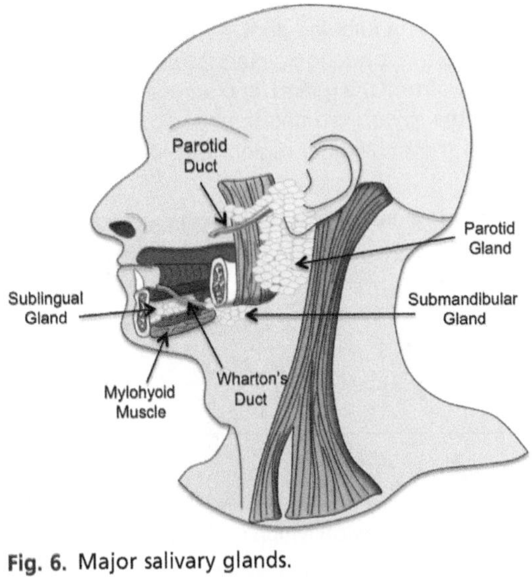

The parotid duct (Stensen's duct) courses over the masseter muscle and then across the buccal muscle before entering the oropharynx at the level of the second upper molar. Unlike Wharton's duct, the parotid duct can be difficult to visualize unless it is pathologically dilated.[4]

The sublingual glands are small and less readily identified, lying adjacent to and between several muscles of the oral cavity floor including the mylohyoid, geniohyoid, genioglossus, and hyoglossus.[4] **Fig. 10** shows the sublingual glands and surrounding anatomy from a coronal view of the submental area.

Thyroid

The thyroid gland is easily visualized by sonography, making this the imaging modality of choice for radiologists and, more recently, for otolaryngologists in the office setting. The gland lies in the midline inferior to the thyroid cartilage, and is composed of right and left lobes and a median isthmus. The posterior surface lies in a semicircle

Fig. 6. Major salivary glands.

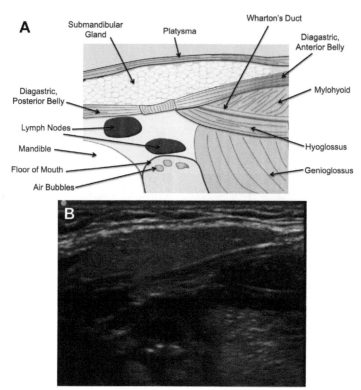

Fig. 7. Normal submandibular gland. (*A*) Diagram. (*B*) Gray-scale image in coronal plane.

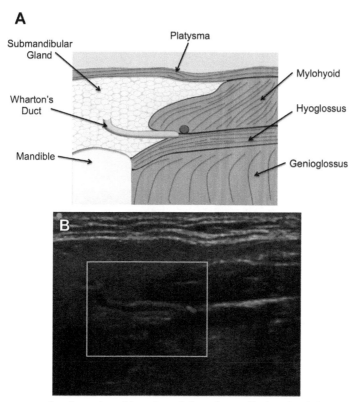

Fig. 8. Wharton's duct emerging from the midportion of the submandibular gland. (*A*) Diagram. (*B*) Gray-scale image with superimposed color Doppler, showing the duct as a nonvascular structure.

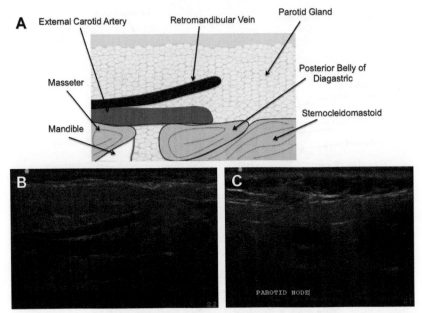

Fig. 9. Parotid overlying mandibular ramus in coronal plane with probe indicator marker pointing upward. (*A*) Diagram. (*B*) Gray-scale image. (*C*) Small lymph node measuring 5 mm within the parenchyma of the parotid gland.

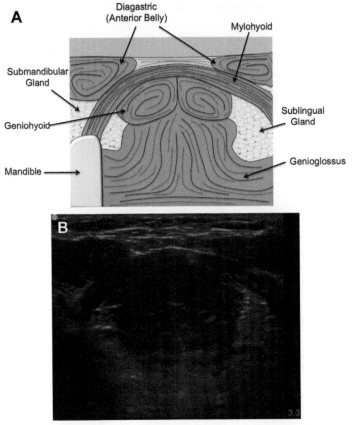

Fig. 10. Submental anatomy including location of sublingual glands. (*A*) Diagram. (*B*) Gray-scale image in coronal plane.

against the inferior larynx and first tracheal rings. The lobes average 4 to 6 cm in cranial-caudal height, with the isthmus averaging 1 to 2 cm in the same dimension. The normal thickness of the lobes is 1 to 2 cm in anterior-posterior diameter. The conical pyramidal lobe is identifiable in some individuals, and projects cranially from the isthmus.[6]

The sonographic appearance of the thyroid is that of a well-encapsulated, homogeneous structure, more hyperechoic in appearance relative to overlying muscle and adipose tissue. The esophagus can usually be visualized lying posterior and medial to the left lobe of the thyroid, and can be identified by its semicircular or ovoid shape and a bull's-eye appearance with a more hyperechoic lumen and less echogenic wall.[6] More inferiorly, the middle thyroid vein can be visualized coursing through each lobe in the axial plain. **Figs. 11** and **12** show normal thyroid anatomy and surrounding structures in the axial plane.

SONOGRAPHY OF THE HEAD AND NECK: PATHOLOGIC CONDITIONS
Soft-Tissue Infections: Cellulitis and Abscess

Although mild cellulitis of the head and neck is often easily recognized clinically without further diagnostic evaluation, any areas of significant swelling and induration should be imaged by the emergency clinician to determine the extent of the infection and the presence or absence of a fluid collection. Clinician-performed ultrasonography is the perfect initial imaging modality in these cases. Investigators have found that when point-of-care sonography is used to evaluate soft-tissue infections in various anatomic locations throughout the body, often those initially thought to be simple cellulitis are found to have a pathologic fluid collection consistent with abscess formation. The contrary case of a clinician suspecting abscess and finding no discernible fluid collection is also a common occurrence.[7–9] **Fig. 13** shows images obtained from a female

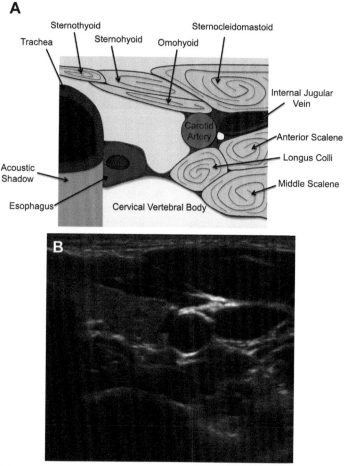

Fig. 11. Left thyroid lobe with esophagus seen between trachea and thyroid at C6 level. (*A*) Diagram. (*B*) Gray-scale axial image at same level.

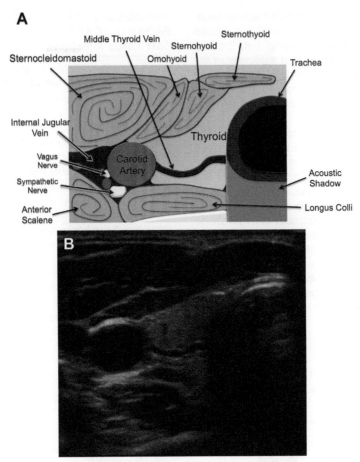

A

Middle Thyroid Vein

Sternothyoid

Sternohyoid

Sternocleidomastoid

Omohyoid

Trachea

Internal Jugular Vein

Thyroid

Vagus Nerve

Carotid Artery

Acoustic Shadow

Sympathetic Nerve

Anterior Scalene

Longus Colli

B

Fig. 12. Inferior aspect of the right lobe of thyroid, showing the middle thyroid vein. (*A*) Diagram. (*B*) Gray-scale axial image at same level.

patient with significant induration and pain to her left cheek. The clinician caring for the patient was concerned she might have an abscess. Point-of-care sonography led to findings consistent with simple cellulitis including thickened subcutaneous tissue, increased echogenicity, and loss of normal tissue plans, but no discernible fluid collection. **Fig. 14** illustrates a similar case whereby clinician-performed sonography revealed an anechoic fluid collection with posterior acoustic enhancement consistent with abscess formation. Incision and drainage confirmed these findings.

The evaluation for an abscess in the head and neck region is complicated by both the density of vital organs in this area and the diversity of structures including major vasculature, lymph nodes, salivary glands, and the thyroid. The sonologist should have an understanding of basic neck anatomy as described earlier, taking note of surrounding structures during the examination. The sonologist should slowly and systematically evaluate the lesion in two orthogonal planes using color Doppler to identify vascular structures. As a general rule, it is important to be aware that inflammatory and malignant conditions of both lymph nodes and salivary glands can mimic abscesses. Familiarity with those conditions as described in subsequent sections is also important.

In addition, congenital cystic structures can also become infected and should be considered in the differential diagnosis when a fluid-filled structure is visualized in the neck. **Fig. 15** shows the normal anatomic distribution of common cystic structures found in the neck.

Fig. 16 and Video 2 demonstrate imaging of an infected thyroglossal duct cyst obtained by a clinician sonographer. If there is any concern that an infected congenital cyst is present, surgical consultation should be accessed.

Peritonsillar Abscess

The palatine tonsils are located in the posterior pharynx, between the anterior and posterior

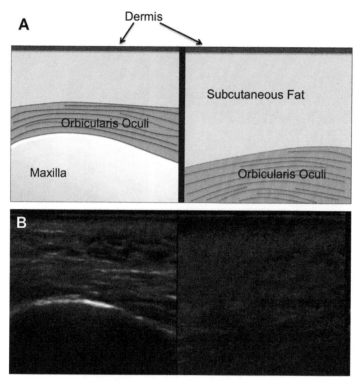

Fig. 13. Cheek cellulitis: side-by-side axial images obtained just below the zygoma on affected side and contra-lateral side. (*A*) Diagram. (*B*) Gray-scale images.

tonsillar pillars formed primarily by the folds of the glossopalatine and pharyngopalatine muscles (**Fig. 17**). Each tonsil is surrounded by a capsule, a remnant of embryologic development. Adjacent to this capsule lies a potential space through which nerves, blood vessels, and lymphatics course, and where peritonsillar cellulitis and abscess formation typically occurs.

Peritonsillar abscess (PTA) can represent a diagnostic and therapeutic challenge for the emergency clinician. PTA can be diagnosed clinically in a patient with pharyngitis who complains of unilateral throat pain and whose oropharyngeal examination reveals bulging of the soft palate with lateral deviation of the uvula. Patients with PTA are classically described as having varying degrees of trismus and drooling, and often will have a fetid, rancid odor to the breath with a muffled

Fig. 14. Gray-scale axial image of a simple cheek abscess.

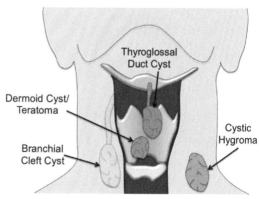

Fig. 15. Common cystic structures in the anterior cervical region.

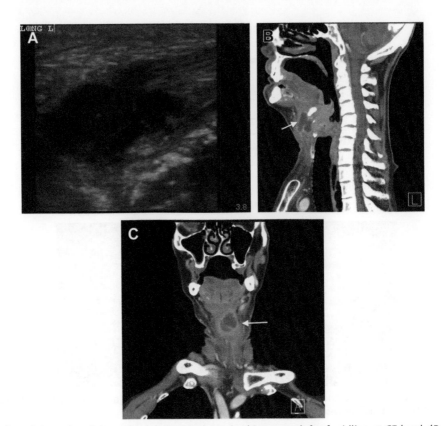

Fig. 16. Infected thyroglossal duct cyst. (*A*) Gray-scale sagittal image to left of midline at C5 level. (*B, C*) Sagittal and coronal computed tomography images of fluid-filled cyst (*arrows*). (*Courtesy of* T. Cook, MD, Palmetto Health Richland, Columbia, SC.)

voice. However, many of these symptoms can be seen in peritonsillar cellulitis (PTC) as well, which exists in a spectrum with PTA, often preceding the development of an abscess.

Without imaging, distinguishing between PTA and PTC requires needle aspiration or scalpel incision of the area of concern. If purulent debris is found, further drainage is performed and the

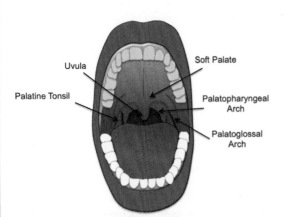

Fig. 17. Regional anatomy of palatine tonsils.

abscess contents evacuated. If no purulent debris is obtained, the patient is prescribed antibiotics and analgesics, and treated as having PTC. As with any aspiration procedure, using this technique to confirm the presence of abscess exposes the patient to risk of injury to surrounding structures in addition to the associated discomfort. The development and increasing use of CT has enabled the clinician to obtain imaging of the posterior pharynx to evaluate for PTA. The presence of a rim-enhancing lesion with central fluid collection on CT can confirm PTA, and limit the risks and discomfort of the procedure to only those patients with fluid collections amenable to drainage. However, CT exposes the patient to ionizing radiation and contrast agents, and is expensive. It also does not allow the clinician performing the drainage to directly visualize the fluid collection during the clinical examination, nor does CT provide any opportunity for dynamic visualization of the intervention.

Clinician-performed sonography has increasingly been used for the bedside diagnosis of PTA versus PTC. First described in the emergency medicine literature in 2003,[10] a recent randomized trial of 28 patients undergoing PTA drainage demonstrated that aspiration performed in conjunction with diagnostic intraoral ultrasonography performed by emergency physicians with basic training in emergency sonography had an overall success rate of 100% (95% confidence interval [CI] = 63%–100%) compared with 50% (95% CI = 24%–76%) using the traditional landmark-based, needle-aspiration approach.[11] This study used a static needle-aspiration approach after identifying the center and depth of the PTA and the relationship of the abscess to the carotid artery. Another prospective study of 14 patients comparing ultrasonography, CT, and clinical examination for the diagnosis of PTA found sensitivities of 89% for ultrasonography, 100% for CT, and 78% for clinical examination. Specificities were 100%, 75%, and 50%, respectively.[12]

Intraoral sonography of the posterior pharynx is performed with a clean endocavitary probe, which is covered by a glove or other nonsterile barrier. A small amount of gel should be placed on the footprint before covering the probe. Additional gel for sound wave transduction is not needed, as the saliva within the mouth is sufficient. Although some studies have reported that intraoral anesthesia is not required to obtain adequate images, intraoral scanning is greatly facilitated by topical anesthesia to decrease patient discomfort and diminish the gag reflex. Anesthesia can easily be accomplished by intraoral nebulization of an amide anesthetic such as lidocaine, or directly spraying the posterior pharynx with a mucosal atomizing device.

Once the patient is appropriately anesthetized, the covered endocavitary probe is inserted into the oropharynx, usually in a transverse orientation with the probe marker oriented to the patient's right. Once sufficient contact is made with the transducer footprint, the structures of the posterior pharynx are easily visualized. Color flow Doppler should be used to identify vascular structures within this area. A PTA will appear as a hypoechoic, often heterogeneous, fluid collection (**Fig. 18**). Peritonsillar cellulitis will have a more homogeneous appearance without a discrete fluid collection (**Fig. 19**). The internal carotid artery is identified by its anechoic ovoid shape posterolateral to the tonsil, and exhibits pulsatile flow on color flow or power Doppler (see **Fig. 18**). See also Videos 3 and 4 for a comparison of an abscess (see Video 3) with a normal palatine tonsil (see Video 4).

Ultrasound-guided needle aspiration can be accomplished using static or dynamic techniques. For the static technique, measure the depth of the

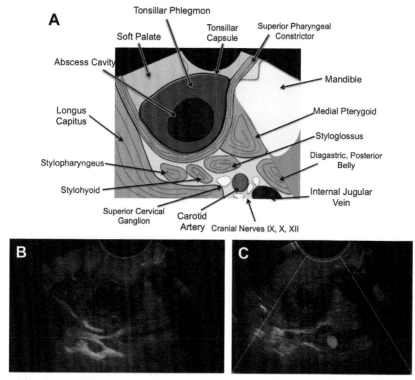

Fig. 18. Peritonsillar abscess (PTA) confirmed by aspiration of pus. (*A*) Diagram. (*B*) Gray-scale image in transverse plane. (*C*) Gray-scale image in transverse plane with color Doppler, showing internal carotid artery.

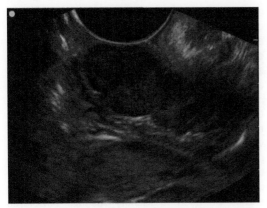

Fig. 19. Clinician-performed sonography obtained on a patient with 2 days of pharyngitis and a clinical examination concerning for PTA, with a bulging soft palate and uvular deviation. Gray-scale image in the sagittal plane shows an enlarged, hypoechoic palatine tonsil without a discrete fluid collection. Based on clinical examination, otolaryngology attempted both needle aspiration and incision and drainage without obtaining purulent fluid. The patient was placed on antibiotics with resolution of peritonsillar cellulitis.

most superficial aspect of the abscess and identify the area of greatest diameter. Measure also the depth of the carotid artery at this location. Using these measurements as a guide, the proceduralist can trim the needle guard of an 18-gauge needle to allow for just enough needle length to penetrate the abscess cavity while avoiding the underlying carotid artery (**Fig. 20**). The needle is then inserted at the site where the measurements were made using the same trajectory as the ultrasound probe.

Alternatively, a dynamic approach can be used to visualize the procedure under direct ultrasound guidance. Once the abscess and surrounding structures have been identified by ultrasound, an 18-gauge needle can be inserted medial to the probe with the tip advanced laterally into the tissues of the soft palate (**Fig. 21**). A trimmed needle guard can be used to prevent overinsertion, similar to the technique for static aspiration (see **Fig. 20**). Once the tip is inserted into the superficial tissues, it should be identified on the ultrasound screen and then advanced into the abscess cavity. In addition to localization of the cavity under ultrasound guidance, the dynamic technique has the added benefit of visualizing evacuation of the abscess contents (Video 5). The dynamic approach should be used whenever possible because of its multiple advantages.

As with any dynamic, ultrasound-guided procedure, it is important that the needle tip is visualized throughout the entire procedure to avoid inadvertent damage to the surrounding structures. The dynamic technique can be more difficult, primarily because of trismus, which limits mouth opening and space for both the probe and needle; however, the real-time guidance of the needle and visualization of surrounding structures has the potential to minimize complications.

Cervical Node Pathology

The basic task of the sonologist should be to recognize the sonographic appearance of normal reactive lymph nodes as well as that of lymphadenitis. In addition, the clinician should be aware of the broad differential of both cervical lymphadenopathy and the overlap between inflammatory nodes and other pathologic conditions including lymphoma.

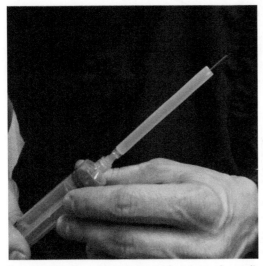

Fig. 20. Needle and syringe with trimmed needle guard.

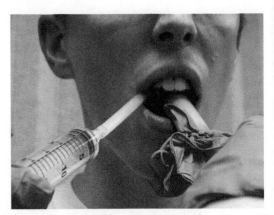

Fig. 21. Dynamic drainage of PTA under ultrasound guidance. Demonstration of relative position of probe and needle during procedure.

Reactive nodes are common in the neck secondary to both local and systemic infections, although they are usually small in size (<2.5 cm) and only mildly painful and palpable. These nodes are often located bilaterally and are usually associated with a viral process or local infection. The inflammation is self-limited, although the lymphadenopathy can persist for several weeks after the resolution of the associated infection. **Fig. 22** shows a normal sonographic appearance and size of a reactive cervical lymph node.

The term lymphadenitis, which literally means "inflamed lymph node," technically can be used interchangeably to describe reactive lymph nodes. However, clinicians typically reserve this term for more clinically obvious, unilateral tender lymphadenopathy with visible swelling believed to be caused by markedly inflamed lymph node(s). This condition is often associated with fever and suppuration.

Although lymphadenitis is found in adult patients, it is far more common in the pediatric population and, thus, most data on the etiology and treatment is found in the pediatric literature. For acute pediatric lymphadenitis in younger children, most investigators cite older studies that demonstrate the causative bacterial agent to be *Staphylococcus aureus* or streptococci, primarily *Streptococcus pyogenes* (group A) or *Streptococcus agalactiae* (group B) species in 40% to 80%, with most other cases being viral.[13,14] More recently, community-acquired methicillin-resistant *S aureus* (MRSA) has emerged as a possible agent.[15] In older children the possible infectious agents are broader

with the addition of anaerobic bacteria, mononucleosis, toxoplasmosis, *Bartonella henselae* (cat-scratch disease), tuberculosis, and nontuberculous mycobacteria. A thoughtful patient history will aid in narrowing the differential diagnosis. Limited data exist for causative agents in adults, but similar to pediatric cases, initial antibiotic therapy should target the most common head and neck bacterial pathogens (*S aureus*, *Streptococcus* species, and anaerobes) unless patient history suggests another causative agent. Although most cases secondary to an infectious cause will resolve with, or even without, antibiotic treatment, a small percentage may require surgical drainage despite a trial of antibiotic therapy.

The sonographic appearance of lymphadenitis is that of either solitary or multiple enlarged (usually >2.5 cm) hypoechoic, rounded structure(s) with a hyperechoic, vascular hilum that has a stalk-like appearance within the lymph node(s). The involved node(s) will usually have increased through transmission, so posterior acoustic enhancement should be seen. Color Doppler will readily show flow through the vascular hilum. **Fig. 23** and Video 6 demonstrate imaging from a case of cervical lymphadenitis. An important point is that the sonographic findings of lymphadenitis are often indistinguishable from lymphomatous nodes in patients with lymphoma.[16] Compare the images from the lymphadenitis case with those of **Fig. 24** and Video 7, which show images obtained from an adult ED patient who presented with tender cervical lymphadenopathy and was later found to have lymphoma on biopsy. These images have a similar sonographic appearance. Thus, one cannot exclude lymphomatous from reactive lymph nodes based on sonographic

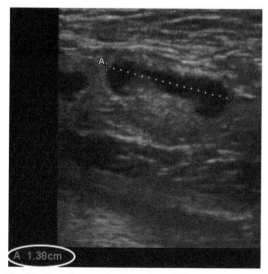

Fig. 22. Reactive cervical lymph node in a patient with a peritonsillar abscess, showing a normal size and appearance.

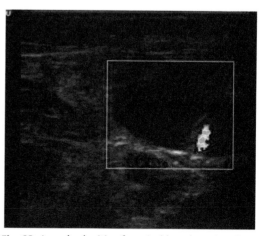

Fig. 23. Lymphadenitis of cervical lymph nodes. Grayscale image with color Doppler showing flow in vascular pedicle of lymph node.

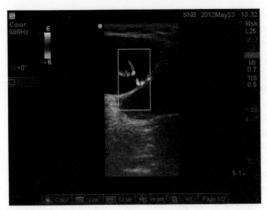

Fig. 24. Lymphomatous cervical lymph node showing a gray-scale and color Doppler appearance similar to that of the cervical lymphadenitis shown in **Fig. 23**. Gray-scale image with color Doppler.

appearance alone. Patients who are suspected of having lymphadenitis and who fail to improve with antibiotics should be referred for biopsy.

Most cases of pediatric cervical lymphadenopathy are secondary to an infectious cause. However, the likelihood that enlarged cervical lymph nodes are due to a malignant process increases significantly with increasing age.[17] Although all patients with lymphadenitis, regardless of age, should be followed up to ensure resolution of lymphadenopathy, the importance of this cannot be overemphasized in the adult patient.

It is also important to recognize that there is considerable overlap in the sonographic appearance of inflammatory and infected lymph nodes with that of abscesses and infected cysts. Nodes may mimic fluid-filled structures by appearing anechoic and demonstrating posterior acoustic enhancement. When imaging what appears to be a fluid-filled structure, the clinician sonographer should look for a hyperechoic vascular hilum on gray-scale imaging and use color Doppler to demonstrate flow in this area. These findings will help to identify this structure as a lymph node. Consideration of additional imaging is prudent if the cause is not clear based on clinical and sonographic findings.

In the case of reactive cervical lymph nodes and lymphadenitis, the patient usually complains of an area of swelling associated with pain or tenderness; however, emergency clinicians are sometimes called on to evaluate patients who present with a nonpainful cervical mass of variable chronicity. Often, many of these patients present to the ED because of fear that they may have a malignancy. A significant number are unable to obtain timely appointments in a primary care setting for evaluation and more definitive testing. In younger

adults, some of these cases may involve benign congenital cysts or other benign growths that have recently increased in size and have become noticeable to the patient.

However, many nontender cervical masses are caused by enlarged lymph nodes, and in the adult patient a malignant process is at the top of the differential, especially if such enlarged nodes have been slowly increasing in size and/or are located in the supraclavicular region.[17] The sonographic features suggestive of metastatic cervical lymph nodes include a more rounded shape with heterogeneous parenchyma. There is often an absence of the echogenic hilum, but they have notable capsular vascularity. These nodes may also show microcalcifications, a cystic component, and indentation of the jugular vein. Most metastatic nodes appear well encapsulated with regular borders, although this feature alone is not reliable as there is considerable overlap with benign processes.[18,19]

Tuberculous nodes deserve special mention because these can resemble malignant nodes, but can often be distinguished from malignant nodes by the presence of surrounding soft-tissue edema and matting.[18]

In summary, although the age of the patient, clinical presentation, and sonographic features can be helpful in determining the causes of cervical lymphadenopathy, the distinction between benign and malignant cervical lymph nodes can be difficult and is beyond the scope of the emergency sonographer. With this in mind, all patients with lymphadenopathy need follow-up with a primary care provider who can ensure resolution or arrange referral for additional testing as indicated.

Dental Abscesses

Dental pulp infections that result in abscess formation usually spread into the vestibular space, which is appreciated clinically by fluctuance overlying the apical area of the involved tooth. These infections can be associated with soft-tissue swelling of the face or neck when involving maxillary and mandibular teeth, respectively. However, the abscess itself is usually localized to the oral cavity, and readily appreciated during the clinical examination and/or Panorex imaging.[20]

In some cases, the abscess can erode either above or below the attachments of the buccinator muscle. These abscesses can be appreciated clinically as swelling, tenderness, and fluctuance either anterior to the maxilla below the zygomatic arch or above the inferior border of the mandible.[20] Sonographic evaluation of these areas of swelling will demonstrate a fluid collection consistent with abscess. Clinical history and examination should reveal an odontogenic source of the infection. These infections are normally treated with simple incision and drainage by a qualified clinician, appropriate antibiotics covering dental flora, and admission or close outpatient follow-up depending on the extent of the associated cellulitis and comorbidities.

The emergency clinician will recognize, however, that when a dental abscess spreads into the sublingual and submandibular spaces involving the tissues on the floor of the mouth, this represents a head and neck emergency. This condition, commonly referred to as Ludwig's angina, can result in elevation of the tongue and airway obstruction. **Fig. 25** and Video 8 show a case of Ludwig's angina demonstrated by point-of-care sonography. If this condition is found or suspected, emergent surgical consultation should be obtained. The astute clinician will also recognize that submandibular or sublingual salivary gland inflammation and/or infection secondary an obstructing stone can mimic Ludwig's angina. Clinician-performed sonography of both the submandibular and submental areas may help in differentiating these two clinical entities (see **Fig. 25C**).

Salivary Glands

In patients presenting with pain and swelling in the area of a major salivary gland, point-of-care sonography should be performed to evaluate the salivary gland and surrounding structures. Akin to a sonographic Murphy's sign, clinician-performed sonography can quickly provide additional information beyond the physical examination to localize the origin of pain and swelling more definitively to the salivary gland. This imaging confirmation enables the provider to focus the differential on diseases that cause salivary gland inflammation.

Salivary gland inflammation, referred to as sialoadenitis, is classified as obstructive and nonobstructive. The obstructive form is usually caused by salivary stones (sialolithiasis), which most commonly occur in the submandibular gland (80%), with the parotid gland affected less commonly (20%)[4] and the sublingual glands rarely affected.[21,22] Predisposing factors include dehydration, medications that decrease salivation,

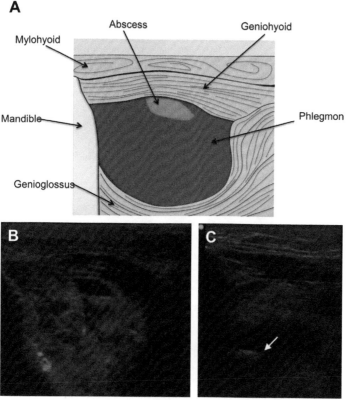

Fig. 25. Ludwig angina with soft-tissue swelling and fluid collection in submental space. Images obtained of the submental space in sagittal plane to the right of midline. (*A*) Diagram. (*B*) Gray-scale image. (*C*) Sagittal gray-scale image obtained from patient with submental swelling, showing submandibular sialolithiasis (*arrow*).

and medical conditions such as disorders of calcium metabolism or Sjögren syndrome. Stones can often cause recurrent symptoms of pain and inflammation of the affected gland around meals secondary to the stimulation of salivary flow, so patients should be queried about prior episodes. In vaccinated adults, sialolithiasis is believed to be the most common disease of the salivary glands.[22,23] In cases of a unilateral, painful swelling in the region of the submandibular gland or parotid gland, the sonologist should first attempt to identify an obstructing stone and dilated, associated salivary ducts as the cause of the symptoms.

Salivary stones appear as hyperechoic lines with posterior acoustic shadowing within a dilated salivary duct. Fig. 26 illustrates a case of sialolithiasis involving the submandibular gland. When performing sonography to evaluate for sialolithiasis, applying additional pressure from inside the oral cavity can aid in visualization.[4] Stones smaller than 2 to 3 mm can be more difficult to identify because they are less likely to cause acoustic

shadowing, although this is less problematic when using newer-generation machines with improved resolution capabilities. Another pitfall is the presence of hyperechoic air bubbles on the floor of the mouth, which may mimic stones.[4] No data exist regarding the test characteristics of clinician-performed sonography in identifying salivary stones in the literature. However, one radiology study from the 1980s found sensitivity of 94% and specificity of 100% with stones identified in 174 of 188 patients with symptomatic sialolithiasis.[21] As with all sonographic studies, sensitivity is limited by operator experience and capabilities; however, the current resolution of most bedside machines equals or exceeds that of the radiology-based machines used during the time period of this study.

Mild sialoadenitis, with or without the identification of small stones, can usually be treated with hydration and massage of the gland as well as sialagogues to increase the flow of saliva. The addition of antibiotics is common practice, as this condition is often complicated by infection with

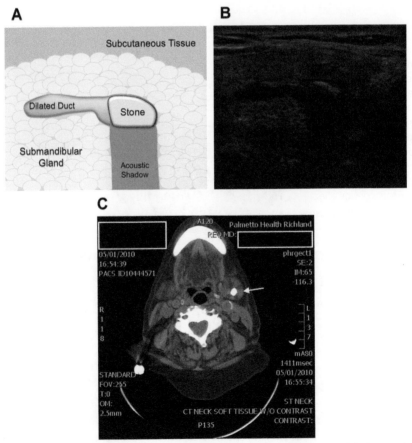

Fig. 26. Obstructing sialolith in the submandibular (Wharton) duct. (*A*) Diagram. (*B*) Gray-scale axial image. (*C*) Computed tomography slice in axial plane showing a stone (*arrow*).

oral flora. Larger stones, especially those causing significant symptoms or complicated by infection, require consultation and removal by a specialist.

Depending on the clinical presentation and the patient's medical history, the etiology of nonobstructive sialoadenitis is broad and includes localized and systemic infection, inflammatory and autoimmune diseases, and malignancy. The nonobstructive form often has a unique sonographic appearance of glandular enlargement and loss of the normal uniform, hyperechoic texture. The parenchyma appears more hypoechoic and heterogeneous with increased Doppler blood flow. The inflamed gland can also contain multiple small, oval, hypoechoic areas without posterior acoustic enhancement (pseudocysts), and enlarged lymph nodes are often visualized within the inflamed glands.[5,24] **Fig. 27** shows the typical sonographic appearance of nonobstructive sialoadenitis of the submandibular gland.

Thyroid

Although many patients in the ED have either a history of thyroid disease or acute complaints that could be related to thyroid gland dysfunction, imaging of this gland acutely is rarely indicated on an emergency basis. However, there are several circumstances whereby the emergency clinician may perform point-of-care sonography of this gland, and recognition of the sonographic appearance of different pathologic conditions can aid in directing clinical care and follow-up treatment.

One emergent presentation whereby clinician-performed thyroid imaging may be helpful is if the patient presents with the signs and symptoms of thyrotoxicosis or thyroid storm. Often, these patients will have clinical presentations that mimic those of other emergency medical conditions, for example, systemic infection or a sympathomimetic toxidrome. The clinician must have a high clinical suspicion to recognize this relatively uncommon condition, especially because the treatment differs markedly from the diseases it mimics and can be associated with significant morbidity and mortality, especially without early recognition and appropriate treatment.[25] Although a thorough physical examination usually discovers an enlarged thyroid, this is not always the case; moreover, the clinical examination can be limited by body habitus and physician inexperience with this particular examination. The most common cause of thyrotoxicosis in areas with adequate iodine supplementation is Graves disease (80% of cases).[26] Thyroid ultrasonography of this condition typically reveals an enlarged thyroid with more heterogeneous and hypoechoic appearance than normal thyroid tissue. Color Doppler shows a marked increase in flow (Videos 9–11).[27–30]

Another instance in which clinician-performed thyroid sonography can be helpful is if the patient complains of anterior neck pain with or without dysphagia. The astute clinician will recognize that this is a common presentation of a relatively uncommon condition, acute thyroiditis. Often these patients will have stable vitals and may not have clinically apparent thyroid disease, because thyroiditis can be associated with normal thyroid hormone levels. Careful physical examination in thinner patients usually enables the clinician to localize the area of pain to the thyroid gland. In patients with a larger body habitus, however, the physical examination can be more limited. In the case of acute thyroiditis, sonography of the involved area allows the emergency provider to localize the area of tenderness to the thyroid. Although some variation exists in the Doppler flow associated with thyroiditis, the gray-scale sonographic appearance is similar to that of Graves disease shown in Videos 9–11.[30] Determining the exact cause of thyroiditis is beyond the scope of the emergency provider, but basic laboratory evaluation including thyroid function tests should be obtained, and close follow-up arranged with an endocrinologist or primary care provider.

In these clinical scenarios the patient is presenting with symptoms that point the clinician toward considering diseases of the thyroid as the cause. However, the sonologist may also encounter thyroid abnormalities incidentally, particularly when performing surveillance for placement of a central venous line in the neck. In these cases, knowledge of the normal sonographic appearance of the thyroid and examples of abnormal findings enables the provider to advise the patient of the incidental finding and the need to be followed up for more definitive testing. Thyroid nodules are

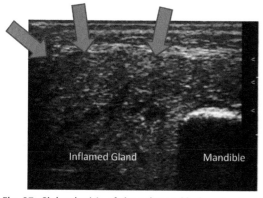

Fig. 27. Sialoadenitis of the submandibular gland.

very common, with one autopsy study from the Mayo Clinic in 1955 demonstrating thyroid nodules in 50.5% of consecutive patients who had clinically normal thyroid glands.[31] More recent population radiology studies from the 1990s using high-resolution ultrasonography report a wide variation in incidence, with nodules occurring in 15% to 72% of normal subjects, the highest prevalence being in older, female patients.[32] **Fig. 28** and Video 12 demonstrate an example of a cystic thyroid nodule found in an ED patient complaining of mild dysphagia. Distinguishing between benign and malignant lesions of the thyroid with ultrasonographic imaging is challenging, even for the most experienced sonographers.[30,33] Of note, the size of the nodule cannot be used to determine the risk for malignancy.[34] All patients with the incidental finding of abnormal thyroid appearance or nodule(s) should be followed up for additional testing.

Internal Jugular Thrombosis

Internal jugular thrombosis has a wide variety of presentations, from an asymptomatic, incidental finding in a patient undergoing surveillance for ultrasound-guided central venous catheter placement to septic thrombophlebitis with distal septic emboli (Lemierre's syndrome). The incidence of deep venous thrombosis (DVT) in this location is less frequent than that reported in the lower extremities.[35] The true incidence is likely underestimated, as this area is not typically evaluated for the source thrombus in patients with pulmonary emboli unless they complain of localizing symptoms or have specific risk factors, such as an upper extremity catheter.

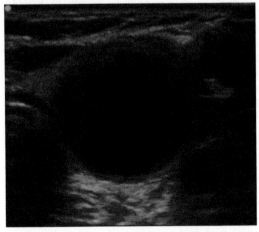

Fig. 28. Point-of-care sonography performed in the emergency department (ED) on a patient complaining of mild dysphagia, showing a complex thyroid nodule. Gray-scale axial image.

Risk factors for internal jugular thrombosis include those typically associated with all DVTs: malignancy, thrombophilia, central venous catheter (particularly dialysis catheters[36]), and, less commonly, pregnancy or use of exogenous estrogens. Other unique risk factors include intravenous drug abuse and neck surgery or trauma.[37,38]

In addition to hypercoagulability and stasis, Virchow's triad also includes endothelial injury from infection or inflammation. Thus, another major risk factor is any head and neck infection in close proximity to the internal jugular vein. When the infection spreads into the internal jugular vein, a septic thrombophlebitis develops. Usually the associated infection is pharyngitis with local extension, but this condition has also been reported with otitis, mastoiditis, dental infections, sinusitis, and parotitis.[39,40] If patients with thrombophlebitis of the internal jugular also have evidence of distal septic emboli, particularly pulmonary or joint involvement, they meet the clinical criteria for having Lemierre's syndrome. This entity was first well described by André Lemierre in a case series of 20 patients published in the *Lancet* in 1936.[41,42] In the postantibiotic era, this syndrome is less common and often overlooked, although more recently there has been a resurgence of case reports in the literature.[39,43–45] The most common causative agent identified is *Fusobacterium necrophorum*.[42] Less commonly, the infection can be caused by gram-negative bacteria or MRSA. Treatment includes anticoagulation and broad-spectrum antibiotics including appropriate coverage for *F necrophorum*.

Internal jugular thrombosis is readily identified by sonologists, especially those already familiar with lower extremity DVT studies and the anatomy associated with placing ultrasound-guided internal jugular catheters. With the increasing utilization of clinician-performed ultrasonography, internal jugular thrombosis and Lemierre's syndrome are being diagnosed in a more expedited fashion by emergency providers.[46–48]

The sonologist should consider evaluation for internal jugular thrombosis in any patient with anterior neck pain and/or swelling, particularly those with the risk factors and the clinical symptoms already described. The sonographer should follow and compress the internal jugular vein along its entire course in the neck in the axial plane. The sonographic findings of thrombosis include a noncompressible vein with or without internal echoes, depending on the age of the clot. Color flow will aid in the identification of vascular structures, but may be absent if the involved vessel is completely occluded. **Fig. 29** and Videos 13 and 14 are axial still images and videos of an internal

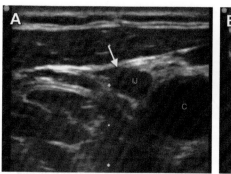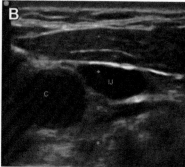

Fig. 29. Images obtained from a female dialysis patient with a tunneled right internal jugular catheter who presented to the ED complaining of neck pain and fever. Clinician-performed ultrasonography showed right internal jugular thrombosis, but clinical examination and ancillary testing did not show evidence of distal septic emboli; therefore, she did not meet criteria for Lemierre syndrome. Her symptoms resolved with anticoagulation and antibiotics. She is asymptomatic and has not required removal of her catheter at 6 months' follow-up. (A) Gray-scale axial image to the right of midline showing an occluded, noncompressible right internal jugular thrombus (arrow). (B) Contralateral side on same patient with normal-appearing internal jugular vein. C, common carotid; IJ, internal jugular.

jugular thrombosis and the normal contralateral side.

Acute Sinusitis

Sinusitis, also referred to as rhinosinusitis, is one of the most common health problems for which Americans seek medical attention. Most cases are attributed to viral infections associated with the common cold, and resolve within 7 to 10 days.[49–51] In patients presenting for care in the ED, the challenge lies in distinguishing between viral and bacterial sinusitis and the appropriate prescribing of antibiotics when indicated.

Multiple different societies have made recommendations regarding clinical criteria to accurately differentiate between these two groups of patients. In 2012, the Infectious Disease Society of America published evidence-based guidelines for the diagnosis and management of acute bacterial rhinosinusitis.[52] Criteria for diagnosis include: (1) persistent symptoms without improvement greater than or equal to 10 days; (2) severe symptoms for 3 to 4 days; or (3) worsening symptoms after 3 to 4 days.

Plain radiographs, CT, and magnetic resonance imaging (MRI) have all been used extensively in evaluating this disease. In cases of acute rhinosinusitis, each of these modalities often show significant abnormalities, but the findings associated with viral infections are indistinguishable from those associated with bacterial infection.[52] Given the limitations as well as the cost, radiation, and time involved in obtaining these imaging studies, imaging with these modalities is rarely indicated

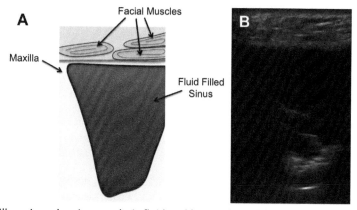

Fig. 30. Right maxillary sinus showing anechoic fluid and hyperechoic debris, and visualization of the posterior wall of the maxillary sinus. (A) Diagram. (B) Gray-scale axial image with probe overlying maxillary sinus inferior to orbital rim.

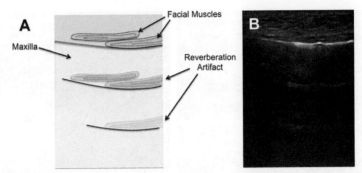

Fig. 31. Normal right maxillary sinus with reverberation artifact deep to the anterior wall and no visualization of the posterior wall. (*A*) Diagram. (*B*) Gray-scale axial image with probe overlying maxillary sinus inferior to orbital rim.

for the evaluation of an ED patient with symptoms of uncomplicated rhinosinusitis.

Several investigators have investigated the utility of ultrasonography in determining the presence or absence of fluid in the maxillary sinuses to aid in the diagnosis of acute sinusitis.[53–57] Ultrasonography has the same limitations as the other imaging modalities, in that the sonographic finding of fluid in the maxillary sinus(es) does not aid the clinician in distinguishing between a viral or bacterial cause. However, unlike the other modalities, clinician-performed ultrasonography is rapid, noninvasive, and does not expose the patient to ionizing radiation. In 2000, Puhakka and colleagues[56] specifically evaluated the sensitivity and specificity of ultrasonography for the detection of maxillary sinusitis in a comparison with MRI, and found that whereas the sensitivity was relatively low at 64%, the specificity was 95%. Because ultrasonography rarely yielded false-positive results, the investigators concluded that this modality could be used to rule in maxillary sinusitis. Given the low sensitivity of ultrasonography in this study, it was also recommended that if the clinician still had a strong clinical suspicion for sinusitis, a single plain radiograph could be added to increase sensitivity.[56]

Point-of-care sonography of the maxillary sinuses is easy to perform using a high-frequency linear array or microconvex probe. Imaging should be done with the patient in the supine position, the probe held in an axial plane, with the transducer overlying the maxillary sinus immediately below the inferior orbital rim.

In the normal air-filled sinus, the posterior wall of the maxilla cannot be seen because of the attenuation of the ultrasound beam. However, reverberation artifact can be seen if enough depth is used. If enough fluid is present to fill the sinus and reach the anterior wall of the maxilla, through-

transmission of the ultrasound beam will allow partial or complete visualization of the posterior sinus wall. **Fig. 30** shows the presence of fluid in the right maxillary sinus in an ED patient presenting with 8 days of congestion, maxillary pain, and fever without improvement. **Fig. 31** displays sonographic findings when a gray-scale image is obtained overlying a normal, aerated maxillary sinus.

SUPPLEMENTARY DATA

Videos related to this article can be found online at http://dx.doi.org/10.1016/j.cult.2014.01.004.

REFERENCES

1. Ying M, Ahuja A. Sonography of neck lymph nodes. Part I: normal lymph nodes. Clin Radiol 2003;58(5):351–8.
2. Lenghel LM. Ultrasonographic identification of the anatomical landmarks that define cervical lymph nodes spaces. Med Ultrason 2013;15(1):29–34.
3. Dudea SM, Lenghel M, Botar-Jid C, et al. Ultrasonography of cervical lymph nodes: benign vs. malignant. Med Ultrason 2012;14(4):294–306.
4. Bialek EJ, Jakubowski W, Zajkowski P, et al. US of the major salivary glands: anatomy and spatial relationships, pathologic conditions, and pitfalls. Radiographics 2006;26(3):745–63.
5. Ching AS, Ahuja AT, King AD, et al. Comparison of the sonographic features of acalculous and calculous submandibular sialadenitis. J Clin Ultrasound 2001;29(6):332–8.
6. Som PM, Curtin HD. Head and neck imaging. In: Chapter 41. 5th edition. St. Louis, MO: Mosby, Inc; 2011. p. 2611–77.
7. Adhikari S, Blaivas M. Sonography first for subcutaneous abscess and cellulitis evaluation. J Ultrasound Med 2012;31(10):1509–12.
8. Squire BT, Fox JC, Anderson C. ABSCESS: applied bedside sonography for convenient evaluation of

superficial soft tissue infections. Acad Emerg Med 2005;12(7):601–6.

9. Tayal V, Hasan N, Norton H, et al. The effect of soft-tissue ultrasound on the management of cellulitis in the emergency department. Acad Emerg Med 2006;13(4):384–8.

10. Blaivas M, Theodoro D, Duggal S. Ultrasound-guided drainage of peritonsillar abscess by the emergency physician. Am J Emerg Med 2003;21(2):155–8.

11. Costantino TG, Satz WA, Dehnkamp W, et al. Randomized trial comparing intraoral ultrasound to landmark-based needle aspiration in patients with suspected peritonsillar abscess: intraoral US for peritonsillar abscess: randomized trial. Acad Emerg Med 2012;19(6):626–31.

12. Scott PM, Loftus WK, Kew J, et al. Diagnosis of peritonsillar infections: a prospective study of ultrasound, computerized tomography and clinical diagnosis. J Laryngol Otol 1999;113(3):229–32.

13. Leung AK, Davies HD. Cervical lymphadenitis: etiology, diagnosis, and management. Curr Infect Dis Rep 2009;11(3):183–9.

14. Peters TR, Edwards KM. Cervical lymphadenopathy and adenitis. Pediatr Rev 2000;21(12):399–405.

15. Thorell EA, Long SS, Pickering LK, et al. Cervical lymphadenitis and neck infections. In: Long SS, editor. Pinciples and practice of pediatric infectious diseases. 4th edition. Philadelphia: Elsevier; 2012. p. 135–47.

16. Giovagnorio F, Galluzzo M, Andreoli C, et al. Color Doppler sonography in the evaluation of superficial lymphomatous lymph nodes. J Ultrasound Med 2002;21(4):403–8.

17. Chen A, Otto KJ. Differential diagnosis of neck masses. In: Flint PW, Haughey BH, editors. Cummings otolaryngology, head and neck surgery. 5th edition. Philadelphia: Mosby, Inc affiliate of Elsevier, Inc; 2010. p. 1636–43.

18. Ahuja A, Ying M. An overview of neck node sonography. Invest Radiol 2002;37(6):333–42.

19. Vaysberg M, Steward DL. Ultrasound imaging of the neck. In: Flint PW, Haughey BH, Lund VJ, editors. Cummings otolaryngology, head and neck surgery. 5th edition. Philadelphia: Mosby, Inc; 2010. p. 1643–55.

20. Read RC. Orocervical and esophageal infection. In: Cohen J, Powderly W, Opal S, editors. Infectious Diseases. 3rd edition. China: Elsevier; 2010.

21. Gritzmann N. Sonography of the salivary glands. AJR Am J Roentgenol 1989;153:161–6.

22. Levy DM, ReMine WH, Devine KD. Salivary gland calculi. JAMA 1962;181:1115–9.

23. Yousem DM, Kraut MA, Chalian AA. Major salivary gland imaging. Radiology 2000;216(1):19–29.

24. Gritzmann N, Rettenbacher T, Hollerweger A, et al. Sonography of the salivary glands. Eur Radiol 2003;13(5):964–75.

25. Goldberg PA, Inzucchi SE. Critical issues in endocrinology. Clin Chest Med 2003;24(4):583–606.

26. Franklyn JA, Boelaert K. Thyrotoxicosis. Lancet 2012;379(9821):1155–66.

27. Donkol RH, Nada AM, Boughattas S. Role of color Doppler in differentiation of Graves' disease and thyroiditis in thyrotoxicosis. World J Radiol 2013; 5(4):178–83.

28. Hankerson M, Seif D, Mailhot T, et al. Thyroid evaluation in a patient with thyrotoxicosis with bedside ultrasound. West J Emerg Med 2012;13(6).

29. Vitti P. Grey scale thyroid ultrasonography in the evaluation of patients with Graves' disease. Eur J Endocrinol 2000;142(1):22–4.

30. Solbiati L, Osti V, Cova L, et al. Ultrasound of thyroid, parathyroid glands and neck lymph nodes. Eur Radiol 2001;11:2411–24.

31. Mortensen JD, Woolner LB, Bennett WA. Gross and microscopic findings in clinically normal thyroid glands. J Clin Endocrinol Metab 1955;15: 1270–80.

32. Ross DS. Nonpalpable thyroid nodules—managing an epidemic. J Clin Endocrinol Metab 2002;87(5): 1938–40.

33. Ahuja A, Evans R. Practical head and neck ultrasound. London: Greenwich Medical Media Limited; 2000.

34. Papini E, Guglielmi R, Bianchini A, et al. Risk of malignancy in nonpalpable thyroid nodules: predictive value of ultrasound and color-Doppler features. J Clin Endocrinol Metab 2002;87(5): 1941–6.

35. Gbaguidi X, Janvresse A, Benichou J, et al. Internal jugular vein thrombosis: outcome and risk factors. QJM 2010;104(3):209–19.

36. Wilkin TD, Kraus MA, Lane KA, et al. Internal jugular vein thrombosis associated with hemodialysis catheters. Radiology 2003;228(3):697–700.

37. Albertyn LE, Alcock MA. Diagnosis of internal jugular vein thrombosis. Radiology 1987;162:505–8.

38. Dimitropoulou D, Lagadinou M, Papayiannis T, et al. Septic thrombophlebitis caused by Fusobacterium necrophorum in an intravenous drug user. Case Rep Infect Dis 2013;2013:1–3.

39. Chirinos JA, Lichtstein DM, Garcia J, et al. The evolution of Lemierre syndrome: report of 2 cases and review of the literature. Medicine (Baltimore) 2002; 81(6):458–65.

40. Karkos PD, Asrani S, Karkos CD, et al. Lemierre's syndrome: a systematic review. Laryngoscope 2009;119(8):1552–9.

41. Lemierre A. On certain septicaemias due to anaerobic organisms. Lancet 1936;227(5874):701–3.

42. Riordan T. Human infection with *Fusobacterium necrophorum* (necrobacillosis), with a focus on Lemierre's syndrome. Clin Microbiol Rev 2007;20(4): 622–59.

43. Righini CA, Karkas A, Tourniaire R, et al. Lemierre syndrome: a study of 11 cases and literature review. Head Neck 2013. [Epub ahead of print].

44. Riordan T. Lemierre's syndrome: more than a historical curiosa. Postgrad Med J 2004;80(944):328–34.

45. Weeks DF, Katz DS, Saxon P, et al. Lemierre syndrome: report of five new cases and literature review. Emerg Radiol 2010;17(4):323–8.

46. Davies O, Than M. Lemierre's syndrome: diagnosis in the emergency department. Emerg Med Australas 2012;24(6):673–6.

47. Nadir NA, Stone MB, Chao J. Diagnosis of Lemierre's syndrome by bedside sonography. Acad Emerg Med 2010;17(2):E9–10.

48. Smith KA, Kibbee NM, Moak JH. Acute internal jugular venous thrombosis from dialysis catheter. J Emerg Med 2012;42(2):e41–2.

49. Piccirillo JF. Acute bacterial sinusitis. N Engl J Med 2004;351:902–10.

50. Hwang PH. A 51-year-old woman with acute onset of facial pressure, rhinorrhea, and tooth pain. JAMA 2009;301(17):1798–807.

51. Aring AM, Chan MM. Acute rhinosinusitis in adults. Am Fam Physician 2011;83(9):1057–63.

52. Chow AW, Benninger MS, Brook I, et al. Executive summary: IDSA clinical practice guideline for acute bacterial rhinosinusitis in children and adults. Clin Infect Dis 2012;54(8):1041–5.

53. Hilbert G, Vargas F, Valentino R, et al. Comparison of B-mode ultrasound and computed tomography in the diagnosis of maxillary sinusitis in mechanically ventilated patients. Crit Care Med 2001; 29(7):1337–42.

54. Varonen H, Mäkelä M, Savolainen S, et al. Comparison of ultrasound, radiography, and clinical examination in the diagnosis of acute maxillary sinusitis: a systematic review. J Clin Epidemiol 2000;53(9): 940–8.

55. Lichtenstein D, Biderman P, Meziere G, et al. The "sinusogram", a real-time ultrasound sign of maxillary sinusitis. Intensive Care Med 1998;24(10):1057–61.

56. Puhakka T, Heikkinen T, Makela MJ, et al. Validity of ultrasonography in diagnosis of acute maxillary sinusitis. Arch Otolaryngol Head Neck Surg 2000; 126(12):1482.

57. Bektas F, Soyuncu S, Yigit O. Acute maxillary sinusitis detected by bedside emergency department ultrasonography. Int J Emerg Med 2010;3(4):497–8.

Ultrasonography in Musculoskeletal Disorders

Eitan Dickman, MD, RDMS[a],*, Marla C. Levine, MD, RDMS[a],
Shideh Shafie, MD[a], John Munyak, MD[b],
Jennifer Hashem, MD[b], Ahmed Saleh, MD[b],
Eric H. Chou, MD[a]

KEYWORDS

- Ultrasonography • Musculoskeletal disorder • Fracture • Dislocation • Effusion • Tendon

KEY POINTS

- Ultrasonography can be useful when assessing patients for joint effusions and occult fractures.
- Anisotropy is a sonographic property of soft tissues that can influence the echogenicity of tendons, nerves, and muscles, and is influenced by the angle of insonation.
- The assessment of tissue stiffness using elastography can complement the information obtained from B-mode and Doppler imaging.
- The ability to assess tendons using dynamic range of motion is a unique advantage of ultrasonography compared with other imaging modalities.
- Visualization of joint dislocation and subsequent reduction can be observed in real time with sonography.

THE NATURE OF THE PROBLEM

Diseases of the musculoskeletal system and connective tissues represent 6.2% of emergency department (ED) visits.[1] Musculoskeletal injuries can often be effectively and efficiently imaged using ultrasonography. Therefore, recent advances in musculoskeletal ultrasonography are pertinent to emergency physicians and emergency patient care and are elaborated in this article. The usefulness of elastography, a method of tissue stiffness assessment, in the evaluation of patients who present with acute musculoskeletal complaints, will also be discussed.

IMAGING PROTOCOLS

Musculoskeletal sonography is typically performed using a high-frequency linear transducer, although a lower-frequency probe may be necessary when imaging deeper structures such as the hip or shoulder joint. Both longitudinal and short-axis images should be obtained of all structures of interest, with the probe held perpendicular to the area of interest. Appropriate training in performing and interpreting musculoskeletal ultrasonography is necessary, particularly because the operator may encounter a variety of tissues and artifacts such as anisotropy, which is a sonographic artifact that is seen less frequently in other areas of sonography.

SONOGRAPHIC DIAGNOSIS OF FRACTURE

Fractures are the most common form of injury among children. The porous nature of children's bones render these structures more pliable and prone to injury, and therefore more vulnerable to fracture. Furthermore, the thick and physiologically active periosteum and associated growth center of

The authors did not receive any financial support for this article and have no conflict of interest.
[a] Division of Emergency Ultrasound, Department of Emergency Medicine, Maimonides Medical Center, 4802 Tenth Avenue, Brooklyn, NY 11219, USA; [b] Department of Orthopaedic Surgery, Maimonides Medical Center, Brooklyn, NY, USA
* Corresponding author.
E-mail address: edickman@maimonidesmed.org

youth is easily stripped from the bony cortex in the context of injury.[2] Although bony fractures are more common in children than injuries of the supporting structures, radiographs have a high false-negative rate.[3–5] In addition to the inherent limitations of radiographic imaging in the evaluation of extremity injuries, there is a growing concern regarding the untoward effects of ionizing radiation exposure. Ultrasonography has emerged as an alternative imaging modality for the diagnosis of fracture. Although sonography is a newer modality for the diagnosis of bony injury, preliminary studies show considerable promise.[3]

IMAGING TECHNIQUE

Regardless of the bone being interrogated, sonographically intact bones appear hyperechoic and uniform in echotexture.[6] The reflection of the incident sound beam off the bone results in the bright echogenic line tracing the cortical surface.[6] The sonographic evaluation of bones is best performed using a high-frequency linear probe. The bone should be imaged in both the long and short axes in order to evaluate for cortical defects. In the long axis, bone tends to have a linear appearance (**Fig. 1**) and, in the short axis (because small bones curve; eg, ribs), it has a rounded appearance (**Fig. 2**). A long bone appears straight and narrow in the diaphysis and widens and flattens as it reaches the epiphysis. To identify long bone fractures, imaging should proceed in the long axis. In this plane of view, fractures appear as a disruption in the hyperechoic cortical surface (**Fig. 3**).[6]

CLAVICLE

Clavicle fractures represent the most common pediatric fracture.[2] Ultrasonography is an accepted modality for the diagnosis of neonatal clavicle fractures secondary to birth trauma,[7–9] but this

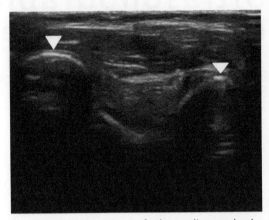

Fig. 2. Transverse view of the radius and ulna (*arrowheads*).

modality is not limited to newborns. In a large prospective study involving 653 children following traumatic injury, ultrasonography had greater accuracy than conventional radiographs in the diagnosis of clavicle fracture (**Fig. 4**).[10] Cross and colleagues[7] performed a prospective study of the diagnostic accuracy of ultrasonography for the diagnosis of clavicle fracture. Ultrasonography had a sensitivity of 95%, a specificity of 96%, a positive predictive value of 95%, and a negative predictive value of 96% for the diagnosis of clavicle fracture among a convenience sample of 100 pediatric patients.[7] A study performed by Chien and colleagues[11] showed similar effectiveness of ultrasonography for the diagnosis of clavicle fracture; in their study of 58 patients, they noted a sensitivity of 89.7%, a specificity of 89.5%, a positive predictive value of 94.6%, and a negative predictive value of 81%. These studies consistently show a usefulness of ultrasonography for the diagnosis of pediatric clavicle fractures; however, ultrasonography has not been well studied for the diagnosis of this type of fracture in adults.

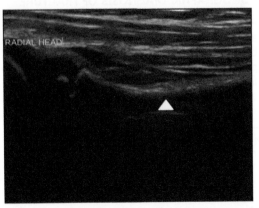

Fig. 1. Long-axis view of the radius. Note the smooth contour of the cortex (*arrowhead*).

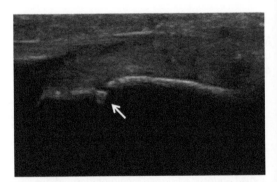

Fig. 3. Fracture of long bone. Note the cortical disruption (*arrow*).

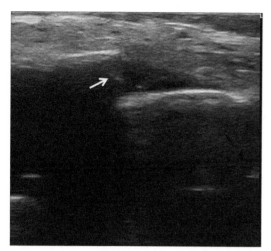

Fig. 4. Fracture of the clavicle (*arrow* points to gap between bony fragments).

EXTREMITY

Forearm fractures are second in frequency only to clavicle fractures in the pediatric population (**Fig. 5**).[2] Pediatric bones are in a state of rapid linear growth and therefore vulnerability exists at the growth plate. When imaged with radiography, Salter-Harris type 1 fractures may appear indistinct from normal bone.[12] Ultrasonography has been shown to identify these occult fractures in cases in which radiographs were negative.[12,13] In a pilot study performed by Williamson and colleagues,[14] radiologists showed comparable diagnostic accuracy in forearm fracture identification using ultrasonography compared with conventional radiographs. Hubner and colleagues[15] compared ultrasonography performed by pediatric surgeons to conventional radiographs. One-hundred and sixty-three patients with findings concerning for extremity fracture underwent both surgeon-performed ultrasonography and radiographic imaging. Surgeon-performed ultrasonography had a sensitivity of 98.3% and a specificity

of 69.3% for detection of long bone fractures. Chen and colleagues[13] and Patel and colleagues[12] performed similar studies of pediatric emergency provider–performed ultrasonography for the diagnosis of forearm fracture. The studies showed comparable diagnostic accuracy for fracture identification by ultrasonography. Chen and colleagues[13] showed a sensitivity of 97% and a specificity of 100%, whereas Patel and colleagues[12] had a sensitivity of 97% and a specificity of 100%. Ultrasonography in these studies was not only comparable with radiographs for the diagnosis of fracture but in several cases ultrasonography was superior to radiographs for fracture identification.[3,12,13] Chen and colleagues[13] also described the usefulness of ultrasonography as an alternative to fluoroscopy for use in fracture reduction. Ultrasonography identified 63 of the 65 radiographically proven fractures. Of these, 26 patients underwent ultrasonography-guided fracture reduction. Only 2 of these required rereduction. The initial success rate for ultrasonography-guided fracture reduction described in this study was 92%.[13]

Supracondylar fracture is a common pediatric fracture, often diagnosed radiographically by an elevation of the posterior fat pad. Rabiner and colleagues[16] evaluated the usefulness of ultrasonography in the diagnosis of this type of fracture. In this prospective study, children with elbow injuries were evaluated both radiographically and sonographically for the presence of fracture. Fracture identification in both imaging modalities was defined as an elevation of the posterior fat pad or evidence of lipohemarthrosis (**Fig. 6**). Ultrasonography had a sensitivity of 98% for the identification

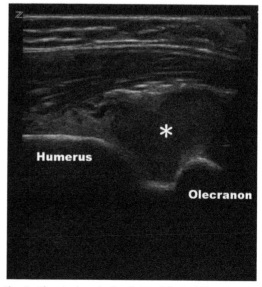

Fig. 6. Elevated posterior fat pad (*asterisk*).

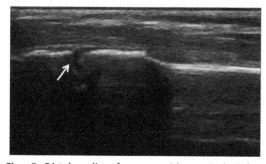

Fig. 5. Distal radius fracture with cortical defect (*arrow*).

of supracondylar fracture, a specificity of 70%, a positive likelihood ratio of 3.3, and a negative likelihood ratio of 0.03.[16]

Ultrasonography has been shown to be an effective imaging modality for the diagnosis of cortical long bone fractures; however, it is a less sensitive modality for diagnosing fractures at the distal aspect of bones. In a prospective observational study by Waterbrook and colleagues,[17] there were 4 false-positive cases among the 147 patients enrolled. All 4 cases involved the distal aspect of long bones: 3 distal radius fractures and 1 of the medial malleolus. The 4 cases of missed fracture were a distal radius buckle fracture, an intertrochanteric femur fracture, an avulsion fracture of the distal fibula, and a lateral malleolus fracture. Marshburn and colleagues[18] reported similar findings in a prospective study of ultrasonography for fracture diagnosis of the upper arm and leg. Ultrasonography misidentified 7 cases: 2 false-negative fractures involving the intertrochanteric line of the femur and 5 false-positive fractures occurring at the hip joint. There were no inaccurate ultrasonography readings below the intertrochanteric line of the femur or along the midshaft of the humerus. McNeil and colleagues[19] performed a longitudinal prospective observational study of the diagnostic accuracy of ultrasonography for fracture diagnosis in a remote medical setting of a military combat zone. Ultrasonography served as a screening modality to determine which patients had fractures and thus needed to be air lifted out of combat to obtain definitive care. Forty-four patients were evaluated, 12 of whom were deemed to have a fracture based on ultrasonography and were therefore evacuated. Radiographs were performed on these patients after arrival at the medical center and 10 patients had radiographic confirmation of the fracture. This number corresponded with a specificity of 94%. The 32 patients who did not show a fracture based on ultrasonography were followed over time and were deemed to not have a fracture at 3 to 7 days following injury based on physical examination. This finding corresponded with a sensitivity of 100%. Based on these studies, ultrasonography should be considered for the diagnosis of fracture in austere settings and for fractures that are radio-occult.

HAND AND WRIST

Wrist fractures can be challenging to identify with radiography. At first, scaphoid fractures often lack radiographic evidence of cortical disruption and are managed as a presumed fracture based solely on the presence of anatomic snuffbox tenderness and other physical examination findings. Senall and colleagues[20] explored the usefulness of ultrasonography in the diagnosis of scaphoid fracture. In this blinded prospective study, patients with snuffbox tenderness and swelling underwent surgeon-performed examination, ultrasonography, and conventional radiographs for the evaluation of scaphoid fracture. Ultrasonography showed 7 of the 9 scaphoid fractures and 8 of the 9 cases in which a fracture was not present (Fig. 7). This finding corresponded with a sensitivity of 78%, a specificity of 89%, a positive predictive value of 88%, and a negative predictive value of 80%. Tayal and colleagues[21] evaluated the diagnostic accuracy of ultrasonography for the diagnosis of hand fractures among adult patients with physical examination findings concerning for fracture. Using ultrasonography, the physicians correctly diagnosed 28 of the 31 fractures identified by radiographs. Ultrasonography had a sensitivity of 90%, a specificity of 98%, a positive predictive value of 97%, and a negative predictive value of 94%. Aksay and colleagues[22] evaluated the sensitivity and specificity of ultrasonography for the diagnosis of fifth metacarpal fractures. A prospective observational study was performed on a sample of 81 patients who sustained a hand injury with tenderness overlying the fifth metacarpal bone. Thirty-nine patients were identified with fifth metacarpal fracture, of which 38 were identified sonographically.[22] One occult fracture, not diagnosed by radiographs but detected by computed tomography (CT), was identified sonographically. There were 3 false-positive cases. The sensitivity, specificity, positive likelihood ratio, and negative likelihood ratio for sonographic diagnosis of fifth metacarpal fracture were 97.4%, 92.9%, 14, and 0.03, respectively,[22]

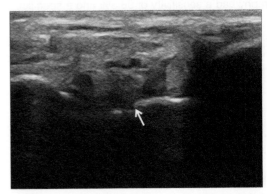

Fig. 7. Scaphoid fracture with small cortical defect (arrow).

showing the usefulness of ultrasonography in these types of fractures.

RIB

Rib fracture can occur following blunt chest trauma (**Fig. 8**). Among the elderly, the presence of rib fracture has been found to correlate with morbidity and mortality.[23] Several radiologist-performed ultrasonography studies have shown improved sensitivity for fracture diagnosis by ultrasonography compared with conventional radiography. Griffith and colleagues[24] performed a prospective observational study among 50 patients with presumed rib fracture. Fracture was defined by a disruption of the anterior margin of the rib, costochondral junction, or costal cartilage.[24] Ultrasonography identified 78% of fractures, as opposed to radiography, which identified 12% of fractures.[24] Kara and colleagues[25] performed a prospective observational study on a subset of patients with nondiagnostic radiographs following blunt chest trauma. Physicians using ultrasonography subsequently diagnosed 40% of patients with rib fracture. Rainer and colleagues[26] compared ultrasonography with clinical acumen and chest radiography. In this prospective study of patients following mild to moderate blunt chest trauma, the sensitivities of ultrasonography, clinical acumen, and chest radiography for the diagnosis of rib and sternal fractures were 80%, 26%, and 24%, respectively.[26] Based on these studies, it seems that ultrasonography is a better test than radiography for the detection of rib fractures. The question of possible rib fracture is frequently raised during emergency care in connection with chest trauma and diagnosis can benefit significantly from sonographic evaluation.

SKULL

The diagnostic evaluation of head injuries among children has long been the source of controversy. Young children, especially infants, can have a normal neurologic examination following even a severe head injury. Approximately 50% of infants with skull fractures and associated intracranial injuries are asymptomatic.[27] Among infants, the presence of a scalp hematoma raises the suspicion of a possible underlying skull fracture,[28,29] which, if present, is associated with a 20-fold increase risk of intracranial injury.[30] Skull radiographs have fallen out of favor because of their poor diagnostic accuracy[31,32] and CT is the gold standard imaging modality for these cases. However, CT delivers ionizing radiation, which may cause untoward effects on the developing brain and may increase lifetime risk of developing malignancy.[33] Ultrasonography was recently explored as an alternative to skull radiographs for the diagnosis of skull fractures. Skull ultrasonography is performed by interrogating the area of injury in 2 orthogonal planes for any cortical defects (**Fig. 9**). Care must be given to distinguish between cranial sutures and fractures, which can have a similar sonographic appearance. When a suspected suture line is encountered, the contralateral area of the scalp should be evaluated to confirm its identification.[34–36] Rabiner and colleagues[34] evaluated point-of-care skull ultrasonography in a prospective sample of pediatric patients scheduled to undergo CT for evaluation of possible intracranial injury. Ultrasonography for the diagnosis of skull fracture had a sensitivity of 88%, a specificity of 97%, a positive likelihood ratio of 27, and a negative likelihood ratio of 0.13. The single false-negative case was that of a

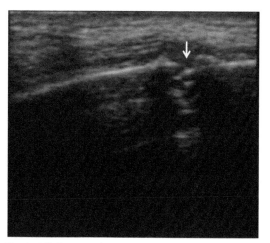

Fig. 8. Rib fracture (*arrow*).

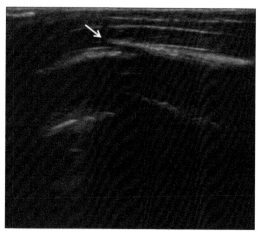

Fig. 9. Skull fracture. Note this clear nondisplaced fracture (*arrow*).

patient with a fracture that was not directly under the hematoma. When results of the Rabiner and colleagues[34] study were combined with other published studies, the sensitivity for sonographic diagnosis of skull fracture was 94% and the specificity was 96%.[35,37,38] Parri and colleagues[38] conducted a similar study in which bedside ultrasonography was compared with CT for the diagnosis of skull fractures. Ultrasonography had 100% sensitivity and 95% specificity for the diagnosis of skull fractures, with a positive predictive value of 97.2% and a negative predictive value of 100%. However, the absence of a skull fracture does not exclude clinically significant head injury. As Rabiner and colleagues[34] showed, 2 children, 1 with an isolated hematoma and 1 with isolated loss of consciousness, had no evidence of skull fracture but had intracranial hemorrhage identified on CT. In specific clinical scenarios, ultrasonography offers an attractive alternative, particularly in the pediatric population, in the evaluation for fracture.

JOINT EFFUSIONS

Joint swelling is a common complaint in the ED with a myriad of possible causes. Delineating the cause allows initiation of appropriate treatment, but can be challenging without the use of imaging. Ultrasonography has been shown to be an excellent modality for the diagnosis of joint effusions, and in many cases is superior to physical examination in this assessment.[39] Adhikari and Blaivas[40] showed the usefulness of emergency physician–performed musculoskeletal ultrasonography in patients presenting with joint-related complaints. In 39 of 54 cases in which there was clinical suspicion of a joint effusion and an arthrocentesis was planned, management was changed in 69.2% of cases after ultrasonography was performed. In the group of patients in which arthrocentesis was not planned, ultrasonography changed the management in 53.3% of cases.[40] In cases in which an arthrocentesis is to be performed, the addition of sonographic guidance has been shown to be of benefit.[41–43]

IMAGING TECHNIQUE

When imaging a joint, the ultrasonography machine's dual screen function can be used to compare the joint of concern with the unaffected contralateral side. Dynamic sonography, in which joint structures are ranged during image acquisition, can be useful in identifying key landmarks. Effusions are detected as hypoechoic or anechoic intraarticular collections that can be compressed and have no Doppler signal. It is important to

image any abnormality noted on ultrasonography in both the longitudinal and transverse planes.

Although ultrasonography cannot reliably distinguish between different types of effusions, characteristics of the fluid collection along with the patient's history may help to narrow the differential and guide the clinician. Effusions that contain internal echoes may indicate a complicated effusion such as fibrinous clot, purulence, or fat from a fracture; the presence of increased color Doppler flow may indicate hyperemia from an inflammatory or infectious process.[44] Septic arthritis may be particularly difficult to identify in patients with chronic joint swelling, but, classically, patients with septic arthritis have a joint effusion with no associated synovial thickening.[40] In addition, sonographic examination of the area surrounding a joint may identify a soft tissue infection, and alert the provider to avoid guiding a needle through infected tissue planes if an arthrocentesis was planned.[45]

ELBOW

The elbow can be sonographically imaged using an anterior or posterior approach. If imaged anteriorly, the elbow is placed in slight flexion, and the probe is moved along the antecubital fossa of the arm, in both the transverse and longitudinal planes. The anterior recess may contain a small amount of fluid, up to 2 mm in thickness, which is considered physiologic.[46] Posterior views can be obtained by holding the arm in 90° of flexion and scanning along the olecranon fossa. An effusion is present if there is displacement of the posterior fat pad that is normally adherent to the bone, similar to the sail sign noted on radiographs. Flexion of the elbow can make small effusions more detectable, because fluid is displaced posteriorly.[47] An effusion in the setting of trauma can indicate an occult elbow fracture. Zuazo and colleagues[48] found that the presence of fat in the effusion was 88% sensitive and 100% specific for the presence of a fracture, using magnetic resonance (MR) imaging as the gold standard (**Fig. 10**). More recently, Rabiner and colleagues[16] found that pediatric emergency physicians were able to identify fracture based on the presence of an elbow effusion. The detection of lipohemarthrosis should raise concern for a fracture (see **Fig. 6**).

KNEE

Because of its large size, the knee can be difficult to evaluate clinically. Ultrasonography has been used to detect a knee effusion more reliably than physical examination alone.[49] The knee can be

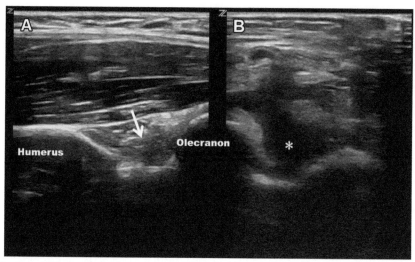

Fig. 10. (*A*) The fat pad (*arrow*) is adherent to the bone in the olecranon fossa, whereas (*B*) shows displacement of the fat pad by an effusion (*asterisk*).

evaluated using an anterior or posterior approach. The anterior approach is best for joint effusion assessment, but the posterior approach may be useful for detecting other disorders, including a Baker cyst. There are multiple different positions in which the knee can be imaged, and there is controversy regarding which is optimal. Hong and colleagues[50] examined 16 cadaveric knees and found that the smallest effusions, 10 mL, were readily visualized with the knee in extension and the probe at the lateral aspect of the knee. If the knee was flexed, the fluid accumulated more readily in the medial aspect. This finding is consistent with those of Hirsch and colleagues,[51] who studied 46 patients with arthritis who were imaged in extension; fluid was most readily noted in the lateral suprapatellar pouch. Mandl and colleagues[52] performed a large multicenter study of 148 knees, and found that fluid was most readily visualized when the knee was positioned in 30° of flexion. It is important to evaluate the entire joint in both the longitudinal and transverse orientations. Because of the size of the knee joint, it may be necessary to examine the area above and below the patella separately. The suprapatellar bursa is just deep to the quadriceps tendon and communicates with the knee joint. Therefore, fluid in this bursa indicates the presence of a joint effusion. The bursa is otherwise a potential space that should contain no sizable amount of fluid. A small amount of fluid may be physiologic and thus obtaining comparison views of the contralateral joint can be helpful. If there is doubt regarding whether an anechoic area is an effusion, the area can be compressed, which causes the fluid to be displaced (**Fig. 11**). A novel technique to increase

detection of an effusion has been recently described. The technique involves cupping the knee such that pressure is applied to the medial infrapatellar pouch with the thumb while the other fingers apply pressure to the lateral lower knee. This cupping maneuver helps to redistribute any fluid, and is thought to make even subclinical effusions readily visible.[53] Another technique, described by Ike and colleagues,[54] showed that when patients voluntarily contracted their quadriceps muscles, otherwise undetectable effusions became visible.

Using ultrasonography, a Baker cyst is readily identifiable as a fluid collection between the medial head of the gastrocnemius muscle and the semimembranosus tendon.[55] A ruptured Baker cyst may be detected as a simple or complex fluid collection tracking into the subcutaneous tissue superficial to the gastrocnemius muscle.[56]

HIP

Hip effusions can be challenging to diagnose based on physical examination alone, and radiography also has limited sensitivity for detection of fluid in this joint.[57] Ultrasonography is a valuable tool when the diagnosis of hip effusion is being entertained. The causes of effusions in the hip can be variable, and include chronic diseases such as osteoarthritis and avascular necrosis, as well as more acute disorders such as a septic hip joint or transient synovitis. Depending on the amount of tissue overlying the hip, a lower-frequency probe may be used. Imaging should be performed along the plane of the femoral neck in the long axis. The optimal positioning of the hip has been

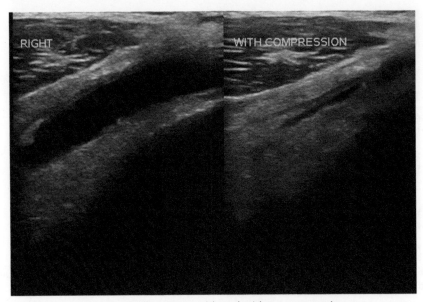

Fig. 11. A knee effusion in the suprapatellar recess, with and without compression.

debated. Some clinicians advocate slight external rotation and extension,[58] whereas others advocate slight hip flexion and internal rotation.[59] When imaging the hip, it is important to be aware of potential pitfalls. The articular cartilage, which appears as a hypoechoic thin stripe, can be mistaken for an effusion. To differentiate between cartilage and effusion, contralateral views can be obtained and compressibility assessed. An effusion is shown as an anechoic or hypoechoic collection between the anterior and posterior synovial layers, and is compressible. In adults, an effusion extends the length of the capsule and measures 5 mm or more in thickness.[60] In children, an effusion is present if the synovial fluid measures 2 mm greater than the contralateral side, or more than 5 mm in thickness (**Fig. 12**).[61] Vieira and

Levy[62] found that pediatric emergency physicians can readily identify hip effusions after focused training sessions. Based on a small case series, ultrasonography can be used to evaluate children with hip pain in a more expeditious manner, which could lead to shorter ED lengths of stay.[63] In a recent case series and a case report of adult patients with native hips, effusions were readily identified with ultrasonography by emergency physicians.[64,65] However, detection of hip effusion by ultrasonography is more challenging if the patient has a prosthetic hip, in which case arthrocentesis may be needed to definitively exclude effusion.[66] Ultrasonography can readily show effusions in a variety of different joints with a higher degree of accuracy than physical examination alone and can be used to guide joint aspiration as well.

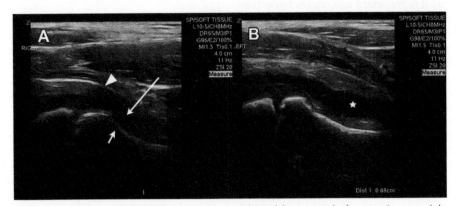

Fig. 12. Components of the hip joint. (*A*) The femoral metaphysis (*short arrow*), the anterior synovial recess (*long arrow*), and the joint capsule (*arrowhead*). (*B*) An effusion is present (*star*).

ULTRASONOGRAPHIC ELASTOGRAPHY

Palpation has been used for millennia as one of the earliest means by which physicians attempted to differentiate healthy from diseased tissue. Elastography harkens back to this type of physical examination and can be conceptualized as a type of sonographic palpation. Ultrasonographic elastography is an application that has been used for more than 20 years. The fundamental concept underpinning this technique is the ability to assess tissue stiffness and to differentiate the hardness of a structure compared with adjacent tissues. An increasing number of ultrasonography equipment manufacturers offer elastography as an option on their machines. The same transducers that are used for B-mode and Doppler imaging are also used when performing elastography; however, additional software is necessary. Different colors are associated with different tissue hardness (**Fig. 13**). Once the area of interest has been assessed, a color-based elastographic map is then generated (**Fig. 14**). This elastogram can be used to quantify the degree of hardness of the area.

Elastography has been used to differentiate malignant from benign lesions, because the former tend to be harder than the latter. Elastography has been successfully used in assessing different types of tissue for possible neoplastic changes, including breast,[67] thyroid,[68] prostate,[69] lymph nodes,[70] and liver.[71] Based on these studies, elastography has been shown to have a high degree of accuracy. Patients benefit from this technology in that a smaller number require an invasive procedure such as a biopsy in order to determine whether a lesion is benign or malignant.

In general, elastography is performed on superficial structures, so a high-frequency linear transducer is used. However, there are situations in which a lower-frequency probe is used, such as when imaging the liver. When imaging the prostate, a transrectal transducer is used. Although both

longitudinal and transverse images of the structure should be obtained, elastography has been shown to be most reliable using a long-axis approach, with the probe held perpendicular to the structure of interest.[72] Multiple images should be obtained, and the sonologist should ensure that the area of interest is in the center of the screen.

Four categories of sonographic elastography have been studied:

1. Compression elastography, also known as strain ultrasound elastography, is the most studied and used type of ultrasound elastography. In order to perform this type of ultrasonography, images are obtained before and after the sonologist manually compresses the tissue using the transducer. Tissue hardness is related to the Young elastic modulus (E) in which E is the stress/strain, and where stress is the force acting on a unit area and strain is the change in size or shape produced by a system of forces. Harder tissue has a lower strain than softer tissue (and therefore a higher Young modulus), and undergoes less change when compressed.[73] The strain information is then superimposed on the B-mode image. In order to maintain reliability of the results of the examination, it is important to avoid excessive variability in the amount of compression exerted. Therefore, one of the limitations of this technique is that, like many other ultrasonography applications, it is operator dependent. Although strain elastography has been successfully used in imaging potentially malignant lesions, there has been recent interest in applying this modality to musculoskeletal conditions.[74]

2. Shear wave elastography. When external compression is applied to tissue, tangential shear waves are produced. The generation and assessment of these shear waves can be studied, and because their production is related to tissue stiffness, the hardness of the tissue can be assessed based on shear wave velocity measurements.[75]

3. Sonoelastography, also known as transient elastography, uses external vibrations to generate an image. This type of elastography is primarily used to assess for liver disease.[74]

4. Acoustic radiation force impulse is a type of elastography in which an ultrasound pulse travels through tissue, causing displacement of the tissue followed by relaxation back to its original configuration. The degree of tissue movement is displayed using different colors on an elastographic map, with softer tissue undergoing a greater amount of displacement than harder tissue.[74]

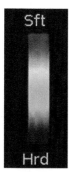

Fig. 13. Elastographic map with different colors representing varying tissue stiffness. (*Courtesy of* R. Gaspari, MD, Worcester, MA.)

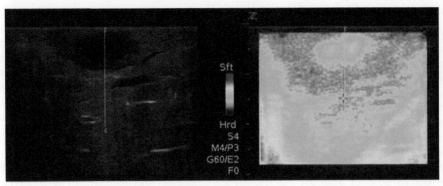

Fig. 14. B-mode (*left*) and elastographic (*right*) representations of an abscess. (*Courtesy of* R. Gaspari, MD, Worcester, MA.)

There is a paucity of emergency medicine–based elastography research. In 2009, Gaspari and colleagues[76] assessed 50 patients with a clinical concern for abscess using both B-mode ultrasonography and elastography. Only 58% of abscesses were identified using elastography (**Fig. 15**), although there were a few instances in which this technique showed abscess cavities that were not visualized with B-mode imaging. However, using elastography, physicians were able to differentiate indurated tissue around an abscess from healthy tissue in 98% of cases. These findings were not always evident with B-mode imaging.

Gaspari and colleagues[77] performed another study with 56 patients who had a documented abscess and underwent incision and drainage. These patients were then followed in an attempt to determine the characteristics of abscesses associated with therapy failure, which was defined as the need for additional surgical drainage. Asymmetry of the area of induration as shown with elastography was the only characteristic studied that predicted treatment failure.

Much of the musculoskeletal research using ultrasound elastography involves the Achilles tendon. Previous studies have shown that tendon disorder is associated with increased softness of the tendon, as shown on an elastogram.[78,79] In a study by De Zordo and colleagues,[78] elastography was 94% sensitive and 99% specific in the diagnosis of pathologic Achilles tendons. In the study by Klauser and colleagues,[79] elastography was more sensitive than B-mode imaging in the detection of tendon disorders (100% vs 86%) when histologic evaluation was used as the criterion standard. Both B-mode imaging and elastography were 100% specific in this study. However, another elastography-based study for assessment of the Achilles tendon showed conflicting results: asymptomatic tendons were softer than those with tendinopathy.[80] These findings confirm the need for additional research in this field.

Another area in which elastography could potentially play a role is in differentiating acute deep venous thrombosis (DVT) from chronic DVT. Although B-mode and Doppler sonography have been shown to be useful in the detection of DVT,[81] these modalities are less accurate when attempting to determine whether a DVT is chronic.[82] With regard to tissue stiffness, chronic DVTs tend to be hard, whereas acute DVTs are usually soft. Rubin and colleagues[83] showed that, when pressure was exerted on veins with thrombosis, there was a statistically significant difference in tissue deformation between acute and chronic DVTs. The acute (soft) DVT had a greater area of deformation than the chronic (hard) DVT.

There have been a limited number of small studies that have focused on other musculoskeletal applications. Bhatia and colleagues[84] studied the use of elastography in the evaluation of neck

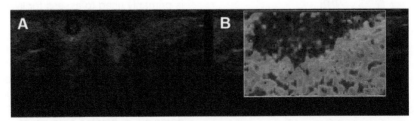

Fig. 15. (*A*) B-mode image of a small abscess. (*B*) Elastogram of the affected area; the abscess is not clearly identified. (*Courtesy of* R. Gaspari, MD, Worcester, MA.)

masses. The investigators found that vascular malformations and thyroglossal cysts were soft, likely because of their fluid content. In contrast, neurogenic tumors were stiff. Abscesses displayed a range of stiffness levels from soft to intermediate. Softer abscesses were associated with a larger amount of purulent fluid aspirated. The greater fluid content likely caused the tissue to be softer.

Orman and colleagues[73] studied 130 wrists of asymptomatic patients and those with carpal tunnel syndrome. The investigators measured tissue strain in the two groups, and found that elastography was useful in differentiating the stiffness of median nerves of patients who had carpal tunnel syndrome from those without the disease.

Both Wu and colleagues[85] and Sconfienza and colleagues[86] found that elastography was helpful in assessing patients with possible plantar fasciitis.[85,86] Wu and colleagues[85] showed that, in patients with plantar fasciitis, this tissue was softer than the corresponding tissue in patients without the disease. In the study by Sconfienza and colleagues,[86] the addition of elastography increased the accuracy of B-mode ultrasonography in the diagnosis of plantar fasciitis. Elastography was particularly helpful in cases in which B-mode imaging was inconclusive.

De Zordo and colleagues[87] used elastography when comparing 44 elbows of healthy patients with 38 elbows of patients with symptoms suggesting lateral epicondylitis. Elastography showed 100% sensitivity, 89% specificity, and an accuracy of 94% when using physical examination findings as the criterion standard. Although these initial results are promising, elastography will likely not be widely adopted until its applicability in an ED setting is more clearly defined.

TENDON INJURY

Emergency physicians can use ultrasonography in the evaluation of acute tendon injury and when there is a suspicion of infectious flexor tenosynovitis. A unique advantage of ultrasonography is that dynamic range of motion of the tendon during the evaluation may assist in the detection of subtle disorders. On sonography, tendons have a fibrillar appearance, with characteristic hyperechoic parallel lines representing collagen bundles (**Fig. 16**); flexor tendons are encased in a hyperechoic sheath.[88] Wu and colleagues[89] compared physical examination findings with emergency physician–performed ultrasonography in the evaluation of tendons, using MR imaging or direct wound exploration as the criterion standard; ultrasonography had a sensitivity of 100% and specificity of 95%,

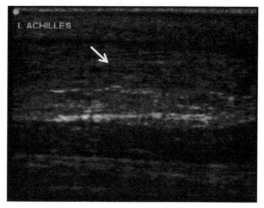

Fig. 16. Achilles tendon: note the characteristic echogenic fibrillar pattern (*arrow*).

whereas physical examination had a sensitivity of 100% and specificity of 76%. Soubeyrand and colleagues[90] studied 26 patients who presented to the ED with penetrating hand injuries, and ultrasonography had 100% sensitivity and specificity in the diagnosis of tendon injuries. There have been several case reports by emergency physicians describing sonographic diagnosis of various tendon ruptures, including the Achilles,[91] flexor digitorum profundus,[92] triceps,[93] and quadriceps tendons.[94] Lee and colleagues[95] assessed 20 flexor tendons, and attempted to differentiate intact tendons from those that had sustained partial or complete lacerations. Ultrasonography was accurate in 18 of the cases (**Fig. 17**).

Complete tendon lacerations can typically be diagnosed based on physical examination. However, partial tendon lacerations can be subtle in presentation because range of motion may be preserved despite a significant tear. With a complete

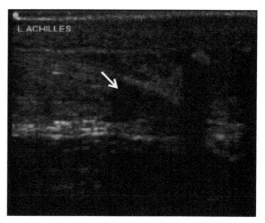

Fig. 17. Tendon laceration: note the disruption of the tendon, with a hematoma around the site of the injury (*arrow*).

tear, a hematoma is often sonographically visualized between both ends of the tendon. A tendon with a partial laceration may show a focal hypoechoic area, discontinuity of some of the collagen fibers, and focal swelling of the tendon.[95,96]

IMAGING TECHNIQUE

When imaging tendons with ultrasonography, it is important to keep the transducer perpendicular to the tendon, otherwise anisotropy may cause the tendon to appear hypoechoic in certain areas (where the ultrasound beam is not perpendicular to the tissue of interest) and raise unnecessary concern about possible disorders. This precaution is particularly important when the tendon runs oblique to the transducer[97] (**Fig. 18**) because even a few degrees of angulation can cause spurious results.[98,99] If anisotropy is encountered, adjusting the angle of insonation and increasing the amount of pressure with which the probe contacts the body can improve the image quality.[100] A water bath can be used when imaging superficial structures such as tendons in the hand. Water is an excellent medium for transmitting sound waves, and the probe can be held 1 to 2 cm away from the hand, avoiding causing an injured patient any additional pain from the transducer.[101]

ROTATOR CUFF

Shoulder injuries are commonly seen in the emergent patient. Patients may present with both acute and chronic pain complaints without radiographic evidence of bony injuries. Sonographic diagnosis of tendon tears has been well studied in the rotator cuff. When assessing the rotator cuff, the patient is seated with the elbow flexed to 90°. The arm is ranged into a variety of positions that allow visualization of the individual tendons surrounding the

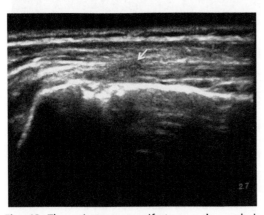

Fig. 18. The anisotropy manifests as a hypoechoic area within the tendon (*arrow*).

shoulder joint.[102] Iannotti and colleagues[102] examined 99 shoulders and compared office-based ultrasonography with MR imaging, using operative findings as the criterion standard. Ultrasonography performed by a physician assistant or nurse clinician in an orthopedist's office accurately revealed 88% of full-thickness or full-thickness and partial-thickness rotator cuff tears, whereas MR imaging led to the correct diagnosis in 95% of cases. Ultrasonography revealed 70% of partial-thickness tears, whereas MR imaging showed 73% of these cases. In addition, 80% of shoulders with normal tendons were correctly detected by ultrasonography, compared with 75% of cases when MR imaging was used. Al-Shawi and colleagues[103] performed a study in which an orthopedic surgeon used a portable ultrasonography machine when evaluating 143 patients with painful shoulders. Using arthroscopy or MR imaging as the gold standard, ultrasonography had a sensitivity of 96.2% and a specificity of 95.4% for the diagnosis of a full-thickness supraspinatus tear. The positive predictive value in this study was 96.2% and the negative predictive value was 95.4%. Sensitivity of ultrasonography for the diagnosis of partial-thickness tears was 95.4%, with a specificity of 84.6%. Sonographic evaluation of patients with shoulder injuries may lead to more accurate diagnosis and efficient referral for definitive management.

ACHILLES TENDON

The Achilles tendon is the largest and strongest tendon in the body; however, Achilles tendinopathy and Achilles tendon ruptures are commonly encountered in the clinical setting. Ultrasonography has also been well studied in the assessment of Achilles tendon disorders. Achilles tendon ruptures tend to occur 3 to 6 cm proximal to the insertion in the calcaneus.[104] The full length of the tendon should be imaged both in a longitudinal and transverse orientation while assessing for any focal swelling, hematoma, or discontinuity in the normal structure. In a study of 30 patients who presented with achillodynia, 34 Achilles tendons were sonographically evaluated. Using surgical evaluation as the criterion standard, ultrasonography had a 96% sensitivity in the detection of Achilles tendon disorders.[105] Kälebo and colleagues[96] studied the usefulness of ultrasonography in the diagnosis of partial tears of the Achilles tendon and found a sensitivity of 94% and a specificity of 95%. Hartgerink and colleagues[106] showed that ultrasonography was able to differentiate full-thickness versus partial-thickness Achilles tendon tears with a sensitivity of 100%, specificity of 83%, positive predictive value of 88%, and a negative predictive value of 100%. In addition, retracted tendon edges, undetectable tendon at the site of injury, and posterior acoustic shadowing at the site of the tear were all associated with a full-thickness tear. The posterior acoustic shadowing was thought to occur because of sound-beam refraction at the torn tendon edges. Because of its superficial position in the body and based on these studies, the Achilles tendon can be accurately evaluated with sonography. In emergency patients with posterior lower leg and ankle injury, few possibilities exist other than physical examination and ultrasonography to evaluate the Achilles tendon.

FLEXOR TENOSYNOVITIS

Jeffrey and colleagues[107] published a small case series that described 2 sonographic findings associated with acute suppurative flexor tenosynovitis: a hypoechoic fluid collection surrounding the tendon, and the affected tendon being 25% greater in diameter than the contralateral tendon. In patients with signs and symptoms concerning for tenosynovitis, these imaging findings may be helpful in confirming the diagnosis (**Fig. 19**). Larger prospective studies are necessary to fully define the role of ultrasonography in the evaluation of this disease process.

JOINT DISLOCATION

Dislocations are usually caused by sudden trauma or direct impact to a specific joint. These injuries cause severe pain and limitation in the range of motion, and can occur in any major or minor joint. The diagnosis is typically made by physical examination and radiography. In general, patients with suspected joint dislocation undergo prereduction and postreduction radiographs, although this process involves radiation exposure and increases the ED length of stay.[108] Several studies have found that ultrasonography is accurate for the early detection of joint dislocation as well as confirmation of successful reduction.[109,110]

TECHNIQUE

Multiple approaches to probe placement, including transverse and longitudinal views, have been described.[111] Bone cortex normally presents as a bright line with posterior shadowing, and the joint space between bones can be measured using ultrasonography. Once the relevant landmarks are identified, the joint can be assessed for any evidence of dislocation. Compared with the unaffected side, dislocation is suspected if the joint space appears abnormally widened or is empty.

SHOULDER

The shoulder is an inherently unstable joint and flexible enough to allow for a wide range of motion. For these reasons, the glenohumeral joint is the most frequently dislocated joint of the body. Shoulder dislocations account for approximately 50% of all major joint dislocations.[112] An anterior dislocation is the most common location, accounting for 95% to 97% of cases, followed by posterior and inferior dislocation.[113]

Ultrasonography of the shoulder can be performed using an anterior, lateral, or posterior approach (**Fig. 20**). The anterior and lateral approaches are preferred for verifying adequate reduction, particularly in a supine patient.[110] In the anterior approach, the transducer is placed in a transverse orientation over the coracoid process at the level of the humeral head (see **Fig. 20A**). In this view, the humeral head is identified by its round echogenic cortex with acoustic shadowing. In this approach, the humeral head is normally located lateral to the coracoid process (see **Fig. 20B**) but is found inferiorly when there is an anterior dislocation.[109] If the probe is placed longitudinally on the anterior shoulder with the indicator aimed superiorly (see **Fig. 20C**), the acromion is visualized on the left side of the screen and the humeral head is on the right (see **Fig. 20D**).[111] Dislocation should be suspected if the humeral head disappears and there is an empty glenoid fossa. In the lateral approach, the transducer is placed longitudinally just inferior to the acromion (see **Fig. 20E**). The humeral head is typically viewed inferior to the acromion process (see **Fig. 20F**). A shoulder dislocation can be identified when the

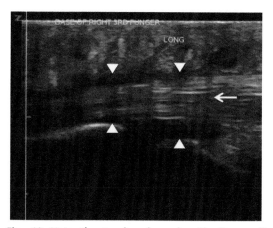

Fig. 19. Note the tendon (*arrow*) with the small amount of fluid around it (*arrowheads*).

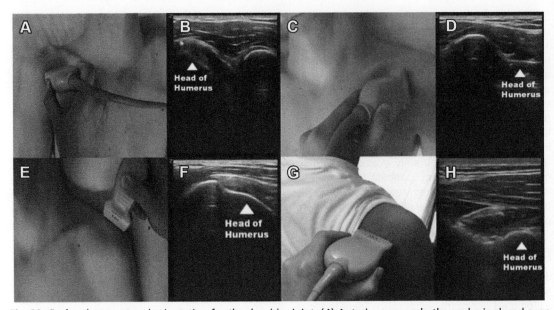

Fig. 20. Probe placement and orientation for the shoulder joint. (*A*) Anterior approach: the probe is placed over the coracoid process at the level of the humeral head with the corresponding sonographic image (*B*). (*C*) Longitudinal view of the anterior aspect of the shoulder with the corresponding sonographic image (*D*). (*E*) Lateral approach: the probe is placed at the level of the acromion and humeral head with the corresponding sonographic image (*F*). (*G*) Posterior approach: the probe is placed on the posterior shoulder parallel to the scapular spine with the corresponding sonographic image (*H*).

space between the acromion and the humeral head widens compared with the unaffected side (**Fig. 21**). The posterior approach can provide a different view of the joint but may not be feasible in a supine patient. In the posterior approach, the transducer is placed in a transverse orientation over the lateral edge of the scapula, parallel to the scapular spine (see **Fig. 20**G, H).[114] Several studies have shown that bedside ultrasonography is accurate for confirming the presence of a dislocation as well as successful joint reduction.[109,110,115] Because postreduction radiographs are usually obtained after the patient has recovered from the procedural sedation, the patient may have to be given additional sedative medications if closed reduction fails. With bedside ultrasonography, clinicians can perform multiple shoulder reduction attempts without the need for repeat sedation.[109] In addition, ultrasonography has the potential to expedite care, reduce costs, and decrease radiation exposure.[116] Posterior shoulder dislocations may be missed with physical examination and radiographs, whereas ultrasonography can be used to accurately diagnose this injury.[114] Although ultrasonography has been shown to be useful, Blakeley and colleagues[115] proposed that ultrasonography should not replace radiography in suspected shoulder dislocations, because associated fractures are more easily

detected on radiographs. Yuen and colleagues[110] also suggested that prereduction radiographs should be performed to rule out any fractures of the proximal humerus before any external rotation maneuver.

A recent observational study with a small sample size showed that ultrasonography achieved 100% sensitivity and specificity in the detection of shoulder dislocation and assessment of joint reduction using radiography as the criterion standard. The mean elapsed time between triage and diagnosis of shoulder dislocation by ultrasonography was only 4.4 minutes compared with 16.5 minutes for patients in the radiography group, thereby showing the significant time advantage of ultrasonography for this diagnosis.[109]

ELBOW

The elbow is the second most commonly dislocated major joint in adults and the most common in children.[117,118] This injury is usually caused by a fall on an outstretched hand. When the elbow joint dislocates, the proximal ulna displaces posterior to the distal humerus, which can be identified sonographically.[119] In the pediatric population, radial head subluxation (also called nursemaid's elbow or pulled elbow) is the most common elbow injury. It usually occurs between the ages of 1 and

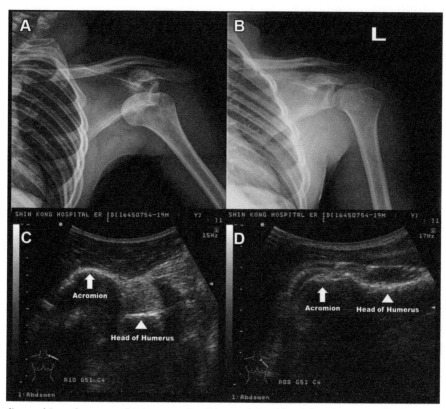

Fig. 21. Radiographic and sonographic images of a dislocated shoulder. (*A*) Radiograph of left shoulder anterior dislocation, and (*B*) after successful closed reduction. (*C*) Ultrasound image of left shoulder dislocation, and (*D*) after successful closed reduction. (*Courtesy of* K. Chen, MD, Taipei, Taiwan.)

4 years, with a peak incidence between 2 and 3 years.[120,121] The diagnosis can be made by characteristic history and physical examination findings. However, it can be difficult to differentiate bone fracture and subluxation if the history of a pull injury is unclear.

For the patient with a suspected elbow dislocation, ultrasonography can play a role in confirming the diagnosis and verifying satisfactory reduction. The transducer is placed on the skin overlying the posterior aspect of the distal humerus with the indicator oriented superiorly.[111] The patient's elbow should be flexed to 90° (**Fig. 22**A). In this view, the distal humerus is on the left side of the screen and the olecranon is on the right, with both bones in the same horizontal plane (see **Fig. 22**D). Elbow dislocation should be suspected if this anatomic relationship is disrupted and the joint space widens compared with the unaffected side (see **Fig. 22**C). A hypoechoic hematoma or interstitial fluid may also be visualized. For detection of radial head subluxation, the transducer is placed longitudinally on the anterior surface of the elbow in the long axis with the elbow extended (see **Fig. 22**B). In a normal radiohumeral joint, the radial head and capitellum can easily be visualized sonographically, and the annular ligament appears as a bright hyperechoic line next to the supinator muscle and radius. An increased distance between the radius and capitellum (ie, radiocapitellar distance) in the affected side compared with the unaffected side suggests a radial head subluxation. Studies have identified the presence of a J-shaped structure as a specific sonographic finding indicating a nursemaid's elbow.[122] The image of the normal annular ligament disappears, and both the supinator muscle and annular ligament are entrapped within the radiohumeral joint to display a J-shaped hypoechoic image (J sign).[122] This J sign disappears after the reduction. In an observational study with 70 patients, the presence of the J sign was 100% sensitive and specific for the diagnosis of nursemaid's elbow.[122] Diab and colleagues[123] reported several sonographic signs associated with the diagnosis of a nursemaid's elbow, including a widened joint space, increased radiocapitellar distance, and increased joint space echogenicity. The radiocapitellar distance in the patients with a nursemaid's elbow was significantly greater than in patients

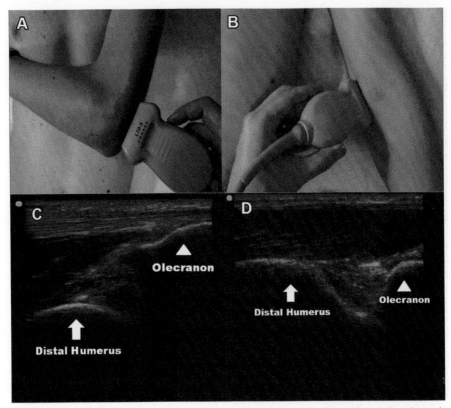

Fig. 22. Probe placement and sonographic images of the elbow joint. (*A*) The probe is placed in a longitudinal orientation on the distal humerus. (*B*) In a patient with suspected radial head subluxation, the probe is placed on the anterior surface of the radiohumeral joint in the long axis. (*C*) Ultrasonography image of elbow dislocation, and (*D*) after successful close reduction. ([*C, D*] *Courtesy of* Dr Turan Saul, MD, New York, NY.)

with normal elbows, measuring 6.4 mm ± 0.8 standard deviation (SD) and 4.3 mm ± 0.6 SD, respectively. Ultrasonography was highly sensitive but not specific in the diagnosis of nursemaid's elbow.[123] However, it achieved high specificity for detection of the dislocation-associated radial annular ligament tear. Based on these studies, ultrasonography seems to be a promising imaging modality for the diagnosis of elbow joint subluxation and dislocation.

SOFT TISSUE ULTRASOUND

Soft tissue infection is a common chief complaint in patients presenting to an ED.[124–126] The usefulness of differentiating cellulitis from abscess with the use of ultrasonography has been well described elsewhere.[127–129] The focus here is on necrotizing fasciitis (NF), which is a rare and life-threatening condition involving aggressive spread of infection along fascial planes. To date, there has been limited research evaluating the usefulness of ultrasonography for the diagnosis of NF, although small studies have identified sonographic features that may be useful.

IMAGING TECHNIQUE

Depth and focal zone adjustments must be made to ensure that the structure of interest takes center position on the screen, which may require the use of abundant ultrasonography gel or an acoustic standoff pad. If feasible, a water bath technique can also be used.[100] On sonography, the anatomy of the skin has a characteristic echotexture. Normal skin is thin, homogeneous, and hyperechoic.[6] Just deep to the skin is the subcutaneous layer, which is primarily composed of fat. On sonography, subcutaneous fat is hypoechoic, with hyperechoic connective tissue strands interspersed between fat lobules.[6,130] Deep to the fat is fascia and connective tissue, which runs parallel to the muscle. Fascia and connective tissue appear hyperechoic on ultrasonography.[6,130] Other structures within the subcutaneous tissue include muscle and blood vessels. Muscle has a hypoechoic appearance with a characteristic pattern of striations in a longitudinal orientation, and a speckled, mosaic appearance in the short axis (**Fig. 23**).[6] Blood vessels appear either circular in the short axis or tubular in the long axis.[6] Arteries have thick

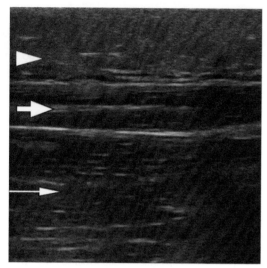

Fig. 23. Normal soft tissue. Note the subcutaneous tissue (*arrowhead*), the fascial layer just deep to the subcutaneous tissue (*short arrow*), and the muscle lying just deep to the fascial layer (*long arrow*). In this image, the muscle is viewed in a longitudinal plane.

hyperechoic outer wall, whereas veins have a thin wall and easily compress if pressure is applied with the probe. To confirm the presence of a blood vessel, Doppler can also be used.

NECROTIZING FASCIITIS

NF represents a rare but life-threatening infection with an associated mortality of approximately 25% to 30%.[131] Characteristic features of NF are rapidly spreading infection of the deep soft tissue with associated signs of severe sepsis.[132] According to an expert panel, NF extends beyond the deep peripheral fascia with involvement of the muscles and intermuscular fascia.[132,133] Given the high morbidity and mortality of this disease entity, prompt diagnosis can be lifesaving. Cross-sectional imaging is usually obtained in the diagnostic evaluation of a patient with presumed NF, with surgical exploration serving as the reference standard for diagnosis.[134] Several studies have used ultrasonography as an imaging modality for the diagnosis of this disease entity. Yen and colleagues[135] noted that, among patients with clinically suspected NF, those with diffuse thickening of the subcutaneous tissue accompanied by fluid accumulation greater than 4 mm in depth along the fascial layer were more likely to have the disease. In this prospective study, ultrasonography had a sensitivity of 88.2%, a specificity of 93.3%, a positive predictive value of 83.3%, and a negative predictive value of 95.4% for the diagnosis of NF.[135] Chao and colleagues[136] described 3 cases in which ultrasonography was performed in the

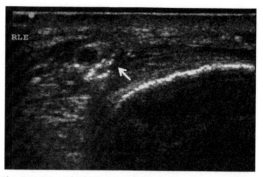

Fig. 24. NF with thickening of the subcutaneous tissue and fascia. Note the thickening of the subcutaneous tissue (*arrow*) with early presence of air within the tissue.

diagnostic work-up of patients with NF. Cutaneous tissue swelling; distorted, thickened fascial planes; and fluid pockets consistent with abscess along the fascia were the sonographic findings noted in this series. In a cadaveric study by Butcher and colleagues,[134] investigators assessed the sonographic identification of iatrogenically instilled air. Their study revealed 100% sensitivity and 87.5% specificity for the sonographic detection of subcutaneous air. Although subcutaneous air is a pathognomonic feature of NF, the incidence of soft tissue air in NF is unknown, although one study estimated this number to be as high as 57%.[137]

SONOGRAPHIC FINDINGS

On sonography, NF initially resembles cellulitis. The soft tissue appears edematous with hypoechoic areas interspersed among the hyperechoic soft tissue. With progression of the disease, there is thickening of the subcutaneous tissue and fascia (**Fig. 24**), abnormal fluid collections along the fascial plane (**Fig. 25**), irregularity of the fascia,

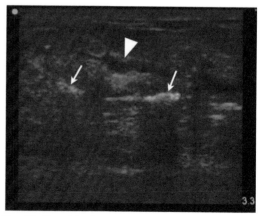

Fig. 25. NF with abnormal fluid collections between fascial planes (*arrowhead*) and air within the soft tissue (*arrows*).

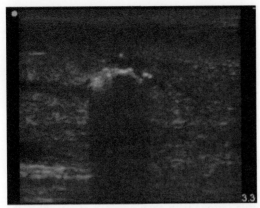

Fig. 26. NF. Note the presence of subcutaneous air and the associated dirty shadowing.

and ultimately air within the subcutaneous tissue (**Fig. 26**).[134,135] These small pockets of air may appear highly echogenic between the soft tissue interfaces.[134] Ultrasonography may have particular usefulness in the diagnosis of NF in children in whom the soft tissue layer is thinner, which allows more effective interrogation of the deep tissue planes.[132] Aside from the presence of subcutaneous gas, most sonographic features of NF are not specific to this disease, because the thick and echogenic hypodermal tissue noted in cases of NF is similar to that observed in soft tissue edema.[132]

SUMMARY

Musculoskeletal sonography has been shown to be a promising imaging modality for the diagnosis of a variety of acute conditions, including fractures, effusions, tendon injuries, dislocations, and soft tissue infections. Ultrasonography avoids the radiation associated with radiography and CT and can often be performed more expeditiously than MR imaging. Assessing the area of concern using dynamic range of motion is also a distinct advantage of this imaging modality. The use of this application of ultrasonography in an ED setting is new, and further work is necessary in order to clarify the role of ultrasonography in the evaluation of patients who present with musculoskeletal complaints.

PEARLS/PITFALLS

Pearls
- Patients should be positioned comfortably with the extremity exposed so that a thorough examination can be performed both statically and with dynamic maneuvers.[98]

- Examine the area in question in 2 orthogonal planes, and ensure that the probe is held perpendicular to the tissue.
- Although ultrasonography has been proved to be accurate for the detection of joint dislocations, radiography is still needed if a dislocation-associated fracture is suspected.

Pitfalls
- Cartilage and effusion can have similar sonographic appearances.
- Anisotropy can be mistaken for a disorder.
- Ultrasonography should not be used to exclude the diagnosis of NF.

ACKNOWLEDGMENTS

The authors appreciate the assistance provided by Dr Romolo Gaspari, Dr Turan Saul, Dr Kuo-Chih Chen, Dr Shree Sharma, and Illya Pushkar, who provided images for this article.

REFERENCES

1. National Hospital Ambulatory Medical Care Survey: 2010 emergency department summary tables. Available at: www.cdc.gov/nchs/data/ahcd/ahcd_products.htm. Accessed November 5, 2013.
2. Fleisher GR, Ludwig S, Henretig FM. Textbook of pediatric emergency medicine. 5th edition. Philadelphia: Lippincott Williams &Wilkins; 2006.
3. Joshi N, Lira A, Mehta N, et al. Diagnostic accuracy of history, physical examination, and bedside ultrasound for diagnosis of extremity fractures in the emergency department: a systematic review. Acad Emerg Med 2013;20(1):1–15.
4. Bentohami A, Walenkamp MM, Slaar A, et al. Amsterdam wrist rules: a clinical decision aid. BMC Musculoskelet Disord 2011;12:238.
5. Heyworth J. Ottawa ankle rules for the injured ankle. Br J Sports Med 2003;37(3):194.
6. Ma O, Mateer JR, Blaivas M. Emergency ultrasound. 2nd edition. New York: McGraw-Hill; 2008. p. 393–445.
7. Cross KP, Warkentine FH, Kim IK, et al. Bedside ultrasound diagnosis of clavicle fractures in the pediatric emergency department. Acad Emerg Med 2010;17(7):687–93.
8. Katz R, Landman J, Dulitzky F, et al. Fracture of the clavicle in the newborn. An ultrasound diagnosis. J Ultrasound Med 1988;7(1):21–3.
9. Kayser R, Mahlfeld K, Heyde C, et al. Ultrasonographic imaging of fractures of the clavicle in newborn infants. J Bone Joint Surg Br 2003;85(1):115–6.
10. Moritz JD, Berthold LD, Soenksen SF, et al. Ultrasound in diagnosis of fractures in children: unnecessary harassment or useful addition to X-ray? Ultraschall Med 2008;29(3):267–74.

11. Chien M, Bulloch B, Garcia-Filion P, et al. Bedside ultrasound in the diagnosis of pediatric clavicle fractures. Pediatr Emerg Care 2011; 27(11):1038–41.

12. Patel DD, Blumberg SM, Crain EF. The utility of bedside ultrasonography in identifying fractures and guiding fracture reduction in children. Pediatr Emerg Care 2009;25(4):221–5.

13. Chen L, Kim Y, Moore CL. Diagnosis and guided reduction of forearm fractures in children using bedside ultrasound. Pediatr Emerg Care 2007; 23(8):528–31.

14. Williamson D, Watura R, Cobby M. Ultrasound imaging of forearm fractures in children: a viable alternative? J Accid Emerg Med 2000; 17(1):22–4.

15. Hubner U, Schlicht W, Outzen S, et al. Ultrasound in the diagnosis of fractures in children. J Bone Joint Surg Br 2000;82(8):1170–3.

16. Rabiner JE, Khine H, Avner JR, et al. Accuracy of point-of-care ultrasonography for diagnosis of elbow fractures in children. Ann Emerg Med 2013;61(1):9–17.

17. Waterbrook AL, Adhikari S, Stolz U, et al. The accuracy of point-of-care ultrasound to diagnose long bone fractures in the ED. Am J Emerg Med 2013; 31(9):1352–6.

18. Marshburn TH, Legome E, Sargsyan A, et al. Goal-directed ultrasound in the detection of long-bone fractures. J Trauma 2004;57(2):329–32.

19. McNeil CR, McManus J, Mehta S. The accuracy of portable ultrasonography to diagnose fractures in an austere environment. Prehosp Emerg Care 2009;13(1):50–2.

20. Senall JA, Failla JM, Bouffard JA, et al. Ultrasound for the early diagnosis of clinically suspected scaphoid fracture. J Hand Surg Am 2004;29(3): 400–5.

21. Tayal VS, Antoniazzi J, Pariyadath M, et al. Prospective use of ultrasound imaging to detect bony hand injuries in adults. J Ultrasound Med 2007;26(9):1143–8.

22. Aksay E, Yesilaras M, Kilic TY, et al. Sensitivity and specificity of bedside ultrasonography in the diagnosis of fractures of the fifth metacarpal. Emerg Med J 2013. http://dx.doi.org/10.1136/emermed-2013-202971.

23. Chan SS. Emergency bedside ultrasound for the diagnosis of rib fractures. Am J Emerg Med 2009;27(5):617–20.

24. Griffith JF, Rainer TH, Ching AS, et al. Sonography compared with radiography in revealing acute rib fracture. AJR Am J Roentgenol 1999;173(6):1603–9.

25. Kara M, Dikmen E, Erdal HH, et al. Disclosure of unnoticed rib fractures with the use of ultrasonography in minor blunt chest trauma. Eur J Cardiothorac Surg 2003;24(4):608–13.

26. Rainer TH, Griffith JF, Lam E, et al. Comparison of thoracic ultrasound, clinical acumen, and radiography in patients with minor chest injury. J Trauma 2004;56(6):1211–3.

27. Greenes DS, Schutzman SA. Clinical significance of scalp abnormalities in asymptomatic head-injured infants. Pediatr Emerg Care 2001;17(2): 88–92.

28. Greenes DS, Schutzman SA. Infants with isolated skull fracture: what are their clinical characteristics, and do they require hospitalization? Ann Emerg Med 1997;30(3):253–9.

29. Kleinman PK, Spevak MR. Soft tissue swelling and acute skull fractures. J Pediatr 1992;121(5 Pt 1): 737–9.

30. Quayle KS, Jaffe DM, Kuppermann N, et al. Diagnostic testing for acute head injury in children: when are head computed tomography and skull radiographs indicated? Pediatrics 1997;99(5):E11.

31. Chung S, Schamban N, Wypij D, et al. Skull radiograph interpretation of children younger than two years: how good are pediatric emergency physicians? Ann Emerg Med 2004;43(6):718–22.

32. Lloyd DA, Carty H, Patterson M, et al. Predictive value of skull radiography for intracranial injury in children with blunt head injury. Lancet 1997; 349(9055):821–4.

33. Brenner D, Elliston C, Hall E, et al. Estimated risks of radiation-induced fatal cancer from pediatric CT. Am J Roentgenol 2001;176(2):289–96.

34. Rabiner JE, Friedman LM, Khine H, et al. Accuracy of point-of-care ultrasound for diagnosis of skull fractures in children. Pediatrics 2013;131(6):e1757–64.

35. Riera A, Chen L. Ultrasound evaluation of skull fractures in children: a feasibility study. Pediatr Emerg Care 2012;28(5):420–5.

36. Ramirez-Schrempp D, Vinci RJ, Liteplo AS. Bedside ultrasound in the diagnosis of skull fractures in the pediatric emergency department. Pediatr Emerg Care 2011;27(4):312–4.

37. Weinberg ER, Tunik MG, Tsung JW. Accuracy of clinician-performed point-of-care ultrasound for the diagnosis of fractures in children and young adults. Injury 2010;41(8):862–8.

38. Parri N, Crosby BJ, Glass C, et al. Ability of emergency ultrasonography to detect pediatric skull fractures: a prospective, observational study. J Emerg Med 2013;44(1):135–41.

39. Kane D, Balint PV, Sturrock RD. Ultrasonography is superior to clinical examination in the detection and localization of knee joint effusion in rheumatoid arthritis. J Rheumatol 2003;30(5):966–71.

40. Adhikari S, Blaivas M. Utility of bedside sonography to distinguish soft tissue abnormalities from joint effusions in the emergency department. J Ultrasound Med 2010;29(4):519–26.

41. Boniface KS, Ajmera K, Cohen JS, et al. Ultrasound-guided arthrocentesis of the elbow: a posterior approach. J Emerg Med 2013;45(5): 698–701.

42. Sibbitt WL Jr, Kettwich LG, Band PA, et al. Does ultrasound guidance improve the outcomes of the arthrocentesis and corticosteroid injection of the knee? Scand J Rheumatol 2012;41(1): 66–72.

43. Wiler JL, Costantino TG, Filippone L, et al. Comparison of ultrasound-guided and standard landmark techniques for knee arthrocentesis. J Emerg Med 2010;39(1):76–82.

44. Nazarian LN. The top 10 reasons musculoskeletal sonography is an important complementary or alternative technique to MRI. AJR Am J Roentgenol 2008;190(6):1621–6.

45. Hadduck TA, van Holsbeeck MT, Girish G, et al. Value of ultrasound before joint aspiration. AJR Am J Roentgenol 2013;201(3):W453–9.

46. Valley VT, Stahmer SA. Targeted musculoarticular sonography in the detection of joint effusions. Acad Emerg Med 2001;8(4):361–7.

47. De Maeseneer M, Jacobson JA, Jaovisidha S, et al. Elbow effusions: distribution of joint fluid with flexion and extension and imaging implications. Invest Radiol 1998;33:117–25.

48. Zuazo I, Bonnefoy O, Tauzin C, et al. Acute elbow trauma in children: role of ultrasonography. Pediatr Radiol 2008;38(9):982–8.

49. Hauzeur JP, Mathy L, De Maertelaer V. Comparison between clinical evaluation and ultrasonography in detecting hydrarthrosis of the knee. J Rheumatol 1999;26(12):2681–3.

50. Hong BY, Lim SH, Cho YR, et al. Detection of knee effusion by ultrasonography. Am J Phys Med Rehabil 2010;89:715–21.

51. Hirsch G, O'Neill T, Kitas G, et al. Distribution of effusion in knee arthritis as measured by high-resolution ultrasound. Clin Rheumatol 2012;31: 1243–6.

52. Mandl P, Brossard M, Aegerter P, et al. Ultrasound evaluation of fluid in the knee recesses at varying degrees of flexion. Arthritis Care Res (Hoboken) 2012;64(5):773–9.

53. Uryasev O, Joseph OC, McNamara JP, et al. Novel joint cupping clinical maneuver for the ultrasonographic detection of knee joint effusions. Am J Emerg Med 2013;31(11):1598–600.

54. Ike RW, Somers EC, Arnold EL, et al. Ultrasound of the knee during voluntary quadriceps contraction: a technique for detecting otherwise occult effusions. Arthritis Care Res (Hoboken) 2010;62(5): 725–9.

55. Alessi S, Depaoli R, Canepari M, et al. Baker's cyst in pediatric patients: ultrasonographic characteristics. J Ultrasound 2012;15(1):76–81.

56. Fananapazir G, Allison SJ. Common applications of musculoskeletal ultrasound in the emergency department. Ultrasound Clin 2011;6(2):215–26.

57. Volberg FM, Sumner TE, Abramson JS, et al. Unreliability of radiographic diagnosis of septic hip in children. Pediatrics 1984;74(1):118–20.

58. Pauroso S, Di Martino A, Tarantino CC, et al. Transient synovitis of the hip: ultrasound appearance. Mini-pictorial essay. J Ultrasound 2011; 14(2):92–4.

59. Berman L, Fink AM, Wilson D, et al. Technical note: identifying and aspirating hip effusions. Br J Radiol 1995;68(807):306–10.

60. Moss SG, Schweitzer ME, Jacobson JA, et al. Hip joint fluid: detection and distribution at MR imaging and US with cadaveric correlation. Radiology 1998; 208:43–8.

61. Zeiger MM, Dor U, Schultz RD. Ultrasonography of the hip joint effusions. Skeletal Radiol 1987; 16:607–11.

62. Vieira RL, Levy JA. Bedside ultrasonography to identify hip effusions in pediatric patients. Ann Emerg Med 2010;55:284–9.

63. Tsung JW, Blaivas M. Emergency department diagnosis of pediatric hip effusion and guided arthrocentesis using point-of-care ultrasound. J Emerg Med 2008;35:393–9.

64. Freeman K, Dewitz A, Baker W. Ultrasound-guided hip arthrocentesis in the ED. Am J Emerg Med 2007;25:80–6.

65. Minardi JJ, Lander OM. Septic hip arthritis: diagnosis and arthrocentesis using bedside ultrasound. J Emerg Med 2012;43:316–8.

66. Weybright PN, Jacobson JA, Murry KH, et al. Limited effectiveness of sonography in revealing hip joint effusion: preliminary results in 21 adult patients with native and prosthetic hips. AJR Am J Roentgenol 2003;181:215–8.

67. Thomas A, Kümmel S, Fritzsche F, et al. Real-time sonoelastography performed in addition to B-mode ultrasound and mammography: improved differentiation of breast lesions? Acad Radiol 2006;13(12):1496–504.

68. Asteria C, Giovanardi A, Pizzocaro A, et al. US-elastography in the differential diagnosis of benign and malignant thyroid nodules. Thyroid 2008;18(5): 523–31.

69. Taylor LS, Rubens DJ, Porter BC, et al. Prostate cancer: three-dimensional sonoelastography for in vitro detection. Radiology 2005;237(3):981–5.

70. Lyshchik A, Higashi T, Asato R, et al. Cervical lymph node metastases: diagnosis at sonoelastography-initial experience. Radiology 2007;243(1):258–67.

71. Ying L, Lin X, Xie ZL, et al. Clinical utility of acoustic radiation force impulse imaging for identification of malignant liver lesions: a meta-analysis. Eur Radiol 2012;22(12):2798–805.

72. Drakonaki EE, Allen GM, Wilson DJ. Real-time ultrasound elastography of the normal Achilles tendon: reproducibility and pattern description. Clin Radiol 2009;64(12):1196–202.

73. Orman G, Ozben S, Huseyinoglu N, et al. Ultrasound elastographic evaluation in the diagnosis of carpal tunnel syndrome: initial findings. Ultrasound Med Biol 2013;39(7):1184–9.

74. Drakonaki EE, Allen GM, Wilson DJ. Ultrasound elastography for musculoskeletal applications. Br J Radiol 2012;85(1019):1435–45.

75. Garra BS. Imaging and estimation of tissue elasticity by ultrasound. Ultrasound Q 2007;23(4):255–68.

76. Gaspari R, Blehar D, Mendoza M, et al. Use of ultrasound elastography for skin and subcutaneous abscesses. J Ultrasound Med 2009;28(7):855–60.

77. Gaspari R, Blehar D, Briones J, et al. Sonoelastographic characteristics of abscess induration associated with therapy failure. J Ultrasound Med 2012;31(9):1405–11.

78. De Zordo T, Chhem R, Smekal V, et al. Real-time sonoelastography: findings in patients with symptomatic Achilles tendons and comparison to healthy volunteers. Ultraschall Med 2010;31(4):394–400.

79. Klauser AS, Miyamoto H, Tamegger M, et al. Achilles tendon assessed with sonoelastography: histologic agreement. Radiology 2013;267(3):837–42.

80. Sconfienza LM, Silvestri E, Cimmino MA. Sonoelastography in the evaluation of painful Achilles tendon in amateur athletes. Clin Exp Rheumatol 2010;28(3):373–8.

81. Douglas MG, Sumner DS. Duplex scanning for deep vein thrombosis: has it replaced both phlebography and noninvasive testing? Semin Vasc Surg 1996;9(1):3–12.

82. Heijboer H, Jongbloets LM, Büller HR, et al. Clinical utility of real-time ultrasonography for diagnostic management of patients with recurrent venous thrombosis. Acta Radiol 1992;33(4):297–300.

83. Rubin JM, Xie H, Kim K, et al. Sonographic elasticity imaging of acute and chronic deep venous thrombosis in humans. J Ultrasound Med 2006;25(9):1179–86.

84. Bhatia KS, Rasalkar DD, Lee YP, et al. Real-time qualitative ultrasound elastography of miscellaneous non-nodal neck masses: applications and limitations. Ultrasound Med Biol 2010;36(10):1644–52.

85. Wu CH, Chang KV, Mio S, et al. Sonoelastography of the plantar fascia. Radiology 2011;259(2):502–7.

86. Sconfienza LM, Silvestri E, Orlandi D, et al. Real-time sonoelastography of the plantar fascia: comparison between patients with plantar fasciitis and healthy control subjects. Radiology 2013;267(1):195–200.

87. De Zordo T, Lill SR, Fink C, et al. Real-time sonoelastography of lateral epicondylitis: comparison of findings between patients and healthy volunteers. AJR Am J Roentgenol 2009;193(1):180–5.

88. Jeyapalan K, Bisson MA, Dias JJ, et al. The role of ultrasound in the management of flexor tendon injuries. J Hand Surg 2008;33(4):430–4.

89. Wu TS, Roque PJ, Green J, et al. Bedside ultrasound evaluation of tendon injuries. Am J Emerg Med 2012;30(8):1617–21.

90. Soubeyrand M, Biau D, Jomaah N, et al. Penetrating volar injuries of the hand: diagnostic accuracy of US in depicting soft-tissue lesions. Radiology 2008;249(1):228–35.

91. Adhikari S, Marx J, Crum T. Point-of-care ultrasound diagnosis of acute Achilles tendon rupture in the ED. Am J Emerg Med 2012;30(4):634.

92. You JS, Chung YE, Kim D, et al. Rupture of the flexor digitorum profundus tendon caused by closed blunt trauma. J Emerg Med 2011;41(4):e91–2.

93. Sisson C, Nagdev A, Tirado A, et al. Ultrasound diagnosis of traumatic partial triceps tendon tear in the emergency department. J Emerg Med 2011;40(4):436–8.

94. LaRocco BG, Zlupko G, Sierzenski P. Ultrasound diagnosis of quadriceps tendon rupture. J Emerg Med 2008;35(3):293–5.

95. Lee DH, Robbin ML, Galliott R, et al. Ultrasound evaluation of flexor tendon lacerations. J Hand Surg 2000;25(2):236–41.

96. Kälebo P, Allenmark C, Peterson L, et al. Diagnostic value of ultrasonography in partial ruptures of the Achilles tendon. Am J Sports Med 1992;20(4):378–81.

97. Campbell RS, Grainger AJ. Current concepts in imaging of tendinopathy. Clin Radiol 2001;56:253–67.

98. Adler RS, Finzel KC. The complementary roles of MR imaging and ultrasound of tendons. Radiol Clin North Am 2005;43(4):771–807.

99. Jamadar DA, Robertson BL, Jacobson JA, et al. Musculoskeletal sonography: important imaging pitfalls. AJR Am J Roentgenol 2010;194(1):216–25.

100. Petranova T, Vlad V, Porta F, et al. Ultrasound of the shoulder. Med Ultrason 2012;14(2):133–40.

101. Blaivas M, Lyon M, Brannam L, et al. Water bath evaluation technique for emergency ultrasound of painful superficial structures. Am J Emerg Med 2004;22(7):589–93.

102. Iannotti JP, Ciccone J, Buss DD, et al. Accuracy of office-based ultrasonography of the shoulder for the diagnosis of rotator cuff tears. J Bone Joint Surg Am 2005;87(6):1305–11.

103. Al-Shawi A, Badge R, Bunker T. The detection of full thickness rotator cuff tears using ultrasound. J Bone Joint Surg Br 2008;90:889–92.

104. Hess GW. Achilles tendon rupture: a review of etiology, population, anatomy, risk factors, and injury prevention. Foot Ankle Spec 2010;3(1):29–32.

105. Lehtinen A, Peltokallio P, Taavitsainen M. Sonography of Achilles tendon correlated to operative findings. Ann Chir Gynaecol 1994;83:322–7.

106. Hartgerink P, Fessel DP, Jacobson JA, et al. Full-versus partial-thickness Achilles tendon tears: sonographic accuracy and characterization in 26 cases with surgical correlation. Radiology 2001; 220(2):406–12.

107. Jeffrey RB, Laing FC, Schechter WP, et al. Acute suppurative tenosynovitis of the hand: diagnosis with US. Radiology 1987;162(3):741–2.

108. Shuster M, Abu-Laban RB, Boyd J. Prereduction radiographs in clinically evident anterior shoulder dislocation. Am J Emerg Med 1999;17(7):653–8.

109. Abbasi S, Molaie H, Hafezimoghadam P, et al. Diagnostic accuracy of ultrasonographic examination in the management of shoulder dislocation in the emergency department. Ann Emerg Med 2013;62:170–5.

110. Yuen CK, Mok KL, Kan PG, et al. Bedside ultrasound for verification of shoulder reduction with the lateral and anterior approaches. Am J Emerg Med 2009;27:503–4.

111. Saul T, Ng L, Lewiss RE. Point-of-care ultrasound in the diagnosis of upper extremity fracture-dislocation. A pictorial essay. Med Ultrason 2013; 15(3):230–6.

112. Zacchilli MA, Owens BD. Epidemiology of shoulder dislocations presenting to emergency departments in the United States. J Bone Joint Surg Am 2010; 92:542–9.

113. Brady WJ, Knuth CJ, Pirrallo RG. Bilateral inferior glenohumeral dislocation: luxatio erecta, an unusual presentation of a rare disorder. J Emerg Med 1995;13:37–42.

114. Beck S, Chilstrom M. Point-of-care ultrasound diagnosis and treatment of posterior shoulder dislocation. Am J Emerg Med 2013;31(2):449. e3–5.

115. Blakeley CJ, Spencer O, Newman-Saunders T, et al. A novel use of portable ultrasound in the management of shoulder dislocation. Emerg Med J 2009;26:662–3.

116. Halberg MJ, Sweeney TW, Owens WB. Bedside ultrasound for verification of shoulder reduction. Am J Emerg Med 2009;27(1):134.e5–6.

117. Kuhn MA, Ross G. Acute elbow dislocations. Orthop Clin North Am 2008;39(2):155–61.

118. Ross G. Acute elbow dislocation: on-site treatment. Phys Sportsmed 1999;27(2):121–2.

119. De Maeseneer M, Marcelis S, Cattrysse E, et al. Ultrasound of the elbow: a systematic approach using bony landmarks. Eur J Radiol 2012;81(5): 919–22.

120. Macias CG, Bothner J, Wiebe R. A comparison of supination/flexion to hyperpronation in the reduction of radial head subluxations. Pediatrics 1998;102:e10.

121. Schunk JE. Radial head subluxation: epidemiology and treatment of 87 episodes. Ann Emerg Med 1990;19:1019–23.

122. Dohi D. Confirmed specific ultrasonographic findings of pulled elbow. J Pediatr Orthop 2013;33(8): 829–31.

123. Diab HS, Hamed MM, Allam Y. Obscure pathology of pulled elbow: dynamic high-resolution ultrasound-assisted classification. J Child Orthop 2010;4(6):539–43.

124. McCaig LF, McDonald LC, Mandal S, et al. *Staphylococcus aureus*-associated skin and soft tissue infections in ambulatory care. Emerg Infect Dis 2006;12(11):1715–23.

125. Pallin DJ, Egan DJ, Pelletier AJ, et al. Increased US emergency department visits for skin and soft tissue infections, and changes in antibiotic choices, during the emergence of community-associated methicillin-resistant *Staphylococcus aureus*. Ann Emerg Med 2008;51(3):291–8.

126. Fergie J, Purcell K. The epidemic of methicillin-resistant *Staphylococcus aureus* colonization and infection in children: effects on the community, health systems, and physician practices. Pediatr Ann 2007;36(7):404–12.

127. Cardinal E, Bureau NJ, Aubin B, et al. Role of ultrasound in musculoskeletal infections. Radiol Clin North Am 2001;39(2):191–201.

128. Robben SG. Ultrasonography of musculoskeletal infections in children. Eur Radiol 2004;14(Suppl 4):L65–77.

129. Loyer EM, DuBrow RA, David CL, et al. Imaging of superficial soft-tissue infections: sonographic findings in cases of cellulitis and abscess. AJR Am J Roentgenol 1996;166(1):149–52.

130. Ramirez-Schrempp D, Dorfman DH, Baker WE, et al. Ultrasound soft-tissue applications in the pediatric emergency department: to drain or not to drain? Pediatr Emerg Care 2009;25(1):44–8.

131. Sarani B, Strong M, Pascual J, et al. Necrotizing fasciitis: current concepts and review of the literature. J Am Coll Surg 2009;208(2):279–88.

132. Malghem J, Lecouvet FE, Omoumi P, et al. Necrotizing fasciitis: contribution and limitations of diagnostic imaging. Joint Bone Spine 2013; 80(2):146–54.

133. Roje Z, Matic D, Librenjak D, et al. Necrotizing fasciitis: literature review of contemporary strategies for diagnosing and management with three case reports: torso, abdominal wall, upper and lower limbs. World J Emerg Surg 2011;6(1):46.

134. Butcher CH, Dooley RW, Levitov AB. Detection of subcutaneous and intramuscular air with

sonography: a sensitive and specific modality. J Ultrasound Med 2011;30(6):791–5.

135. Yen ZS, Wang HP, Ma HM, et al. Ultrasonographic screening of clinically-suspected necrotizing fasciitis. Acad Emerg Med 2002;9(12): 1448–51.

136. Chao HC, Kong MS, Lin TY. Diagnosis of necrotizing fasciitis in children. J Ultrasound Med 1999; 18(4):277–81.

137. Elliott DC, Kufera JA, Myers RA. Necrotizing soft tissue infections. Risk factors for mortality and strategies for management. Ann Surg 1996;224(5):672–83.

Ultrasound Protocol Use in the Evaluation of an Unstable Patient

Danielle Hallett, MD[a], Parisa P. Javedani, MD[a],
Jarrod Mosier, MD[a,b,*]

KEYWORDS

- Ultrasound • Hemodynamically unstable • Resuscitation • Protocol • Emergency • Shock

KEY POINTS

- Bedside ultrasound has been shown to facilitate faster and more accurate diagnoses in unstable patients in the emergency department.
- Rapid ultrasound examination of the unstable patient allows physicians to detect reversible causes, such as pericardial tamponade, decreased cardiac contractility, right heart strain, hypovolemia, pleural effusion, pulmonary edema, pneumothorax, and abdominal aortic aneurysm, with reasonable accuracy.
- The ultrasound examination can be repeated frequently to determine a patient's response to therapy.
- In patients with pulseless electrical activity or asystole, lack of cardiac motion on echocardiography correlates with a poor likelihood of survival.
- Many ultrasound protocols have been proposed for the evaluation of the unstable patient but few have been validated.

 Videos related to pertinent ultrasound findings accompany this article at http://www.ultrasound.theclinics.com/

CASE 1

A 63-year-old woman with a history of atrial fibrillation, asthma, rheumatoid arthritis, and hypertension arrives in the emergency department (ED) via ambulance for shortness of breath and cough. On initial evaluation, her heart rate is 120 beats per minute (bpm), blood pressure is 87/50 mm Hg, temperature is 38.4°C, respiratory rate is 28 breaths per minute, and oxygen saturation is 85% on 15 liters per minute (lpm) via a nonrebreather mask. The patient's heart and lung examination reveals crackles throughout all lung fields. Her electrocardiogram shows ST elevation in leads aVR and V_1, with diffuse ST depression in the other leads.

Discussion of the Problem/Introduction

This case describes a common diagnostic and therapeutic dilemma when treating a patient in the ED with undifferentiated hypotension. An immune-suppressed middle-aged woman presents febrile, hypotensive, and tachycardic with shortness of breath and electrocardiographic findings concerning for myocardial ischemia. The

Disclosures: None.
[a] Department of Emergency Medicine, University of Arizona, 1609 North Warren Avenue, FOB 122C, Tucson, AZ 85719, USA; [b] Section of Pulmonary, Critical Care, Allergy and Sleep, Department of Medicine, University of Arizona, 1609 North Warren Avenue, Room 122C, PO Box 245057, Tucson, AZ 85724-5057, USA
* Corresponding author. Department of Emergency Medicine, University of Arizona, 1609 North Warren, FOB 122C, Tucson, AZ 85719.
E-mail address: jmosier@aemrc.arizona.edu

Ultrasound Clin 9 (2014) 293–306
http://dx.doi.org/10.1016/j.cult.2014.01.006
1556-858X/14/$ – see front matter © 2014 Elsevier Inc. All rights reserved.

physician must determine whether this is severe sepsis requiring fluid resuscitation or a cardiogenic or obstructive cause of shock, in which fluid resuscitation might be detrimental. In this case, a bedside ultrasound is performed and the echocardiogram shows an enlarged right ventricle with septal flattening (Video 1). The inferior vena cava (IVC) measures 2.2 cm and has no respiratory variation (**Fig. 1**).

All findings were consistent with elevated right heart pressure and suspected pulmonary embolism. The emergency physician evaluated the veins of the lower extremities and found a thrombus in the popliteal vein (Video 2). Treatment with tissue plasminogen activator was given in the ED and the patient was admitted to the intensive care unit (ICU).

When critically ill patients arrive in the ED, the initial evaluation can be limited by a variety of factors, leaving practitioners to sift through the vast possibilities for the patient's deteriorating condition. Traditionally, physicians depend on physical examination to guide diagnosis and initiate resuscitation in these critical first minutes. The scarcity of information can lead to inaccurate diagnosis or unnecessary and potentially harmful therapeutic interventions, which could be detrimental to the patient's care. Using the case described as an example, administering intravenous fluids to a patient believed to be in septic shock could cause further decompensation if the patient were actually experiencing obstructive shock from a pulmonary embolism.

Point-of-care ultrasound provides the ability to quickly narrow the differential diagnosis and guide appropriate resuscitation of critically ill patients. Early ultrasound evaluation of critically ill patients has been shown to increase the accuracy of and decrease the time to diagnosis, and change the disposition of many patients.[1–3]

In the evaluation of unstable patients, ultrasound has several advantages. First, it is performed at the bedside, allowing tenuous patients to remain where they can be aggressively treated and carefully monitored. Second, it is the only readily available modality that allows real-time dynamic imaging to occur at the same time as an intervention or diagnostic maneuver, such as passive leg raise. Finally, the examination can be repeated frequently to assess the patient's response to therapies without concern for additional radiation.

Several ultrasound protocols have been developed for the evaluation and resuscitation of unstable patients, both medical and traumatic.[3–10] Few of these protocols have been studied or validated in their entirety, but good evidence supports the individual components within these protocols. Each protocol is unique in the views obtained and level of complexity of image interpretation. Despite that, all protocols evaluate some combination of the following structures: heart, IVC, aorta, abdomen, pleura, and lower extremity veins. The following is a review of how each of these structures is evaluated with ultrasound and how the evaluation guides resuscitation of an unstable patient. This review will describe and compare ultrasound use and protocols in the undifferentiated unstable patient. **Table 1** describes the common ultrasound findings in the shock state.

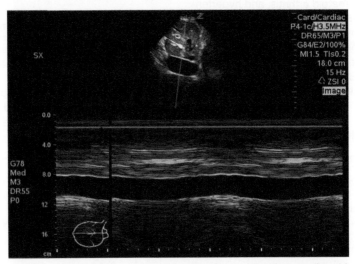

Fig. 1. An M-mode image through the inferior vena cava showing a dilated, noncollapsible inferior vena cava.

Table 1
Common ultrasound findings in the shock state

		Hypovolemia		Obstructive			Cardiogenic	Distributive
		Dehydration	Hemorrhage	Pulmonary Embolism	Tamponade	Tension Pneumothorax	Heart Failure/ Acute MI	Sepsis
Cardiac	Pericardial effusion	—	—	—	Present	—	—	—
	Contractility	Increased	Increased	Increased	Increased	Increased	+/− WMA	Increased
	Right atrium	Collapse	Collapse	Enlarged	Collapse	Collapse	+/− Enlarged	Collapse
	RVDC	—	—	—	Present	Present	—	—
	Ventricular size	—	—	Enlarged RV	—	—	+/− Enlarged ventricles	—
IVC		>50% collapse	>50% collapse	Plethoric	Plethoric	Plethoric	Plethoric	>50% collapse
Aorta		—	+/− AAA	—	—	—	—	—
Abdomen		—	+/− Peritoneal hemorrhage	—	—	—	—	—
Pleura	Lung sliding	—	—	—	—	Absent	—	—
	Comet tails	—	—	—	—	Absent	+/− Pulmonary edema	+/− Pneumonia
	Pleural effusion	—	+/− Hemothorax	—	—	—	+/−	—
Lower extremity veins		—	—	+/− DVT	—	—	—	—

Abbreviations: AAA, abdominal aortic aneurysm; DVT, deep vein thrombosis; MI, myocardial infarction; RV, right ventricle; RVDC, right ventricular diastolic collapse; WMA, wall motion abnormality.

COMPONENTS OF POINT-OF-CARE ULTRASOUND PROTOCOLS AND THEIR INTERPRETATION

Cardiac: Evaluate for Pericardial Effusion, Tamponade, Assess Contractility, Chamber Size

Every protocol includes cardiac imaging, and varies in the number of views obtained, goals of evaluation, and level of interpretation. A bedside echocardiogram traditionally consists of 4 views (subxiphoid, parasternal long axis, parasternal short axis, and apical 4 or 5 chamber). The subxiphoid view (Video 3) provides a reliable view of all 4 chambers of the heart, using the liver as an acoustic window, and is optimal for determining the presence of cardiac effusion and tamponade (Video 4). The subxiphoid view can also provide a general idea of overall contractility. From the subxiphoid view, the IVC can be quickly evaluated for volume responsiveness (Video 5). The parasternal long axis (Video 6) is most useful for evaluating the left ventricle (LV) and LV outflow tract for contractility, wall motion, and outflow obstruction. Additionally, right ventricular (RV) diastolic collapse seen in tamponade is assessed in the parasternal long axis view. The parasternal short axis view (Video 7) assesses contractility, wall motion, relative ventricular diameter, and signs of RV pressure or volume overload. Finally, an apical view (Video 8) provides a 4-chamber longitudinal view of the heart for assessment of contractility, relative chamber size, and the valves, and allows hemodynamic measurements.

In the assessment and resuscitation of unstable patients, comprehensive echocardiography is often impractical to obtain in a timely manner. Focused point-of-care echocardiography provides information through quickly addressing some basic yes/no questions (ie, "Is a pericardial effusion present?"). Basic applications of point-of-care echocardiography evaluate for the presence of pericardial effusion, assess overall contractility, and evaluate relative chamber size.[4,10,11] More-advanced protocols provide a more detailed evaluation of chamber contractility and motion, valvular integrity, and hemodynamic measurements.[3,5,6,12]

In patients at high-risk for pericardial effusion, ultrasound-trained emergency physicians (EPs) are able to detect pericardial effusion on bedside ultrasound with excellent accuracy.[11] In the setting of an unstable patient, the presence of a pericardial effusion suggests pericardial tamponade as a possible cause of hypotension or dyspnea. Pericardial effusions are best visualized using the subxiphoid or parasternal long axis views (Fig. 2).[6] If a pericardial effusion is seen, further evaluation for signs of pericardial tamponade should be pursued, including RV diastolic collapse and IVC plethora.[13]

RV diastolic collapse is often difficult to visualize in patients with tachycardia, and using M-mode can help differentiate the status of the ventricle in various phases of the cardiac cycle. In the parasternal long axis view, M-mode can be adjusted to include the anterior leaflet of the mitral valve and the free wall of the RV. The motion of the ventricle can then be correlated with the phase of the cardiac cycle based on the open or closed position of the mitral valve.[13] Additionally, using a cine loop function allows the sonologist to review cardiac movement frame by frame, better detailing chamber changes of the RV. In the setting of pericardial effusion, any collapse of the RV when the mitral valve is open is highly suggestive of tamponade.

Assessing overall cardiac contractility and wall motion abnormalities are important components of the point-of-care echocardiogram performed on hypotensive patients. A hyperdynamic LV as assessed by an emergency physician has a high

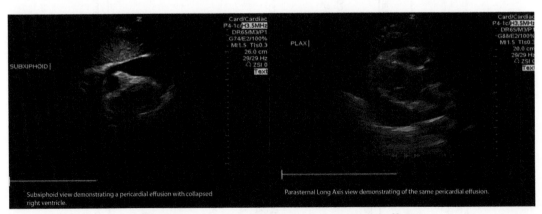

Subxiphoid view demonstrating a pericardial effusion with collapsed right ventricle.

Parasternal Long Axis view demonstrating of the same pericardial effusion.

Fig. 2. Subxiphoid and parasternal long axis views showing a large pericardial effusion.

specificity for sepsis as the underlying cause for hypotension.[14] In addition, with proper ultrasound training, EPs are capable of detecting wall motion abnormalities and hypokinesis that suggest cardiogenic causes for hypotension.[12,15] For the emergent evaluation, a global estimate of contractility is sufficient rather than the normal 17-segment evaluation performed on comprehensive echocardiography. Estimated ejection fraction can also be assessed on the parasternal long axis view with reasonable accuracy. Randazzo and colleagues[16] showed that ultrasound-trained EPs were able to categorize LV ejection fraction (LVEF) on bedside ultrasound as poor (<30%), moderate (30%–55%), or normal (>55%) with an 86.1% agreement with a formal echocardiogram.

The parasternal short axis is useful for comparing ventricular chamber size, pressures, and contractility. A dilated, hypodynamic LV suggests a cardiogenic origin. However, a hyperdynamic LV with cavitary obliteration on systole suggests volume depletion and sepsis as the cause. Further, LV cavitary obliteration in systole correlates with hypovolemia and suggests the patient would be responsive to intravenous fluid resuscitation.[17] An enlarged RV suggests right heart failure or obstructive disease, such as pulmonary embolism. Septal motion evaluated on the parasternal short axis view indicates relative chamber pressures; septal flattening with systole suggests RV pressure overload, whereas septal flattening in diastole suggests RV volume overload (**Fig. 3**).[18]

The apical view provides a longitudinal view of either 4 chambers or 5 chambers, if it includes a cross-section of the left ventricular outflow tract (LVOT). This view provides a qualitative estimate of relative chamber size and contractility and of valvular function, and allows for quantitative hemodynamic measurements of chamber pressures, stroke volume, and cardiac output. In the apical 5-chamber view, the pulse-wave Doppler can be placed over the LVOT, which creates a visual representation of stroke volume by measuring the LVOT velocity-time integral (VTi) (**Fig. 4**).[19] In addition to stroke volume measurement, respiratory variation in the LVOT VTi suggests hypovolemia and volume responsiveness (**Fig. 4**).[20–22] More advanced valvular and hemodynamic assessments are possible on bedside ultrasound but are beyond the scope of this review.

IVC: Collapsibility and Plethora

In addition to, or as part of the cardiac examination, evaluation of the IVC is important for assessing volume responsiveness and evidence of elevated right heart pressures. Appreciating volume responsiveness is of extreme importance in the resuscitation of a hypotensive patient and is often very challenging. Frequently, resuscitation efforts result in volume overload, which correlates with poor outcomes.[23–25] IVC collapsibility with respiration provides a view of the volume responsiveness of the patient and has been shown to be useful in spontaneously breathing and mechanically ventilated patients.[26,27]

The IVC is best evaluated using a subcostal approach as an extension of the subxiphoid cardiac view. When visualized in the long axis, M-mode may be used to determine the end-inspiratory and end-expiratory diameter of the IVC. Collapsibility of the IVC suggests the patient may be intravascularly depleted and responsive to intravenous fluids (**Fig. 5**). Most protocols consider clinically significant collapsibility to be 50% or greater because this correlates with a central venous pressure of less than 10 mm Hg.[28] However, significant controversy exists over the utility of central venous pressure, and lower thresholds (20%) of IVC collapsibility have been shown to correlate with fluid responsiveness.[26,29–32]

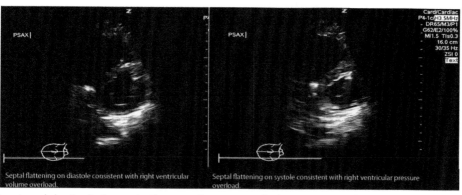

Septal flattening on diastole consistent with right ventricular volume overload.

Septal flattening on systole consistent with right ventricular pressure overload.

Fig. 3. Parasternal short axis demonstrating septal movement during pressure and volume overload of the right ventricle.

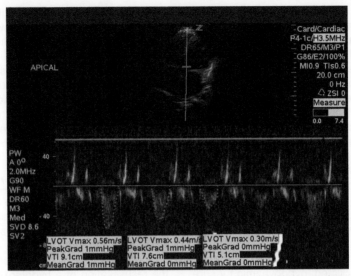

Fig. 4. Respiratory variation of the left ventricular Velocity-Time integral indicating volume responsiveness.

IVC plethora is described as an IVC measuring greater than 2 cm in diameter with little or no respiratory variation. This finding is suggestive of elevated right heart pressures, as seen with pulmonary embolism, tamponade, RV infarct, and fluid overload. Taken in combination with a large RV seen on the cardiac images and septal flattening seen on the parasternal short axis view, pulmonary embolism is the likely cause of this patient's instability (Video 9).

CASE 2

A 59-year-old man with a history of myocardial infarction and end-stage renal disease on dialysis arrives in the ED via ambulance for shortness of

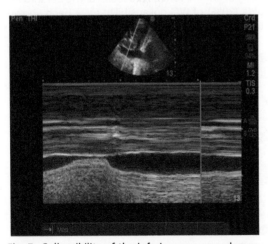

Fig. 5. Collapsibility of the inferior vena cava demonstrating volume responsiveness.

breath and altered mental status. His heart rate is 110 bpm, blood pressure is 67/42 mm Hg, temperature is 35.7°C, respiratory rate is 24 breaths per minute, and oxygen saturation is 90% on 2 lpm via nasal cannula. The patient opens his eyes to verbal stimulus, groans and mumbles incoherently to questions, and follows simple commands. His Glasgow coma score is 11. The remainder of his examination reveals crackles at the right lung bases and a normal heart and abdomen examination. An electrocardiogram shows a left bundle branch block. No old electrocardiogram results are available for comparison. A chest radiograph shows bilateral basilar opacities, worse on the right, concerning for pulmonary edema or infection. The physician suspects septic shock but cannot rule out cardiogenic shock, and is hesitant to initiate aggressive intravenous fluid resuscitation in the setting of renal failure and possible cardiogenic shock.

A bedside ultrasound is performed, which shows a hyperdynamic LV with no clear wall motion abnormality. The IVC is 100% collapsible with inspiration. The physician rapidly administers 1 L of normal saline along with broad-spectrum antibiotics and uses ultrasound to reevaluate the patient. The IVC now collapses 70% with inspiration and the blood pressure improves to 78/50 mm Hg. Fluids are bolused in increments of 500 mL and physical and ultrasound examinations are repeated frequently. After 2.5 L, the IVC is 10% collapsible, his heart rate is 86 mm Hg, his blood pressure is 94/60 bpm, and his mental status has improved. He is admitted to the ICU for further management.

Aorta: Abdominal Aortic Aneurysm

Many point-of-care ultrasound protocols include evaluation of the abdominal aorta, which consists of a single transverse sweep of the aorta from the subxiphoid position to the umbilicus to identify aortic dilation, false lumen, or clot. Studies have shown that EPs are capable of detecting abdominal aortic aneurysms (AAA) on ultrasound with high sensitivity and specificity.[33,34] Aortic dilation greater than 3 cm or evidence of dissection or rupture in an unstable patients warrants further investigation or emergent surgical consultation, depending on the clinical situation. However, a 3.5 cm classic AAA is unlikely to rupture and be the cause of instability (**Fig. 6**).

Abdomen (Free Fluid/Hemoperitoneum)

Although the abdominal examination is most often used for patients with blunt trauma, it may also be applicable in some medically unstable patients. The examiner can quickly examine the hepatorenal, splenorenal, and pelvic areas for free fluid in the abdomen (**Fig. 7**). Depending on the clinical situation and the physician's level of suspicion, free fluid found in any of these locations could signify aortic aneurysm rupture, ectopic pregnancy rupture, perforated colon, or other visceral abdominal injury.

Pleura: Sliding Lung Sign, B-Lines, Pleural Effusion

Lung ultrasound can be very helpful when evaluating unstable patients, particularly those presenting in respiratory distress. Using a vertically oriented linear probe to survey the anterior or lateral intercostal spaces, an examiner can often find evidence of pulmonary edema, pleural effusion, pneumonia, and pneumothorax.

A normal lung ultrasound will demonstrate the parietal and visceral pleura sliding beneath the chest wall with every respiration, known as the *sliding lung sign*. This function can be seen more easily when applying M-mode, which will create the classic seashore sign in which the sand-like appearance of moving normal lung appears below the linear appearance of the chest wall (Video 10). In radio-occult pneumothorax, absence of a lung sliding sign has been shown to be 100% sensitive and 78% specific.[35] Moreover, the transition point at which lung sliding is no longer visualized can sometimes be identified, known as the *lung point*. This finding is 66% to 79% sensitive and 100% specific for pneumothorax.[35,36]

A pleural effusion or hemothorax may appear as a hypoechoic fluid collection, particularly when evaluating the dependent lung portions (Video 11). Ultrasound can also be useful when evaluating lung parenchyma. Lung tissue may demonstrate "A-lines" or "B-lines," which can help support certain diagnoses. A-lines are artifactual, motionless, regularly spaced repetitive horizontal lines arising from pleura.[35] B-lines, or "comet tails," are artifacts that run vertically starting from the pleural surface. In normal lung, B-lines efface A-lines and run the depth of the screen without attenuation. In pneumothorax, ultrasound beams cannot be transmitted and lung sliding is absent because of the air between pleural layers. Furthermore, B-lines are no longer visible, and horizontal and A-lines are exclusively seen; this is called the *A-line sign*, which is 95% to 100% sensitive and 60% to 94% specific for diagnosing pneumothorax.[35] More than 3 B-lines in one intercostal space suggests interalveolar congestion, seen in conditions such as pulmonary edema and acute respiratory distress syndrome (ARDS), with a sensitivity of 93% and specificity of 93% compared with chest radiograph.[37,38]

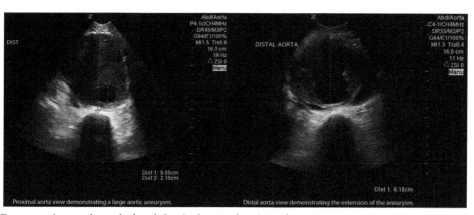

Fig. 6. Transverse image through the abdominal aorta showing a large aneurysm.

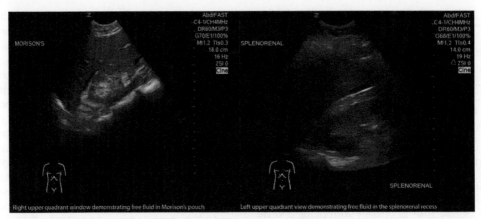

Right upper quadrant window demonstrating free fluid in Morison's pouch   Left upper quadrant view demonstrating free fluid in the splenorenal recess

Fig. 7. Free fluid seen in the right and left upper quadrants on a FAST exam.

Lower Extremity Veins: Deep Venous Thrombosis

Some protocols include a rapid assessment of the lower extremity veins for signs of thrombosis. Multiple studies show that bedside deep venous thrombosis (DVT) studies performed by EPs have reasonable sensitivity and specificity.[39–43] An abbreviated DVT study that assesses only the femoral and popliteal veins can be performed in emergent situations and still have a high correlation with comprehensive DVT ultrasound.[39,40] Evidence of DVT in either the femoral or popliteal vein might suggest pulmonary embolism as a source of hypotension, particularly in patients with a plethoric IVC or those showing signs of right heart strain on a cardiac examination.

ULTRASOUND EVALUATION OF THE MEDICALLY UNSTABLE PATIENT

Many bedside ultrasound protocols have been developed for evaluating unstable patients. Although the individual components comprising the protocols are supported by evidence, very few of the protocols have been evaluated in their entirety for feasibility or efficacy. The following summarizes key published protocols. **Table 2** provides a brief comparison of the existing protocols.

Undifferentiated Hypotensive Patient Protocol

One of the first protocols developed to assess patients with hypotension is the undifferentiated

Table 2
Comparison of ultrasound protocols

| Protocol | Cardiac | | | | | Abdomen | | | | | Formally Studied | Comments |
	Subx	PS	Apical	IVC	Aorta	HR	SR	Pelvic	Pleura	DVT		
UHP	X				X	X					No	
FATE	X	X	X						X		Yes	Studied in ICU setting[45]
Jones	X	X	X	X	X	X		X			Yes	Studied in ED setting[1]
BEAT		X	X	X							No	Intended for ICU application[6]
ACES	X	a	a	X	X	X	X	X			No	
RUSH	X	X	X	X	X	X	X	X	X	X	No	
FEEL	X	a	a								Yes	Code and peri-code situations[5]
eFAST	X					X	X	X	X		Yes[b]	Trauma patients

Abbreviations: DVT, deep vein thrombosis; ED, emergency department; HR, hepatorenal; ICU, intensive care unit; IVC, inferior vena cava; PS, parasternal; SR, splenorenal; Subx, subxiphoid.
  [a] Views may be added if subxiphoid view is inadequate.
  [b] eFAST has not been studied formally.

hypotensive patient (UHP) ultrasound protocol, which uses 3 views to evaluate the heart, aorta, and abdominal cavity using a small-footprint 3.5-MHz probe.[4] The UHP protocol assesses for intra-abdominal free fluid in the hepatorenal space (Morison pouch) with a single image, followed by a subxiphoid cardiac view to assess qualitative cardiac activity and the presence of a pericardial effusion, and a transverse sweep of the abdominal aorta to the bifurcation of the iliac arteries. Although the protocol only uses 3 views, the authors hypothesize that the source should be seen easily if present, overcoming the limitations of single-image evaluations. Based on level of suspicion or initial ultrasound findings, other images can be obtained for further diagnostic accuracy.

Although the UHP protocol provides a simple diagnostic maneuver to evaluate for pericardial effusion with tamponade; aortic aneurysm rupture; or intra-abdominal free fluid as the cause of hypotension, this abbreviated protocol has several limitations. Single images of Morison pouch to assess for intraperitoneal fluid have been shown to have a much lower sensitivity for detecting intraperitoneal hemorrhage than the traditional 3-view approach that includes splenorenal and pelvic views (51% vs 87%, respectively).[44] In addition, the protocol includes no evaluation of the pleura to investigate pulmonary causes of hypotension, such as pneumothorax. Finally, the protocol also does not include assessment of volume responsiveness (ie, evaluation of the IVC), limiting its ability to help guide resuscitation rather than just providing a simple diagnostic maneuver.

Focus Assessed Transthoracic Echocardiographic Protocol

The Focus Assessed Transthoracic Echocardiographic (FATE) protocol proposed by Jensen and colleagues[45] was initially intended for and studied in an intensive care unit (ICU) setting; however, it has utility in the ED because of its similarity to other existing protocols. This protocol involves obtaining 3 cardiac views (subxiphoid, parasternal, and apical) and bilateral lung views from the lateral thoracic wall using a phased array probe. In 233 FATE examinations performed on 210 patients in the ICU, at least one cardiac image was obtained in 97.0% of patients, and provided decisive information in 24.5% of patients and supplemental or supportive information in 73.0%. The cardiac window with the highest percentage of usable images was the apical position (79.8%). For the 4 examinations without obtainable cardiac images, a transesophageal echocardiogram was performed.

Although potentially helpful in the ICU, transesophageal echocardiography is usually not available for unstable patients in the ED. Additionally, the FATE protocol is limited in that it does not evaluate the IVC for volume status, abdominal compartment/aorta for hemorrhage, or anterior pleural windows for pneumothorax, or evaluate for lower extremity DVT.

Bedside Echocardiographic Assessment for Trauma/Critical Care Examination

The bedside echocardiographic assessment for trauma/critical care (BEAT) examination was initially established to evaluate cardiac function and volume status in a surgical ICU.[6] Although designed for the ICU, it does have some usefulness in the ED and, unlike the FATE examination, assesses volume status in addition to cardiac function. This protocol uses cardiac windows to obtain specific pieces of information: beat (cardiac output), effusion (pericardial or pleural effusion), area (ventricular size and contractility), and tank (preload).

First, with the patient in the left lateral decubitus position, the examiner uses the fractional shortening method to estimate cardiac output through measuring LV end systolic and end diastolic diameter in the parasternal long axis view. The ultrasound software can then estimate end systolic and diastolic volumes, and thus stroke volume, which is multiplied by the heart rate to estimate cardiac output. Next, the examiner may use any window to evaluate for pericardial effusion followed by parasternal short axis and apical 4-chamber views to assess relative ventricular size and contractility.

The last step involves assessing volume status using 2 separate methods. In the parasternal long axis view, the mitral valve is evaluated with M-mode or pulse-wave Doppler. An E wave corresponds to early diastolic filling, whereas the A wave corresponds to atrial contraction. The authors propose that a prominent E wave suggests hypervolemia, whereas an A wave that is more dominant suggests hypovolemia. Lastly, the IVC is visualized and measured in inspiration and expiration. An IVC collapse of greater than 50% is suggestive of hypovolemia or diminished preload.

Like the FATE examination, the BEAT protocol is highly focused on cardiac function and avoids assessing the abdomen for AAA or free fluid. However, it does provide a more quantitative analysis of hemodynamics, allowing practitioners to assess response to therapies in addition to using this protocol as a diagnostic maneuver to answer the 4 BEAT questions.

Abdominal and Cardiac Evaluation with Sonography in Shock Protocol

The Abdominal and Cardiac Evaluation with Sonography in Shock (ACES) protocol, proposed by Atkinson and colleagues,[7] uses 6 common ultrasound windows to investigate causes of hypotension. The first view is the subxiphoid window to assess overall contractility, compare chamber size, and evaluate for the presence of pericardial effusion. If a subxiphoid view is unattainable, a parasternal long axis or apical 4-chamber view is used to gain similar information. The second view is of the IVC to measure IVC diameter in inspiration and expiration, thus offering information about volume status and preload. From the IVC view, the third view is obtained by sliding the probe transversely down the abdominal aorta to the bifurcation, evaluating for AAA as the cause of shock. The remaining 3 views assess for peritoneal free fluid. The right upper quadrant view includes the hepatorenal space and the right lung base, allowing the examiner to see abdominal or pleural fluid. Similarly, a left upper quadrant or splenorenal view may show abdominal or left-sided pleural fluid. Finally, a transverse view of the pelvis allows evaluation of the bladder and surrounding fluid. Although its provides the most systematic method for evaluating the common causes of hypotension and shock among all of the protocols described, the ACES protocol has not been formally studied.

Rapid Ultrasound in Shock Protocol

In the Rapid Ultrasound in Shock (RUSH) protocol, complex physiologic possibilities for shock are simplified into 3 major categories with several yes or no questions. The 3 main categories evaluated are "the pump, the tank, and the pipes."[10]

The pump refers to examination of the heart for pericardial effusion, global contractility, and relative chamber size that would suggest tamponade, cardiogenic shock, or obstructive shock.

The tank is broadly applied to the assessment of volume status and preload. This step evaluates the diameter of the IVC and its variation with respiration to assess volume status. Similarly, Perera suggests also evaluating the internal jugular vein for respiratory variation. This step also includes using a linear probe to evaluate lung parenchyma. Absence of a sliding lung sign could suggest pneumothorax, which, in patients who are hypotensive, could represent a tension pneumothorax and impede venous return. One may also see B-lines, which would suggest pulmonary edema (ie, volume overload or "the tank is too full"). Finally, in this step, views of the abdomen are used to assess for free fluid in the peritoneal cavity.

The pipes are representative of the large vessels. In this step, the examiner performs a survey of the thoracic and abdominal aorta, looking for aneurysm, dissection, or intimal flap. In addition, the veins of the lower extremity are evaluated for evidence of thrombus, which might suggest a pulmonary embolism in patients who are hypotensive. Like the ACES protocol, the utility of RUSH has not yet been studied in practice, but the latter represents the most comprehensive of all the undifferentiated hypotension ultrasound protocols.

Jones and colleagues[1] studied a comprehensive protocol consisting of 7 windows for patients with hypotension arriving to the ED. This protocol used the subxiphoid view to assess for pericardial effusion, whereas the parasternal long axis and apical 4-chamber views were used to evaluate chamber size and contractility. The IVC was assessed to estimate volume status, and hepatorenal and pelvic views were obtained to evaluate for intra-abdominal free fluid. Finally, the abdominal aorta was examined for signs of AAA. In this randomized controlled trial, which compared ultrasound performed immediately on arrival to the ED versus standard care followed by ultrasound at 15 minutes for the management of adult nontrauma patients with hypotension presenting with shock, the investigators showed that physicians achieved a narrower differential (4 vs 9) and a more accurate diagnosis (80% vs 50%) for the patients undergoing an ultrasound examination immediately on presentation.

CARDIAC ARREST

Several studies have demonstrated the utility of cardiac ultrasound as a prognostic indicator in patients who arrive to the ED in cardiac arrest.[8,46–48] A brief cardiac view to check for cardiac motion can be obtained between compressions during standard pulse checks. In both traumatic and nontraumatic cardiac arrest, the absence of cardiac motion on echocardiogram correlates to a poor likelihood of survival to hospital admission.

Focused Echocardiography Entry Level Protocol

Breitkreutz and colleagues[5] designed the focused echocardiography entry level (FEEL) protocol particularly for the rapid evaluation of patients with profound hypotension in a periresuscitation state or undergoing active cardiopulmonary resuscitation (CPR). FEEL involves obtaining a single cardiac view using a 3.5- to 5.0-MHz curved array probe. Either the subxiphoid, parasternal, or apical view may be used to evaluate the presence or absence of cardiac motion, ventricular function, RV dilation, and pericardial effusion.

The protocol was studied in the prehospital setting where EPs evaluated patients undergoing active CPR or in the periresuscitation period. Usable cardiac views were obtained in 95 of 104 patients who did not undergo CPR and all 100 patients who did. The physicians perceived that use of the FEEL protocol resulted in a change in therapy in 66% of patients who did not undergo CPR and 89% of patients who did. Patients with an electrocardiographic diagnosis of asystole or pulseless electrical activity were more likely to survive to hospital admission if cardiac activity was seen on echocardiogram than if there was not (34% vs 6%, respectively).[5]

ULTRASOUND EVALUATION OF THE UNSTABLE TRAUMA PATIENT

Ultrasound for initial evaluation of trauma patients has become standard of care because it is a mobile and reliable method of detecting fluid collections requiring immediate operative management in unstable patients for whom transport out of the trauma room for imaging is particularly dangerous.[49] In addition to identifying intra-abdominal free fluid, ultrasound is useful for detecting specific conditions, including cardiac injury, pneumothorax, hemothorax, and traumatic dissection.

Focused Assessment with Sonography in Trauma and Extended Focused Assessment with Sonography in Trauma Protocols

The most widely used protocol for evaluation of trauma in adult patients is the Focused Assessment with Sonography in Trauma (FAST) and the modified extended FAST (eFAST) protocols. In the traditional FAST examination, 4 standard views are obtained: (1) longitudinal view of the right upper quadrant with demonstration of the right lobe of the liver, right kidney, and Morison pouch; (2) longitudinal view of the left upper quadrant demonstrating the spleen, left kidney, and splenorenal fossa; (3) transverse and longitudinal views of the suprapubic region with views of the urinary bladder and rectouterine or retrovesicular pouch; and (4) subxiphoid view.[50] The eFAST has 4 additional views: (1) right anterior axillary line demonstrating the right hemidiaphragm, (2) longitudinal view of the right anterior hemiclavicular line between the third and fifth intercostal spaces, (3) left anterior axillary line showing the left hemidiaphragm, and (4) longitudinal view of the left anterior hemiclavicular line between the third and fifth intercostal spaces.

The FAST examination is useful for detecting fluid collections greater than 200 mL, and women of reproductive age may present with up to 45 to 50 mL of physiologic free fluid.[51–53] Studies evaluating the utility of the FAST examination yield conflicting results, although consensus suggests that positive FAST results are valuable in evaluating blunt abdominal trauma, whereas negative FAST results are thought to be less helpful in clinical decision-making.[53–55]

Fewer studies exist regarding the use of the FAST examination in evaluating penetrating torso trauma. In a review of studies evaluating this indication, Quinn and Sinert[56] concluded that the FAST examination is useful for rapid, initial evaluation of penetrating torso trauma, because positive results necessitate the need for immediate laparotomy, whereas negative results require further diagnostic evaluation.[57] Several studies comparing the FAST examination with computed tomography and diagnostic peritoneal lavage (DPL) showed that the FAST protocol had high specificity (0.86–1.00) and variable sensitivity (0.64–0.98), which was attributed to varying levels of experience.[58]

When evaluating all organ injuries, the FAST examination has a high specificity (0.84–1.00) and variable sensitivity (0.44–0.95) for evaluation of all organ injuries.[58] Although the FAST examination has high specificity (0.99–1.00) for detecting traumatic liver injury, its sensitivity is highly variable and its performance requires too much time to be useful in acute trauma evaluations.[58] Evaluation of the liver is particularly challenging because hepatic lacerations evolve over time and appearance on ultrasound is highly variable.[59] Although the spleen is the most frequently injured organ in blunt abdominal trauma, its evaluation is limited because the left lung frequently obscures a complete view, and thus ultrasound alone is not sufficient for evaluation.[60] The FAST examination is highly specific (0.98–1.00) for evaluation of renal injuries; however, the anatomic location of the kidneys, particularly the left kidney, and the variable sensitivity of this examination prevent it from being the only method needed to evaluate for kidney injuries.[58] Although pelvic images are obtained, no studies have been published on the utility of the FAST examination for evaluating intraperitoneal or extraperitoneal bladder rupture; furthermore, results will be negative for free fluid in the setting of an extraperitoneal bladder rupture. The FAST examination is highly sensitive (0.97–1.00) for injuries to the heart and pericardium; thus, the subxiphoid view is 1 of the 4 essential views. Evaluation for solid organ injuries to the pancreas, bowel, and mesentery are missed by the FAST examination, and therefore many of these patients still require further imaging in the setting of a suspicious mechanism of injury.

The FAST and eFAST examinations use indirect signs to evaluate for pneumothorax, diaphragm rupture, pericardial tamponade, and pleural effusion. Some studies suggest that ultrasound is superior to chest radiograph for detecting pneumothorax, making ultrasound a useful modality for diagnosing this condition in trauma patients.[61,62] Kirkpatrick and colleagues[63] found the sensitivity and specificity of the eFAST examination (58.9 and 99.1, respectively) to be superior to both chest computed tomography (48.8 and 98.7, respectively) and chest radiography (20.9 and 99.6, respectively) for detecting pneumothorax. Evaluation of the FAST examination for diagnosing acute diaphragmatic rupture is mostly limited to case reports. Findings include disruption of the diaphragm, poor diaphragmatic movement, elevation of the diaphragm, absence of liver sliding, herniated loops of bowel or the liver through the defect, and spleen visualization in the thorax, whereas nonvisualization of the spleen or heart, pleural effusion, and subphrenic fluid collections indirectly suggest possible diaphragmatic rupture.[64–67]

CONCLUSION

While no one ultrasound protocol has been studied rigorously, there are many protocols in existence to assist the emergency physician in the evaluation of the undifferentiated patient in shock. While no single protocol may adequately evaluate every patient, the physician should familiarize themselves with the basic principles of evaluating the causes of shock: cardiac failure or tamponade, volume depletion, hemothorax or pneumothorax, and ruptured aortic aneurysm.

SUPPLEMENTARY DATA

Videos related to this article can be found online at http://dx.doi.org/10.1016/j.cult.2014.01.006.

REFERENCES

1. Jones AE, Tayal VS, Sullivan DM, et al. Randomized, controlled trial of immediate versus delayed goal-directed ultrasound to identify the cause of nontraumatic hypotension in emergency department patients. Crit Care Med 2004;32(8):1703–8.
2. Manno E, Navarra M, Faccio L, et al. Deep impact of ultrasound in the intensive care unit: the "ICU-sound" protocol. Anesthesiology 2012; 117(4):801–9.
3. Schmidt GA, Koenig S, Mayo PH. Shock: ultrasound to guide diagnosis and therapy. Chest 2012;142(4):1042–8.
4. Rose JS, Bair AE, Mandavia D, et al. The UHP ultrasound protocol: a novel ultrasound approach to the empiric evaluation of the undifferentiated hypotensive patient. Am J Emerg Med 2001;19(4): 299–302.
5. Breitkreutz R, Walcher F, Seeger FH. Focused echocardiographic evaluation in resuscitation management: concept of an advanced life support-conformed algorithm. Crit Care Med 2007; 35(Suppl 5):S150–61.
6. Gunst M, Sperry J, Ghaemmaghami V, et al. Bedside echocardiographic assessment for trauma/critical care: the BEAT exam. J Am Coll Surg 2008;207(3):e1–3.
7. Atkinson PR, McAuley DJ, Kendall RJ, et al. Abdominal and Cardiac Evaluation with Sonography in Shock (ACES): an approach by emergency physicians for the use of ultrasound in patients with undifferentiated hypotension. Emerg Med J 2009; 26(2):87–91.
8. Breitkreutz R, Price S, Steiger HV, et al. Focused echocardiographic evaluation in life support and peri-resuscitation of emergency patients: a prospective trial. Resuscitation 2010;81(11):1527–33.
9. Volpicelli G, Lamorte A, Tullio M, et al. Point-of-care multiorgan ultrasonography for the evaluation of undifferentiated hypotension in the emergency department. Intensive Care Med 2013;39(7):1290–8.
10. Perera P, Mailhot T, Riley D, et al. The RUSH exam: Rapid Ultrasound in SHock in the evaluation of the critically Ill. Emerg Med Clin North Am 2010;28(1): 29–56, vii.
11. Mandavia DP, Hoffner RJ, Mahaney K, et al. Bedside echocardiography by emergency physicians. Ann Emerg Med 2001;38(4):377–82.
12. Moore CL, Rose GA, Tayal VS, et al. Determination of left ventricular function by emergency physician echocardiography of hypotensive patients. Acad Emerg Med 2002;9(3):186–93.
13. Nagdev A, Stone MB. Point-of-care ultrasound evaluation of pericardial effusions: does this patient have cardiac tamponade? Resuscitation 2011; 82(6):671–3.
14. Jones AE, Craddock PA, Tayal VS, et al. Diagnostic accuracy of left ventricular function for identifying sepsis among emergency department patients with nontraumatic symptomatic undifferentiated hypotension. Shock 2005;24(6):513–7.
15. Kerwin C, Tommaso L, Kulstad E. A brief training module improves recognition of echocardiographic wall-motion abnormalities by emergency medicine physicians. Emerg Med Int 2011;2011:483242.
16. Randazzo MR, Snoey ER, Levitt MA, et al. Accuracy of emergency physician assessment of left

ventricular ejection fraction and central venous pressure using echocardiography. Acad Emerg Med 2003;10(9):973–7.

17. Scheuren K, Wente MN, Hainer C, et al. Left ventricular end-diastolic area is a measure of cardiac preload in patients with early septic shock. Eur J Anaesthesiol 2009;26(9):759–65.

18. Haddad F, Doyle R, Murphy DJ, et al. Right ventricular function in cardiovascular disease, part II: pathophysiology, clinical importance, and management of right ventricular failure. Circulation 2008; 117(13):1717–31.

19. Lewis JF, Kuo LC, Nelson JG, et al. Pulsed Doppler echocardiographic determination of stroke volume and cardiac output: clinical validation of two new methods using the apical window. Circulation 1984;70(3):425–31.

20. Slama M, Masson H, Teboul JL, et al. Respiratory variations of aortic VTI: a new index of hypovolemia and fluid responsiveness. Am J Physiol Heart Circ Physiol 2002;283(4):H1729–33.

21. Dinh VA, Ko HS, Rao R, et al. Measuring cardiac index with a focused cardiac ultrasound examination in the ED. Am J Emerg Med 2012;30(9): 1845–51.

22. Levitov A, Marik PE. Echocardiographic assessment of preload responsiveness in critically ill patients. Cardiol Res Pract 2012;2012:819696.

23. Rosenberg AL, Dechert RE, Park PK, et al. Review of a large clinical series: association of cumulative fluid balance on outcome in acute lung injury: a retrospective review of the ARDSnet tidal volume study cohort. J Intensive Care Med 2009;24(1): 35–46.

24. Stewart RM, Park PK, Hunt JP, et al. Less is more: improved outcomes in surgical patients with conservative fluid administration and central venous catheter monitoring. J Am Coll Surg 2009;208(5): 725–35 [discussion: 735–7].

25. Boyd JH, Forbes J, Nakada TA, et al. Fluid resuscitation in septic shock: a positive fluid balance and elevated central venous pressure are associated with increased mortality. Crit Care Med 2011; 39(2):259–65.

26. Barbier C, Loubieres Y, Schmit C, et al. Respiratory changes in inferior vena cava diameter are helpful in predicting fluid responsiveness in ventilated septic patients. Intensive Care Med 2004;30(9): 1740–6.

27. Feissel M, Michard F, Faller JP, et al. The respiratory variation in inferior vena cava diameter as a guide to fluid therapy. Intensive Care Med 2004; 30(9):1834–7.

28. Kircher BJ, Himelman RB, Schiller NB. Noninvasive estimation of right atrial pressure from the inspiratory collapse of the inferior vena cava. Am J Cardiol 1990;66(4):493–6.

29. Kumar A, Anel R, Bunnell E, et al. Pulmonary artery occlusion pressure and central venous pressure fail to predict ventricular filling volume, cardiac performance, or the response to volume infusion in normal subjects. Crit Care Med 2004;32(3):691–9.

30. Osman D, Ridel C, Ray P, et al. Cardiac filling pressures are not appropriate to predict hemodynamic response to volume challenge. Crit Care Med 2007;35(1):64–8.

31. Marik PE, Baram M, Vahid B. Does central venous pressure predict fluid responsiveness? A systematic review of the literature and the tale of seven mares. Chest 2008;134(1):172–8.

32. Marik PE, Cavallazzi R. Does the central venous pressure predict fluid responsiveness? An updated meta-analysis and a plea for some common sense*. Crit Care Med 2013;41(7):1774–81.

33. Tayal VS, Graf CD, Gibbs MA. Prospective study of accuracy and outcome of emergency ultrasound for abdominal aortic aneurysm over two years. Acad Emerg Med 2003;10(8):867–71.

34. Dent B, Kendall RJ, Boyle AA, et al. Emergency ultrasound of the abdominal aorta by UK emergency physicians: a prospective cohort study. Emerg Med J 2007;24(8):547–9.

35. Lichtenstein DA, Mezière G, Lascols N, et al. Ultrasound diagnosis of occult pneumothorax. Crit Care Med 2005;33(6):1231–8.

36. Lichtenstein D, Mezière G, Biderman P, et al. The "lung point": an ultrasound sign specific to pneumothorax. Intensive Care Med 2000;26(10): 1434–40.

37. Lichtenstein D, Mézière G, Biderman P, et al. The comet-tail artifact. An ultrasound sign of alveolar-interstitial syndrome. Am J Respir Crit Care Med 1997;156(5):1640–6.

38. Lichtenstein D, Mezière G. A lung ultrasound sign allowing bedside distinction between pulmonary edema and COPD: the comet-tail artifact. Intensive Care Med 1998;24(12):1331–4.

39. Blaivas M, Lambert MJ, Harwood RA, et al. Lower-extremity Doppler for deep venous thrombosis–can emergency physicians be accurate and fast? Acad Emerg Med 2000;7(2):120–6.

40. Frazee BW, Snoey ER, Levitt A. Emergency Department compression ultrasound to diagnose proximal deep vein thrombosis. J Emerg Med 2001; 20(2):107–12.

41. Jang T, Docherty M, Aubin C, et al. Resident-performed compression ultrasonography for the detection of proximal deep vein thrombosis: fast and accurate. Acad Emerg Med 2004; 11(3):319–22.

42. Burnside PR, Brown MD, Kline JA. Systematic review of emergency physician-performed ultrasonography for lower-extremity deep vein thrombosis. Acad Emerg Med 2008;15(6):493–8.

43. Kline JA, O'Malley PM, Tayal VS, et al. Emergency clinician-performed compression ultrasonography for deep venous thrombosis of the lower extremity. Ann Emerg Med 2008;52(4): 437–45.
44. Ma OJ, Kefer MP, Mateer JR, et al. Evaluation of hemoperitoneum using a single- vs multiple-view ultrasonographic examination. Acad Emerg Med 1995;2(7):581–6.
45. Jensen MB, Sloth E, Larsen KM, et al. Transthoracic echocardiography for cardiopulmonary monitoring in intensive care. Eur J Anaesthesiol 2004; 21(9):700–7.
46. Blaivas M, Fox JC. Outcome in cardiac arrest patients found to have cardiac standstill on the bedside emergency department echocardiogram. Acad Emerg Med 2001;8(6):616–21.
47. Blyth L, Atkinson P, Gadd K, et al. Bedside focused echocardiography as predictor of survival in cardiac arrest patients: a systematic review. Acad Emerg Med 2012;19(10):1119–26.
48. Cureton EL, Yeung LY, Kwan RO, et al. The heart of the matter: utility of ultrasound of cardiac activity during traumatic arrest. J Trauma Acute Care Surg 2012;73(1):102–10.
49. American College of Surgeons. ATLS: Advanced Trauma Life Support Student Manual. 9th edition. Hearthside Publishing Services; 2012.
50. Bahner D, Blaivas M, Cohen HL, et al. AIUM practice guideline for the performance of the focused assessment with sonography for trauma (FAST) examination. J Ultrasound Med 2008;27(2):313–8.
51. Branney SW, Wolfe RE, Moore EE, et al. Quantitative sensitivity of ultrasound in detecting free intraperitoneal fluid. J Trauma 1995;39(2):375–80.
52. Sirlin CB, Casola G, Brown MA, et al. Us of blunt abdominal trauma: importance of free pelvic fluid in women of reproductive age. Radiology 2001; 219(1):229–35.
53. Beck-Razi N, Gaitini D. Focused assessment with sonography for trauma. Ultrasound Clin 2008;3(1): 23–31.
54. Soudack M, Epelman M, Maor R, et al. Experience with focused abdominal sonography for trauma (FAST) in 313 pediatric patients. J Clin Ultrasound 2004;32(2):53–61.
55. Fox JC, Boysen M, Gharahbaghian L, et al. Test characteristics of focused assessment of sonography for trauma for clinically significant abdominal free fluid in pediatric blunt abdominal trauma. Acad Emerg Med 2011;18(5):477–82.
56. Quinn AC, Sinert R. What is the utility of the Focused Assessment with Sonography in Trauma (FAST) exam in penetrating torso trauma? Injury 2011;42(5):482–7.
57. Udobi KF, Rodriguez A, Chiu WC, et al. Role of ultrasonography in penetrating abdominal trauma: a prospective clinical study. J Trauma 2001;50(3): 475–9.
58. Korner M, Krotz MM, Degenhart C, et al. Current role of emergency US in patients with major trauma. Radiographics 2008;28(1):225–42.
59. McGahan JP, Wang L, Richards JR. From the RSNA refresher courses: focused abdominal US for trauma. Radiographics 2001;(21 Spec No): S191–9.
60. Scalea TM, Rodriguez A, Chiu WC, et al. Focused Assessment with Sonography for Trauma (FAST): results from an international consensus conference. J Trauma 1999;46(3):466–72.
61. Zhang M, Liu ZH, Yang JX, et al. Rapid detection of pneumothorax by ultrasonography in patients with multiple trauma. Crit Care 2006;10(4):R112.
62. Soldati G, Testa A, Pignataro G, et al. The ultrasonographic deep sulcus sign in traumatic pneumothorax. Ultrasound Med Biol 2006;32(8): 1157–63.
63. Kirkpatrick AW, Sirois M, Laupland KB, et al. Handheld thoracic sonography for detecting post-traumatic pneumothoraces: the Extended Focused Assessment with Sonography for Trauma (EFAST). J Trauma 2004;57(2):288–95.
64. Gangahar R, Doshi D. FAST scan in the diagnosis of acute diaphragmatic rupture. Am J Emerg Med 2010;28(3):387.e1–3.
65. Kim HH, Shin YR, Kim KJ, et al. Blunt traumatic rupture of the diaphragm: sonographic diagnosis. J Ultrasound Med 1997;16(9):593–8.
66. Blaivas M, Brannam L, Hawkins M, et al. Bedside emergency ultrasonographic diagnosis of diaphragmatic rupture in blunt abdominal trauma. Am J Emerg Med 2004;22(7):601–4.
67. Speight J, Sanders M. Pericardial tamponade with a positive abdominal FAST scan in blunt chest trauma. J Trauma 2006;61(3):743–5 [discussion: 745].

Index

Note: Page numbers of article titles are in **boldface** type.

Ultrasound Clin 9 (2014) 307–312
http://dx.doi.org/10.1016/S1556-858X(14)00023-1
1556-858X/14/$ – see front matter © 2014 Elsevier Inc. All rights reserved.

Printed and bound by CPI Group (UK) Ltd, Croydon, CR0 4YY

08/06/2025

01896870-0020